DATE DUE

12/4/97	9-13-02
3-24-98	9-30-02
4/16/98	4-25-03
6/5/98	3-12-04
6/22/98	
9/26/98	
11/18/98	
5-21-99	
10-1-99	
11-18-99	
5-5-00	
2-1-02	
4-22-02	

PLEASE RETURN IN TWO WEEKS

ALZHEIMER'S®
ASSOCIATION

Alzheimer's Association
1650 NW Naito Pkwy, #190
Portland, OR 97209

24-Hour Helpline
1-800-733-0402
TDD/TTY (503) 413-7374

DEMCO

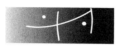

Designing for Alzheimer's Disease

Wiley Series in Healthcare and Senior Living Design

Elizabeth C. Brawley
Designing for Alzheimer's Disease: Strategies for Creating Better Care Environments

Sara O. Marberry
Healthcare Design

Alfred H. Baucom
Hospitality Design for the Graying Generation: Meeting the Needs of a Growing Market

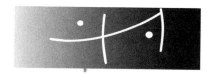

Designing for Alzheimer's Disease

STRATEGIES FOR CREATING BETTER
CARE ENVIRONMENTS

Elizabeth C. Brawley

JOHN WILEY & SONS, INC.

New York • Chichester • Weinheim • Brisbane • Singapore • Toronto

Copyright © 1997 by John Wiley & Sons, Inc.

Library of Congress Cataloging in Publication Data:

Brawley, Elizabeth C.
    Designing for Alzheimer's Disease: strategies for creating better
care environments / by Elizabeth C. Brawley.
        p.   cm. — (Wiley series in healthcare and senior living
design)
    Includes bibliographical references and index.
    ISBN 0-471-13920-3 (alk. paper)
    1. Alzheimer's disease — Patients — Dwellings.   2. Senile dementia-
-Patients--Dwellings.   3. Long-term care facilities--Design and
construction.   4. Architecture--Psychological aspects.   5. Interior
decoration — Psychological aspects.   I. Title.   II. Series.
RC523.B73   1997
362.1'96831 — dc20   96-33457

With gratitude and great respect, this book is dedicated to the members of the Alzheimer's Association, who work so hard to assure quality care, and to the many individuals who contribute so much to improving special care environments and the quality of life for people with Alzheimer's disease and other related illnesses.

I am constantly touched by the remarkable courage and strength of so many people, who in quiet, unassuming ways make such a difference in the lives of others. It is their respect for all human beings that allows people a chance to live in dignity.

Contents

SECTION III
Special Care Settings

SECTION IV
Implementing Effective Interior Design

SECTION V
The Design Process

Foreword

One of the surprising and underappreciated aspects of dealing in the pain-wracked world of Alzheimer's disease falls into a category probably best described as "unexpected fringe benefits." For those of us who have survived the excruciating experience of being a caregiver or simply of losing a loved one to this cruel thief, the notion of any kind of benefit accruing from this awful time is difficult to grasp, much less convey, but it is in this universe of shared pain that we are wont to find hidden treasures.

Such a one is the book brought to us by Betsy Brawley, *Designing for Alzheimer's Disease: Strategies for Creating Better Care Environments.* Betsy is herself one of the treasures of which I speak, as will be clear to readers of this book, but the especially important contribution made here is the wedding of her special talents in the area of interior design with her experience as a caregiver for her mother, Helen Carlton Brawley.

In her unique and generous way, Betsy takes us through her personal grief and allows us all to profit from it by bringing to bear the remarkable and practical insights drawn from her artistry as a designer and focusing them on the way in which we can and should consider the environment in which the Alzheimer's victim spins out her or his final years, months, weeks, days, or hours. Things that few of us who are not professionals in the area of design or architecture ever take into consideration are pointed out in this loving work, with the great care that could only come from one who has lived both lives: the design professional and the compassionate caregiver.

Because of this unique combination of knowledge and experience, Betsy is able to lay out here facts and experiences that will provide insight and comfort to the layperson on the same page as she presents ideas that are of great value to the architect and design professional. Concern for all five of the senses of the Alzheimer's victim is shown, concern that many might assume unnecessary given the people with whom she's dealing, yet it is here presented with great care given to the explanation of why such is not only necessary, but beneficial—even therapeutic.

Color, lighting, design, texture, exterior as well as interior—nothing, it seems, escapes her unsparing eye—and all of it is handled with an absolute fealty to the single most important tenet that undergirds this invaluable book: an absolute commitment to the recognition of the dignity of the individual Alzheimer's sufferer.

We are richer for this work.

SHELLEY FABARES
Los Angeles, CA
September, 1996

Preface

As our population ages, the incidence of Alzheimer's disease is increasing dramatically, as is the need for long-term care. Almost all people with dementia—now estimated to number well over four million—are likely to reside in a residential care setting or a nursing home during the course of their illness.

Special care environments did not exist 25 years ago, yet today they are being built at a remarkable rate. Through a better understanding of the aging process, the challenges posed by frailty and dementia, and Alzheimer's disease and the unique problems associated with its dependent population, we can better identify problems, explore appropriate solutions, and provide more responsive and responsible care environments.

Studies have shown that the environment strongly influences the behavior of individuals with Alzheimer's disease and related dementing illnesses, and that well-designed physical environments can maintain and enhance the ability to function and improve quality of life.[1] Diminished memory and reasoning capacities cause such individuals to respond more intensively to the immediate environment than the cognitively unimpaired. Existing care settings still too often resemble a hospital care setting, an inappropriate design model for persons with Alzheimer's disease or care of the frail elderly. Designing a residential long-term care setting for persons with Alzheimer's disease is different from designing for those with acute or skilled nursing care needs.

---

[1] Congress of the United States Office of Technology Assessment. *Special Care Units for People with Alzheimer's and Other Dementias* references Powell Lawton's research in this area.

Mildly to moderately impaired people—those whose quality of life can be most improved—are made particularly vulnerable by existing environments that inhibit movement, stimulation, and a sense of personal safety. More severely impaired people, whose physical needs predominate over their mental needs, are also significantly affected by the environment. For example, the presence of glare, noise, odors, and insufficient access to safe and secure outside areas are particularly difficult for these residents.

Architects and design professionals, even those who specialize in healthcare, have little training in the physiological changes of aging, Alzheimer's disease, or the special needs of the elderly—particularly residents with Alzheimer's. *Designing for Alzheimer's Disease* provides information for architects, facility planners, interior designers, and other design and healthcare professionals who plan and design environments for the elderly and for residents with Alzheimer's disease. For those who are unfamiliar with Alzheimer's disease, it is discussed in understandable language. What is it? How does it affect a person's cognitive and functional skills? How does Alzheimer's influence the ability to interpret, understand, and act within the physical environment? And most importantly, how can a well-designed environment be therapeutic, and how can quality of life be enhanced?

Too many planners have been content to provide generic healthcare buildings that look and operate just as they always have. Today we are facing new challenges and healthcare providers are looking for design professionals who have the insight to "diagnose" current problems and the vision to creatively and practically solve them. Innovative designers can do more than create new buildings; they can build awareness and raise the level of consciousness for healing design.

In my experience, design professionals have relied heavily on healthcare professionals to define needs. Necessary questions for better design solutions have gone unasked, because of an inadequate understanding of these special populations and their needs. On the other hand, critical information was routinely never conveyed to designers by healthcare providers. It was not that information was intentionally withheld; quite the contrary, in fact. These healthcare professionals, having dealt with difficult situations for so long, could no longer see the problems, and, invariably, no longer expected better solutions. Yet many of these situations are quite "fixable" to someone with a praticed eye, a different perspective, and very different expertise.

Environmental features often contribute to unsatisfactory responses or behaviors in cognitively impaired people and, regrettably, the average facility conspires to reinforce dependency and to immobilize residents. Just as a carefully planned setting may reduce agitation, incontinence, and wandering, a poorly designed environment can contribute to disorientation and confusion, and precipitate agitation.

The expertise of innovative design professionals, armed with practical knowldge of Alzheimer's disease, results of the latest research, the ability to ask questions that identify problem areas, and the design skills to develop better solutions gives rise to hope and a real expectation for better care environments.

This book is meant to provide the information necessary to understanding the realities of aging, in order to help identify the problems of aging and Alzheimer's disease more easily, to make the residents and their needs more real, and to assist in finding better solutions. Aging covers a large age range and many personality distinctions. Though our training teaches us there are many solutions to a problem, our downfall as design professionals comes when we forget we are designing for indivivduals—real people. Individuals with Alzheimer's disease are our mothers, our fathers, grandmothers and grandfathers, sisters, brothers, uncles, aunts, relatives, neighbors, and best friends. We must constantly keep in mind that an identified solution that meets a need is certainly not the only solution, and may not be the best one. While successful solutions for specific problems are illustrated, they are only examples. We need to continually explore better and more appropriate ways to solve problems, be open to new ways of doing things, and work together with a strong spirit of mutual cooperation.

Aging and Alzheimer's special care design is an emerging field, ripe for responsible, sensitive design professionals and creative design thinking. Care settings today cry for design that looks beyond the obvious (the aesthetics) and addresses the more complex needs of physically, mentally, and emotionally challenged residents. These are not problems without solutions.

The single largest missing ingredient in healthcare facilities for the elderly, for example, is light. Understanding light and aging vision, why it is so important, how it affects mobility, the level of function and the level of stress for residents—and staff—should create dramatic improvements. Bathing environments, another source of extreme difficulty for residents and staff, are another area that can benefit from the creative expertise of sensitive designers.

Open communication and cooperative planning between design professionals and healthcare providers is fundamental to creating better care environments. We have so much to learn from each other and everyone stands to benefit, especially the residents. While design for Alzheimer's special care is a challenging task, it offers the opportunity to make a difference. If there is a silver lining to the terrible tragedy of Alzheimer's disease, it is the humanity we learn to express under the most difficult circumstances. Imagine, in carefully planned and thoughtfully designed care environments, how the quality of life might be enhanced for those afflicted with Alzheimer's disease.

ELIZABETH C. BRAWLEY

Acknowledgments

This book is a reality because of the generosity and contribution of many, with special acknowledgment of my mother, Helen Carlton Brawley, who fought Alzheimer's disease with grace and dignity for too many years. It is my hope that this book will be a resource of information and inspiration for designing better care environments for Alzheimer's disease and long-term care, and that it will motivate others to find better solutions for the needs and many challenges of this special population.

Thank you to the many friends and associates who have been so supportive, especially Cynthia Leibrock, who encouraged me to write this book and was relentless with her support.

Special thanks to colleagues who volunteered their time to review portions of this book. Ruth Fangmeier of The Lighthouse, Inc., helped enormously with the challenges of aging vision. Eunice Noell, Center of Design for an Aging Society, is gratefully acknowledged for her generosity and her contributions to the discussions of the complexities of lighting and hearing. Thank you to Dr. Philip Sloane of the University of North Carolina, to Uriel Cohen of the University of Wisconsin–Milwaukee, and to Margaret Calkins for reviewing material on Alzheimer's special care.

I am grateful to the Alzheimer's Association for their continued support of individuals with Alzheimer's disease and their families, and their constant efforts to insure better quality care and better quality care environments. To the many healthcare professionals who care and contribute so much, and to design professionals who are proving that we can improve quality of life through better design, thank you.

I would like to gratefully acknowledge the Hall Family Foundation, The Helen Bader Foundation, and Parke-Davis for funding.

Thank you to Linda Watson, and to the Alzheimer's Association, Greater San Francisco Bay Area Chapter, for their kindness in helping to gather the many photographs, and to each individual and facility who contributed them.

A very special thanks to Anastasia Dellas and Martha O'Connell Dawdy, whose special talents and generosity of spirit enabled the completion of this book.

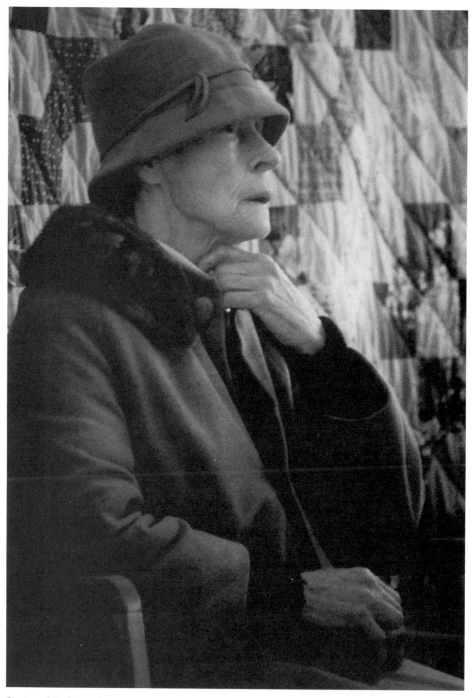

Courtesy of the Greater San Francisco Bay Area Alzheimer's Association. Photographer: Anna M. Ross.

In a society where youth is glorified and perpetuated with virtually every advertisement, it's tough to admit you're getting on in years and tougher still to prepare for it.

Introduction

The nation's entire aged population is increasing rapidly. In the 10- year period between 1980 and 1990, the population over age 65 increased by 22.3 percent and it is estimated that by 2050, the United States will have 67.5 million people over the age of 65, compared with 25.5 million today. By the year 2000—in just 4 years—this same age group will represent 13 percent of the U.S. population, and that number is projected to double by the year 2030 according to census data.[1] These numbers are of no small concern. Texas, followed by Pennsylvania, New York, Florida, California, Illinois, and Ohio, are the states with the highest percentage of residents over 65.[2]

The most rapid leap, however, will come in the population 85 years or older. This age group which requires a disproportionate share of long-term care, will number over 8 million by the year 2030—just 35 years from today. According to the U.S. Administration on Aging, the number of disabled elderly also is expected to grow rapidly, and because of the higher proportion of people 85 years and older, will be a larger percentage of the total elderly population.[3]

One of the major consequences of this dramatic restructuring of the population, occurring as a result of the aging revolution, is the growing demand for long-term care services. This takes on added significance when we realize that the demand for these services is likely to increase considerably as the baby boom generation begins to enter the ranks of the elderly shortly after the turn of the century. With increased life expectancy, more people will be needing help in their final years.

1

For many of us, the scariest aspect about old age is not wrinkles and gall bladder operations, but where we'll be living. There is no question that most older people want to live out their lives at home. The negative image of the nursing home, the image many people once had of housing for seniors, has been largely responsible for consumer surveys where seniors consistently say that they would rather die than live out their last years in a nursing home.

Those who design and deliver services to older people recognize that meaningful changes in long-term care mean moving away from the medical models we have used in the past, to provide more holistic care, especially for those with cognitive impairment. Whether designing housing for seniors or healthcare setting for the elderly, we must focus on maintaining the individual's ability to function as much as possible, in a familiar setting, in ways that keep that individual confident and comfortable. Indeed, studies have shown that the environment strongly influences the behavior of individuals with Alzheimer's disease and related dementing illnesses.

The elderly have eagerly welcomed the recent expansion of services in home healthcare and assisted living, which has allowed many seniors to stay out of nursing homes. In 1992, 900,000 seniors lived in assisted living settings, and the demand is expected to grow to as much as 7 million by 1996.[4]

There are more than 30,000 residential and skilled care facilities in the United States today,[5] and more than 50 percent of the residents are estimated to be victims of Alzheimer's disease or a related disorder,[6] some 637,000 to 922,000 people.[7] As our population ages, the incidence of Alzheimer's disease increases, as does the need for long-term care facilities. After their families' ability to provide round-the-clock care at home is exhausted, almost all people with dementia are likely to reside in a residential care setting or a nursing home during the course of their illness. This number is currently estimated at over 4 million, and by the middle of the next century, 14 million Americans will have Alzheimer's disease.[8]

With the current and prospective need for residential care for the elderly fueling a boom in assisted living, in Alzheimer's disease special care settings, and in the renovation of existing nursing home space, architects and interior designers who specialize in healthcare design are recognizing how little they know about the elderly. The traditional design curriculum does not include geriatric information or training relevant to age-related changes, Alzheimer's disease, the physiological changes and special needs of residents with dementia, or the impact of the environment on elderly residents' ability to function.

There is no doubt that architects and designers want to do a good job. However, overwhelmed and out of frustration, they frequently rely on models commonly used in designing for acute care, models neither adapted for care of the frail elderly nor appropriate as settings for those with cognitive impairments such as Alzheimer's disease. Consequently, many facilities are not designed to tolerate exploration and movement, access to the outside, or walking in safe and interesting areas—activities necessary to most residents.

With increased practical knowledge of the elderly and Alzheimer's disease, the ability to ask the right questions to identify problem areas, and the design skills to begin developing better solutions, design professionals can make a greater contribution in reforming long-term care with better and more sensitively designed care environments.

The problems of facility administrators, who must cope with growing needs and budgetary constraints, are quite different from those of design professionals. They often must function as designers by default. These healthcare professionals know the aging process well and understand the special problems of dementia, but many have dealt with difficult situations for so long they no longer identify them as problems. They may be reluctant to expect the possibility of better solutions. Many of these situations, however, are quite "fixable" to someone with a practiced eye, a different perspective, and very different expertise.

Because design is not the primary area of expertise for these care providers, their job is made increasingly difficult. They may be unaware of products recently developed to address the needs of an aging and often cognitively impaired population, and they are unfamiliar with criteria that should be applied in making appropriate selections.

This forces caring, intelligent people to make critical design choices without sufficient information to make *good* choices. As a consequence, precious resources are expended on products that may not work. The choice then becomes to live with a poor or inappropriate selection or to replace it at additional cost.

The problem of product selection is magnified by the number of products carrying labels "made for healthcare." It can be quite confusing when selecting furniture, for example, to determine what really meets special needs and what is being sold for use in healthcare setting with no special criteria applied.

The term "healthcare," in this context, is a broad, generic term. With no distinction made between the vastly different needs in designing for pediatrics, geriatrics, or the multitude of special needs groups in between, the term is, for the most part, meaningless.

Promoting independence and dignity in long-term care settings is extremely important, as is the crucial need to provide an atmosphere that takes into consideration the individual needs of each resident. With better understanding of the unique problems associated with aging, dependent populations, and the challenges posed by Alzheimer's disease and dementia, architects, facility planners, interior designers, and administrators can better define problems, explore appropriate solutions, and create care environments that better serve human beings in need of support during the final years of life.

Careful design planning for the environments we create may prove to be one of the most valuable interventions in allowing individuals to function more independently and improving quality of life. With this in mind, *it benefits healthcare design professionals and residents alike to develop a philosophy where the environments we create speak about life and the living, about vitality and the dignity of a human being.*

We must get serious about functional design and begin integrating gerontological research into design rather than focusing only on aesthetics in a few visible areas. Designers can bridge the gap between the many diverse and complex needs of residents and providers, in ways that go beyond surface treatments and soothing color palettes, to address meaningful changes.

Aging and Alzheimer's Disease

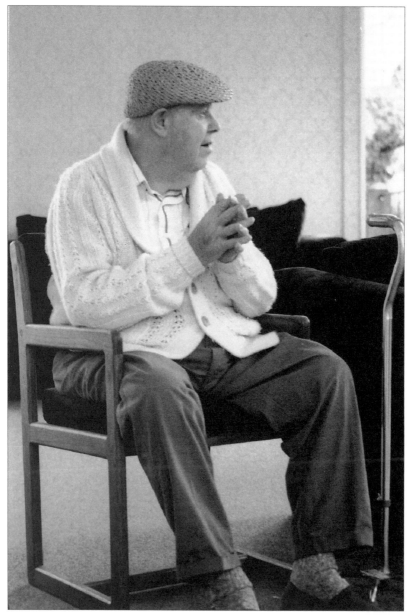

Courtesy of the Greater San Francisco Bay Area Alzheimer's Association. Photographer: Anna M. Ross.

"Contrary to popular opinion, people do not suddenly become old at a particular age. Aging occurs throughout one's lifetime, and it does not depend on chronology. Each person ages differently, at his or her own pace."1

James Pirkl, Chairman, Department of Design
at Syracuse University, retired.

1

Aging and Age-Related Changes

During the twentieth century, life expectancy in the United States has increased from 49 years to 75 years. Through research and public health programs, we have eliminated many of the major causes of death at the turn of the century, diseases such as diphtheria and cholera that killed during infancy and midlife. In the second half of the twentieth century, we have seen a continuous drop in deaths from two of the three current major killers—heart disease and stroke. As a result, more people than ever before are surviving to live into their 70s, 80s, and 90s.

The 65-and-older population in 1993 was 13 percent of the total population, but by 2050, 80 million Americans—more than one in five—will be in the senior category. By midcentury the 85-and-older population will zoom to 19 million, almost 5 percent of the United States population. At the same time the image of aging is also changing, from one of illness and frailty to one of increased vigor and vitality into much later years. Clearly we will need more healthcare settings and other facilities for an older population with greater emphasis on both aging and "wellness"—maintenance of health and productivity in later years.[2]

Aging Is a Process, Not a Disease

The greatest fear of an aging person is the prospect of loss of independence, not only the loss of physical function, the ability to care for one's self, but even more so the fear of cognitive decline. Alzheimer's disease and Parkinson's disease, the most common chronic diseases, slowly rob us of our most valuable possessions—our minds and our memories. They are devastating to individuals, to their dignity, and to their families. As we age we are at increasing risk of the chronic diseases and disorders of aging, diseases that cause long-term disability and dependency. For too many people, chronic disease and disability are constant companions in late life. Osteoarthritis, the thinning of bone, is also extremely debilitating, leading to hip fractures; it is one of the most frequent reasons for hospitalization in the elderly.[3]

People of many ages are living with chronic conditions for a much longer period of time, because the age group at greatest risk for these conditions, the 70s and 80s, are the fastest growing age groups in America. The result is a large and growing population of people needing assistance in meeting basic daily needs—preparing meals, cleaning the house, doing the shopping.

Age-Related Changes

What's Normal?

There is much misunderstanding on the part of elders, their care providers, and their caregivers regarding changes in health due to "aging" versus "disease." The normal aging process produces sensory losses, visual impairment, and hearing loss, as well as mobility loss with decreased muscle strength and reflex time, and diminished energy levels. Without making special effort to compensate, these changes compromise the ability of the older person to cope with the environment.

Architects and interior designers have an obligation and a responsibility to understand the changes that occur in the aging process and the special needs resulting from those changes. It is difficult to provide quality environments if the needs are not thoroughly understood. Those with Alzheimer's disease or other dementias and cognitive impairments are particularly vulnerable.

The reality of our frailties becomes more apparent as we age. Reduced eyesight, arthritis, and broken bones can happen at every age, not just when we're old, but they make us uniquely vulnerable as we age. Other chronic diseases such as heart disease, hypertension, stroke, diabetes and vascular disease also contribute to altered physical function. The special needs of the elderly, rather than being determined by the number of years they have lived, should be defined by the range of things they

> *Architects and interior designers have an obligation and a responsibility to understand the changes that occur in the aging process and the special needs resulting from those changes.*

can do and the number of things they can no longer do. The key question then is, how can we best accommodate the elderly and maintain their independence and dignity?

Vision

Vision is by far our most important sensory channel. In fact, we receive a wider range of information through sight than through all our other senses combined — approximately 90 percent of the information most of us learn in a lifetime enters through the eyes. The sensory aspect receives information, the integrative aspect compares that visual input with our past experience and processes it through the mind's filters, and the motor aspect is the final outcome — our speech, movements, and actions. So vision is our primary channel for learning as well as the navigational system that enables us to move through and influence our world.[4]

WHAT ARE THE NORMAL CHANGES TO THE HEALTHY AGING EYE?

Just as the body ages, so the eye ages. Normal age-related changes in the visual system that disrupt the capacity to see include:

- Impaired ability to adapt to changes in light levels
- Extreme sensitivity to glare
- Reduced visual acuity (the ability to discern detail)
- Restricted field of vision, depth perception
- Reduced contrast sensitivity
- Restricted color recognition

Changes to the healthy aging eye differ from loss of visual function due to specific eye diseases. Presbyopia, the significant loss of focusing power, may begin in the 40s and is one of the changes that can be corrected with glasses.

The normal aging eye adjusts more slowly than the young eye to changes in levels of illumination and sudden junctures of light and dark. After 50, it may become harder to see in conditions of glare or in low levels of light. Visual acuity is reduced and many older adults experience increasing difficulty perceiving patterns and require greater contrast for recognition. Fine details become harder to spot in the 70s. Color perception may be affected, as well as the ability to perceive depth.

Age-related visual deficits make it more difficult to read and interpret the environment correctly, making it more difficult to carry out productive activities. It is useful from a design standpoint to divide the partially sighted population into two categories based on the primary reasons for vision loss: (1) people who cannot form a clear image on an otherwise normal retina and (2) people with retinal or optic nerve disease.[5]

FUNCTIONAL VISION LOSS

There is a difference between the reduced function in the healthy eye and the loss of visual function from specific eye diseases. The change in visual function, known as low vision, is not correctable by ordinary glasses, contact lenses, medical treatment, or surgery. This condition typically results from cataracts, diabetic retinopathy, macular degeneration, glaucoma, and stroke. The three common functional vision losses are: (1) overall blurred vision, (2) central vision loss, and (3) peripheral (side) vision loss.

With a better understanding of vision loss it is easier to understand the importance of adapting the environment to accommodate for changing abilities. We may also find that interventions designed to cope with vision loss ease the agitation and confusion of the cognitively impaired who are also experiencing some of the same losses.

A resident's vision should be evaluated at the time of admission to a healthcare facility, and the vision status should be included in the medical information used to create the resident's care plan. The presence of a vision problem, the diagnosis, medications prescribed, and the resident's sensitivity to light should be noted.

Hearing

In addition to sight, one of the first senses to be affected by age is hearing, and this begins to occur by the age of 40. High frequency pitches are the first to become less audible, with a lesser sensitivity to lower frequency pitches. Contrary to popular thought, this situation is not corrected by speaking loudly. Increased volume doesn't enhance the ability to hear, it only heightens the register of the voice, making it more difficult for the older person to hear.

The ability to understand normal conversation is usually not disturbed at first, but when combined with the presence of background noise, comprehension may be affected. Background noise can be offensive to those with hearing loss, particularly to residents who use hearing aides. "Normal" background sounds are magnified and distorted by a hearing aid, making some environments unbearable.

Hearing less can affect self-esteem, producing self doubt. The constant strain of trying to hear is physically tiring and emotionally fatiguing and that fatigue can quickly produce agitation and anger. Loss of hearing results in not being able to hear everything and may, in fact, account for some fear of memory loss. Assessing and reviewing the hearing capacities of aged persons is a step toward creating better and more appropriate communications. This is especially true when trying to communicate with a dementia resident.

Smell and Taste

The inability to smell can be destructive, both physically and emotionally. We've all heard stories of houses blowing up because gas was undetected by the inhabitants, but a more common problem associated with olfactory loss is dietary. As we pass 65, the odds increase that we'll have a harder time smelling. And while losing the sense of smell may not be fatal, it certainly can deprive us of the pleasure of fragrance and good food. The enjoyment of eating is, physiologically, mostly smell. Flavor is taste — sweet, sour, bitter, salty — plus aroma, along with certain visual and tactile clues, but it's 90 percent aroma.[6] People often don't eat well because food doesn't taste as good as it used to. This can lead to depression.

According to Richard L. Doty, Ph.D., director of the Smell and Taste Center at the University of Pennsylvania, "Men often think they can't smell because their wives smell things they don't. But most men have less sense of smell than women."[7]

Touch

As adults we need and seek touch, which can be provided in many ways — holding a hand, giving a pat on the shoulder, being more generous with our hugs. Massage can calm breathing. Hand massage, foot massage, or rubbing a back or shoulders can be relaxing and very beneficial for older persons who may not enjoy body massage. Touch is a means of communication and we should learn to rely on it more often.

As the skin becomes drier and less elastic with advanced age, sensitivity to touch naturally and normally declines. Subtle changes in environmental texture can go unnoticed by the older resident.

Immediate sensitivity to pain and temperature are among the most important tactile losses of aging. Because the elderly can be both less aware of dangerous changes in temperature and less able to tolerate such changes, they have an increased susceptibility to hypothermia and frostbite, as well as less ability to recover from these conditions.

Older adults generally prefer more warmth in the winter, and are less able to endure extreme heat in summer. Complaints are not uncommon when there is a draft, especially for those who are seated beside windows and immobile.[8]

Mobility

As Americans advance in age, their level of physical activity typically declines. Motor skills directly affect options in getting around and in performing simple tasks of daily life. Studies have shown that regular exercise not only improves flexibility, strength, endurance, bone mass, and cardiovascular fitness, but it can also reduce anxiety and fatigue, and even alleviate depression. Getting fit and staying fit should be a top priority.

Those with stronger muscles are less likely to fall as a result of being too frail to balance well. A major benefit of exercise is that it develops muscle tissue, helping to maintain balance and avoid falls and fractures. Brisk walking is the simplest form of weight-bearing exercise. Tai Chi and weight lifting have also proved to be good balance and strength training.[9]

Range of motion exercises and strength activities, such as weights and isometric exercises, keep muscles that support joints strong. Aerobic activities keep the heart, lungs, and bones fit, and if the body is fit, it is better able to support efforts to improve joint fitness.[10]

Arthritis

Arthritis ranks second only to heart disease in the number of disability claims filed each year in the United States. It affects one out of seven people, 40 million Americans, making it the nation's most common crippling condition. It strikes three times as many women as men and by age 70 about 85 percent of the United States population suffers from arthritis to some degree, particularly in the hands and weight-bearing joints, such as knees and hips.[11]

Two types are most common — rheumatoid arthritis (RA) and osteoarthritis (OA). Rheumatoid arthritis, which often strikes people in their 40s and 50s, is an autoimmune disease that attacks the body's own tissue as if it were foreign. Osteoarthritis is more directly related to age and involves the deterioration of cartilage, the spongy tissue at the tips of bones that functions as a shock absorber. As cartilage wears away, bone begins to rub against bone. Apart from aging, OA may be prompted by improperly treating joint injuries and by being overweight. Heredity also plays a role.

Not only does arthritis produce loss of mobility, but it is painful. Weight loss or regular exercise may significantly relieve joint pain and stiffness and can improve or maintain joint mobility. For those who are able, walking can be one of the best exercises.

Osteoporosis

Osteoporosis is a silent disease, subtle but devastating, sneaking up on apparently healthy people—especially women—as they age. It is a bone thinning disease that affects millions of older people, making them subject to painful fractures, often of the hip, wrist, or spine, or to the stooped posture so often seen in older women.

> *The single most important risk factor for fractures associated with age is low bone density.*

The single most important risk factor for fractures associated with age is low bone density. Of the 6.5 million bone fractures that occur each year in the United States, forearms are the most frequent fractures of adults under age 75, when hip fractures become more frequent.

Women are more at risk after age 45, and over age 65 they suffer three times as many fractures as men.[12] Women, on average, lose up to 6 percent of their bone mass per year after the onset of menopause and at the age when it is most critical, most women do not get enough calcium in their daily diet or enough vitamin D to insure the calcium is absorbed.

Depression

Depression, loss of self-esteem, loneliness, anxiety, and boredom become more common in the elderly as they deal with retirement, the deaths of spouses, relatives, and friends, and other crises. Attempting to cope with more than one crisis at the same time can easily become overwhelming. Recent research demonstrates that clinically significant depression is present in 15 to 50 percent of nursing facility residents.[13] It can be severe enough to produce cognitive problems that may be successfully reversed with treatment. Depression is present with other causes of dementia, especially Alzheimer's diease.

Cognitive Impairment and Dementia

Dementia is not a normal part of aging. In the adult population dementia is a major and growing medical and social problem. It occurs at all ages, but its highest rate is in the population over age 85, the age group that is increasing faster than any other.

A certain increase in forgetfulness seems to be a normal by-product of aging. Mild changes in memory are thought to be normal at age 50 in some people. Slight changes in spatial perception and attention are similarly regarded as normal at age 60. Small changes in abstract thinking and language are considered normal at age 70.[14] These changes may be a result of the gradual loss of brain cells over a lifetime and the accompanying 15 to 20 percent reduction in blood flow to the brain that occurs between the ages of 30 and 70.[15] Regardless of age, everyone experiences occasional episodes of forgetfulness. Slight confusion or occasional forgetfulness throughout life may only signify an overload of facts in the brain—our storehouse of information—but many people fear that a growing number of such lapses is a sure sign of Alzheimer's disease. There are, however, important differences between simple forgetfulness and dementia.[16] Persons suffering from a dementing illness lose cognitive abilities; this manifests itself in changes in behavior and losses of function.[17] It is important to distinguish the early stages of dementia from the nonprogressive cognitive changes known to occur in otherwise normal aging.

Everyone forgets things at some time—the keys, where the car is parked, or the name of an acquaintance. Most memory problems are likely to occur when a person is under stress, fatigued, ill, distracted, or trying to remember too many details at one time, but we usually dismiss such brief memory lapses as something of little importance and eventually the information is remembered.[18] In dementia, memory of important information, such as names of close family members or the way to get home from a familiar place, may be lost.

Normal forgetfulness is neither progressive nor disabling.

The most distinguishing characteristic of dementia is impairment of memory, which differs from normal forgetfulness in healthy individuals. Normal forgetfulness is neither progressive nor disabling.

Dementia begins with minor forgetfulness, restlessness, or apathy, an increasing tendency to misplace things, small inconsistencies in some of the ordinary tasks of daily living, and repetitiousness of words or actions. As it progresses, the memory loss eventually becomes severe enough to interfere with a person's work and social life.

In most cases, there are significant difficulties with one or more other intellectual functions such as language, learning, thinking, and reasoning. Persons with dementia may fail to recognize people familiar to them and become lost in their own neighborhoods.

Some retain the shadows of their personalities even into severe dementia; others behave inappropriately and even antisocially.

There may be hallucinations, delusions, or overt paranoid behavior.[19] Dementia can be caused by a multitude of different dementing diseases. The important thing to remember is that some of the problems can be arrested or reversed, and many are preventable. Brain tumor or any infection involving the brain is capable of producing a dementing illness. Metabolic and nutritional disorders can cause symptoms that may be reversible with a physician's care.

Medications, especially multiple drugs in combination, and virtually all of the chemicals used in substance abuse from heroin to glue are capable of producing dementia.

Alzheimer's disease is by far the most prevalent of the more than 70 diseases that are thought to manifest in dementia, accounting for 55.6 percent of the cases of irreversible dementia.[20] Another 20 percent are caused by hypertension, especially severe hypertension or stroke, the most common cause of multi-infarct dementia. Parkinson's disease, Huntington's disease, Pick's disease, and AIDS are other diseases of the nervous system where dementia may occur.[21] Because it affects dignity and independence, dementia causes widespread suffering, not only for the person affected but also for families, friends, and caregivers.

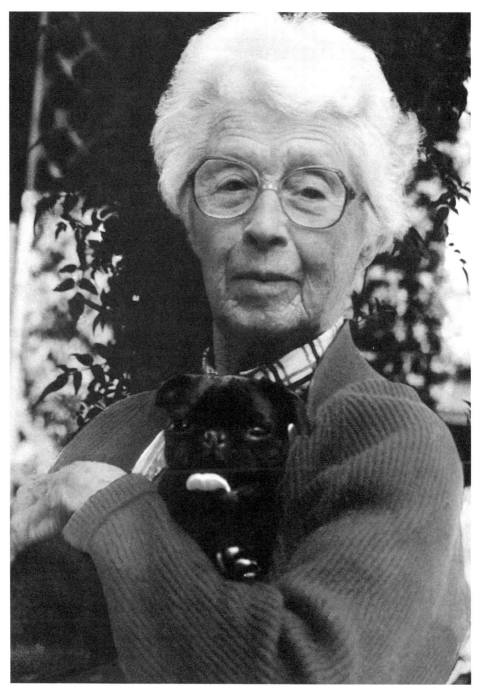

Courtesy of Grace DeVincenzi

"*You have to begin to lose your memory, if only in bits and pieces, to realize that memory is what makes our lives. Life without memory is no life at all. Our memory is our coherence, our reason, our feeling, even our action. Without it we are nothing.*"

LUIS BUÑUEL, *Spanish filmmaker*

CHAPTER 2

A Discussion of Alzheimer's Disease

Today a great fear haunts people as they age—the fear of losing their mental capabilities, their memory—the loss of self. The fear is real. For millions of Americans approaching retirement, Alzheimer's disease is the greatest threat to their health and financial security. It will deny them the rewards of a lifetime of work.[1] It will steal their memories, their judgment, their language, and eventually their lives. It is a serious and growing problem. With the graying of America it is clear that an increasing number of people will be at risk for the various disorders that cause dementia.

Most of us expect our bodies and our reflexes to slow down with age, but physicians are now recognizing that many healthy individuals are less able to remember certain types of information as they get older. The term "age-associated memory impairment" (AAMI) is used to describe minor memory difficulties that come with age.

   Most people with AAMI can compensate for memory loss with reminders and notes. It is neither progressive nor disabling and may

What Is "Normal" Memory Loss?

What is the difference between AAMI and Alzheimer's disease?		
Activity	*Alzheimer Patient*	*Age-Associated Memory Impairment*
Forgets	whole experience	parts of an experience
Remembers later	rarely	often
Follows written or spoken directions	gradually unable	usually able
Able to use notes	gradually unable	usually able
Able to care for self	gradually unable	usually able

Figure 2-1 The Difference Between AAMI & Alzheimer's Disease. Derived from *Care of Alzheimer's Patients: A Manual for Nursing Home Staff* by Lisa P. Gwyther, ACSW (1985). Reprinted by permission of the Alzheimer's Association.

remain unchanged for years. Minor memory difficulties are often most noticeable when a person is under pressure, and once relaxed, the same person is able to remember the forgotten information without difficulty. Figure 2-1 shows graphically the major differences between AAMI and Alzheimer's disease.

"Age-related memory impairment" may also be caused by fatigue, depression, grief, illness, medication, alcohol, vision or hearing loss, lack of concentration, or an attempt to remember too many details at once. How often are you doing several things at once? While working on the computer or mixing a recipe for dinner, you answer the telephone, carry on a conversation, look up to visually acknowledge someone else who walked into the room, and wonder later why you have difficulty recalling the details of the conversation.

Memory loss associated with dementia, however, will begin to interfere with the normal activities of daily life—the ability to use words, work with figures, solve problems, and use reasoning and judgment. Dementia is progressive, and when "forgetfulness" begins to affect the ability to carry on daily life, it is cause for concern. Even in advanced old age, memory loss that interferes with everyday life is not normal.[2]

What Is Alzheimer's Disease?

When it was first described by German physician Alois Alzheimer in 1907, Alzheimer's disease was considered a rare disorder. It has recently gained heightened awareness and today it is recognized as the most common cause of dementia.

It is a progressive and relentlessly degenerative disease that attacks the brain, causing brain cells to die; they are not replaced.[3] Over time this causes impaired memory, impaired thinking, and changes in behavior, resulting in the affected individual becoming less able to function independently and more dependent on others for care.

Stages of Alzheimer's Disease

It is difficult to place a patient with Alzheimer's in a specific stage. However, symptoms seem to progress in a recognizable pattern, and these stages provide a framework for understanding the disease. It is important to remember they are not uniform in every patient and the stages often overlap.

1. FIRST STAGE — two to four years leading up to and including diagnosis;

Symptoms. Recent memory loss begins to affect job performance.

- What was he or she just told to do?
- Confusion about places—gets lost on way to work.
- Loses spontaneity, the spark or zest for life.
- Loses initiative—can't start anything.
- Mood/personality changes patient becomes anxious about symptoms, avoids people.
- Poor judgment—makes bad decisions.
- Takes longer with routine chores.
- Trouble handling money, paying bills.

Examples. Forgets which bills are paid and phone numbers that are called frequently.

- Loses things. Forgets grocery list.
- Arrives at wrong time or place, or constantly rechecks calendar.
- "Mother's not the same- she's withdrawn, disinterested."
- She spent all day making dinner and forgot to serve several courses
- She paid the bills three times over, or didn't pay for 3 months.

2. SECOND STAGE — two to ten years after diagnosis (longest stage);

Symptoms increasing memory loss and confusion —shorter attention span.

- Problems recognizing close friends and/or family.
- Repetitive statements and/or movements.
- Restless, especially in late afternoon and at night.
- Occasional muscle twitches or jerking.
- Perceptual-motor problems.
- Difficulty organizing thoughts, thinking logically.
- Can't find right words—makes up stories to fill in blanks.
- Problems with reading, writing, and numbers.
- May be suspicious, irritable, fidgety, teary, or silly.
- Loss of impulse control—sloppy—won't bathe or afraid to bathe—trouble dressing.
- Gains and then loses weight.
- May see or hear things that are not there.
- Needs full-time supervision.

Examples: Memory loss—can't remember visits even though the visitor just left.

- Repetitive movements or statements.
- Sleeps often; awakens frequently at night and may get up and wander.
- Perceptual-motor problems difficulty getting into a chair, setting the table for a meal.
- Can't find the right words.
- Problems with reading, numbers—can't follow written signs, write name, add, or subtract.
- Suspicious—may accuse spouse of hiding things, infidelity; may act childish.
- Loss of impulse control sloppier table manners; may undress at inappropriate times or in the wrong place.
- Huge appetite for junk food and other people's food; forgets when last meal was eaten, then gradually loses interest in food.

3. TERMINAL STAGE — one to three years;

Symptoms Can't recognize family or self in mirror.

- Loses weight even with good diet.
- Little capacity for self care.
- Can't communicate with words.
- May put everything in mouth or touch everything.
- Can't control bowels, bladder.
- May have seizures, experience difficulty with swallowing, skin infections.

Examples:

- Looks in mirror and talks to own image.
- Needs help with bathing, dressing, eating, and going to the bathroom.
- May groan, scream, or make sounds.
- May try to suck on everything.
- Sleeps more.

Figure 2-2 Stages Of Alzheimer's Disease. Derived from *Care of Alzheimer's Patients: A Manual for Nursing Home Staff* by Lisa P. Gwyther, ACSW (1985). Reprinted by permission of the Alzheimer's Association.

The onset of Alzheimer's disease can be so gradual that it is only when reasoning problems and memory losses can no longer be ignored that help is sought. Trouble remembering recent events and difficulty accomplishing familiar tasks are early symptoms that may signal the onset of a dementing illness. The person with Alzheimer's disease may also experience confusion and personality and behavioral changes, such as gradual withdrawal from friends, social events, and activities.

When we realize that someone is increasingly unable to process new information, it becomes easier to understand the reasoning difficulties and impaired judgment, and the difficulty finding words, finishing thoughts, or following directions. The person with Alzheimer's disease is losing the ability to retrieve and use information that has been accumulated throughout a lifetime. How quickly these changes occur will vary from person to person.

Today people are living longer—which means they are living long enough to develop Alzheimer's disease. It was once thought that persons severely demented with Alzheimer's disease could not live very long, but while the course of the disease varies enormously from one individual to another, it can run anywhere from 2 to more than 20 years.[4] The stages of the disease are shown in Figure 2-2.

The relentlessness of Alzheimer's disease makes it a nightmare for families who watch their loved ones experience an unending series of losses as their minds and memories fade.[5] Eventually the disease leaves its victims totally unable to perform even the simplest tasks and incapable of caring for themselves. The overall costs, both to individual families and to society as a whole, are staggering. A recent study estimated that the cost of caring for one person with Alzheimer's disease is $47,000 each year. The disease is always fatal.

What Causes Alzheimer's Disease?

It would be far easier to detect and treat Alzheimer's disease if doctors knew what caused it. In recent years researchers have discovered much about Alzheimer's disease, but the cause is still unknown. Some of the suspected causes being investigated are genetic predisposition, a slow virus or other infectious agents, environmental toxins, and immunologic changes. It is probably not a single disorder with a single cause; there is currently no cure.

The initial diagnosis is made after a thorough medical and psychological evaluation has ruled out all the other possible causes of dementia. There has been enormous progress in recent years, and today there is 80 to 90 percent accuracy by highly qualified physicians in diagnosing Alzheimer's disease. Currently there is no single, or simple test, and definitive diagnosis is only possible with an autopsy.

An estimated 4.5 million Americans are afflicted with Alzheimer's disease and another 20 million family members must care for them. It is the fourth leading cause of death among adults. As medical technology advances and lifestyles improve, the number of people living to very old age—and, therefore, the number of people at risk for Alzheimer's disease—is likely to increase dramatically.[6] Over the next 50 years, by the time the last of the baby boomers reaches old age, the number is projected to increase threefold and it is estimated in the year 2040, at least 14 million Americans will have the disease and that 70 million people will be enlisted in their care.[7]

How Prevalent Is the Disease?

Alzheimer's disease is almost exclusively a disease of the elderly. It knows no social or economic boundaries; Alzheimer's disease strikes equally at men and women, all races and all socioeconomic groups. The risk rises with increasing age. Ten percent of those over 65, and almost half of those over age 85 have the disease.[8] While less than 5 percent of those diagnosed with the disease are younger than 65,[9] physicians are seeing an increase in patients in their 40s and 50s.

Who Gets Alzheimer's Disease?

The tragic impact of Alzheimer's disease, however, extends beyond its victims. Families usually provide the bulk of care in the early stages as the loss of mental function, personality changes, and troublesome behavior translate into years of constant supervision and care. Caring for a person with Alzheimer's disease can be emotionally, physically, and financially stressful. Regardless of how carefully one tries, there is no way to prepare for the awful reality of Alzheimer's disease.

Few health issues pose greater challenges than Alzheimer's disease.

As the illness progresses, and the behavior includes confusion, wandering, and outbursts of aggression, at some point, the stress and burden of providing care becomes overwhelming. When the strain takes its toll, caregivers must seek an alternative arrangement, and often this alternative is institutionalization. Few health issues pose greater challenges than Alzheimer's disease.[10]

Memory loss, confusion and disorientation are common symptoms of dementing illness, not a normal part of the aging process. Symptoms of Alzheimer's disease may develop gradually, and go unnoticed for a long time. Unfortunately, many people fail to recognize that these symptoms indicate something is wrong.[11] Families of dementia patients may live with a growing sense of unease for months, or even years, while the evidence that something is wrong accumulates and becomes harder to deny. Figure 2-3 lists the warning signs of Alzheimer's disease.

*A*lzheimer's disease is a degenerative disease of the brain. Its causes are unknown, and there currently is no cure. ⚐ To help you know what warning signs to look for, the Alzheimer's Association has developed a checklist of common symptoms of Alzheimer's disease (some of these symptoms also may apply to other dementing illnesses). ⚐ Review the following list and make a check mark next to symptoms that seem to be a matter of concern to you. If, when you've completed the list, you have made several check marks, you should make an appointment with a physician for a complete examination of the individual with the symptoms.

RECENT MEMORY LOSS AFFECTS JOB SKILLS
It's normal to occasionally forget assignments, colleagues' names or a business associate's telephone number, and remember them later. Those with a dementia, such as Alzheimer's disease, may forget things more often, and not remember them later. They repeatedly may ask the same question, not remembering the answer.

DIFFICULTY PERFORMING FAMILIAR TASKS
Busy people can be so distracted from time to time that they may leave the carrots on the stove and only remember to serve them at the end of the meal. People with Alzheimer's disease could prepare a meal and not only forget to serve it, but also forget they made it.

PROBLEMS WITH LANGUAGE
Everyone has trouble finding the right word sometimes, but can finish the sentence with another appropriate word. A person with Alzheimer's disease may forget simple words, or substitute inappropriate words, making their sentence incomprehensible.

DISORIENTATION OF TIME AND PLACE
It's normal to forget the day of the week or your destination for a moment. But people with Alzheimer's disease can become lost on their own street or in a familiar shopping mall, not knowing where they are, how they got there or how to get back home.

Figure 2-3 "Is It Alzheimer's? Ten Warning Signs". Courtesy of the *Alzheimer's Association, 1994*

5 POOR OR DECREASED JUDGMENT

People can become so immersed in an activity or telephone conversation they temporarily forget the child they're watching. A person with Alzheimer's disease could forget entirely the child under their care and leave the house to visit a neighbor. They may dress inappropriately, wearing several shirts or blouses.

6 PROBLEMS WITH ABSTRACT THINKING

People who normally balance their checkbooks may be momentarily disconcerted when the task is more complicated than usual, but will eventually figure out the solution. Someone with Alzheimer's disease could forget completely what the numbers are and what needs to be done with them.

7 MISPLACING THINGS

Anyone can misplace their wallet or keys, but eventually find them by reconstructing where they could have left them. A person with Alzheimer's disease may put things in inappropriate places: an iron in the freezer, or a wristwatch in the sugar bowl.

8 CHANGES IN MOOD OR BEHAVIOR

Everyone has a bad day once in a while, or may become sad or moody from time to time. Someone with Alzheimer's disease can exhibit rapid mood swings for no apparent reason: e.g., from calm to tears to anger to calm in a few moments.

9 CHANGES IN PERSONALITY

People's personalities ordinarily change somewhat at different ages, as character traits strengthen or mellow. But a person with Alzheimer's disease can change drastically, becoming extremely confused, irritable, suspicious or fearful.

10 LOSS OF INITIATIVE

It's normal to tire of housework, business activities or social obligations, but most people regain their initiative. The person with Alzheimer's disease may become passive and require cues and prompting to get them involved in activities.

Figure 2-3 *Continued.*

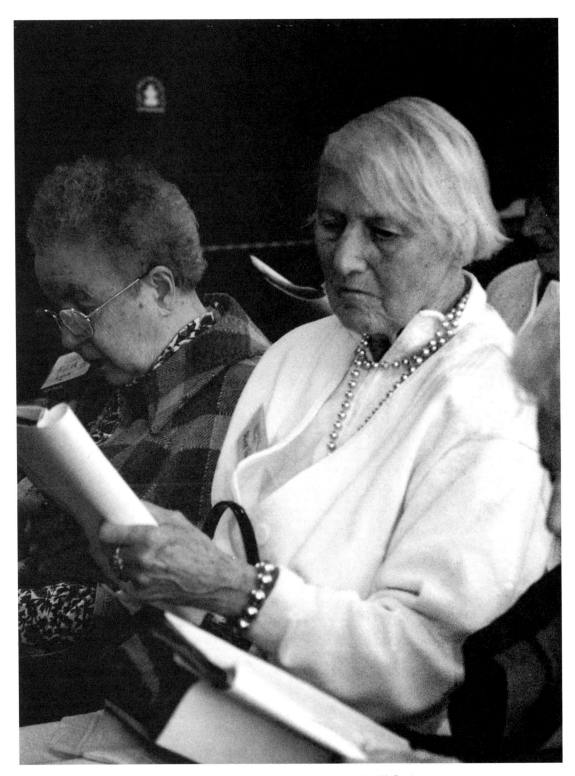

Courtesy of the Greater San Francisco Bay Area Alzheimer's Association. Photographer: Anna M. Rossi.

CHAPTER 3

Impact of Environmental Design

L iving environments influence our quality of life—including our health. If we are to have humane living environments that support independence and emphasize dignity and personal choice, we must recognize that the way we design and build these settings does, in fact, have a significant impact on health and well-being.

The same environment means different things to different people. Depending on a person's background, culture, experience, age, and position in life, the same social and spatial conditions are perceived differently and will probably stimulate different reactions. But a "healthy environment" provides a range of opportunities for its residents to participate in activities that affect their lives.

In today's fast-paced world, we have created a higher standard of living in material goods, but we are paying a very high price. The constant movement required in the job market has separated families and, in many cases, disrupted the ties between nuclear and extended families. In addition, current busy lifestyles make social relationships difficult.[1]

As a consequence, the family unit looks quite different. The elderly, frequently left to fend for themselves, often end up in retirement communities or in nursing homes. When supportive ties between people are interrupted, without attention and compassionate care, good health can be compromised by loneliness and depression. There is considerable evidence to suggest that these interrupted social ties are associated with increased rates of disease and ill health.

The concept of "active participation" is an important factor in strengthening resistance to disease, but the elderly may have less opportunity to derive satisfaction and feelings of usefulness by participating in the primary concerns of life: work, building a home, growing food, and caring for another in birth, old age, and death. Disease rates are higher among people with less opportunity to participate in the activities of life, and with less control over conditions affecting their lives they respond in various ways. Some feel angry, some humiliated and degraded, others have feelings of low self-esteem and self-worth, and some even feel their lives are without value.[2] Being "connected" with others, and with one's biological and cultural heritage helps define a person's sense of self and place in the world. Isolation from the life cycle affects our sense of identity, and it is these connections with one another and with the environment that are important to health.[3] Even families who want aged parents to live with them find it socially, economically, and spatially difficult.

> *Isolation from the life cycle affects our sense of identity, and it is these connections with one another and with the environment that are important to health.[3]*

The impact of the most demanding situation may be softened if one has chosen to be in that situation, but that is often not the case when the move is to a nursing care setting. The decision is seldom accompanied with enthusiasm and excitement. The change of lifestyle is enormous and difficult for most, but when it is the result of dementia or Alzheimer's disease it is even more difficult.

The importance of living in harmony with biological laws and having connections with a personal and historical past cannot be overemphasized. Many of us are living most of our lives in artificial environments, ignoring lunar and seasonal rhythms. The health consequences can be neuropsychiatric disorders including depression, anxiety, confusion, drug abuse, and sleep disturbance.

Effective Design Planning

Without a good understanding of the resident population's functional characteristics, environmental design cannot meet its needs. The first step in designing effective care settings is to get to know the people who live there—for design purposes this must include the mobility and abilities of the residents.

There may be a substantial difference between what residents are currently doing and what they could be doing with the assistance of good programming and effective design. Many residents would be less dependent on staff members with the right environment, opportunities, equipment, and help.[4] The more responsive the environment is to the needs of older residents, by addressing the lengthy walking distances, the need for good seating, and access to safe and stimulating outside spaces, the more likely it is that the environment will also serve those who are cognitively impaired. Effective design is quite often just a case of sensitivity, good planning, and design for all people. The presence of glare, noise, and odors in the environment is particularly aggravating, and significantly affects comfort levels.

Mildly to moderately impaired people tend to be more vulnerable to the weaknesses of existing long-term care design; for example, long corridors distance residents from essential activities such as dining, and distance staff, making them less readily available. Impaired residents are particularly vulnerable to the cueing effects of the environment—windows, access to sunlight and secure, safe outdoor spaces, as well as, the lack of culturally meaningful cues or objects. For design planning to succeed in remedying existing problems and to avoid creating new problems, it must be based on a clear understanding of the population. Design professionals need to forge a close and cooperative relationship with the care staff.

Mobility

In the typical nursing home 66 percent of the residents require assistance with walking.[5] The Alzheimer's population is generally much more active and only about a third of these residents need assistance. Sedentary activities cannot replace ambulation nor fulfill the need for physical activity in the mobile person and every effort should be made to maintain mobility levels.

The average older person is capable of standing, walking, and using their hands and coordinating the muscles to smile or grip a hand. Medical research suggests that many difficulties, such as circulatory problems, agitation, and depression, which could be prevented or delayed, are caused by lack of motion. Regrettably, the average facility and common management practice conspire to reinforce dependency and immobilize residents.

Using tools, manipulating fingers, and upper body exercise are all significant motions, but because it is so difficult to manipulate eating utensils, clothing, and grooming aids, people are often encouraged to simply stop doing so for themselves. The challenge is to offer the right tools—items that can be safely handled—and to train staff in encouraging older people to continue to exercise manual dexterity and coordination skills.[6]

It's amazing that we don't see how handicapping many traditional institutional environments are and how successfully we restrain residents — inadvertent as it may be — in what are proudly referred to as "restraint free environments." The fear of falling, for example, conspires to keep many people immobile, resulting in further debilitation. Residents might feel more comfortable moving about if objects that lead to imbalance were better designed or more secure. The risk of injury from a fall could be diminished by using carpet, which provides a slightly softer surface, instead of hard surface flooring.

> *It's amazing that we don't see how handicapping many traditional institutional environments are and how successfully we restrain residents—inadvertent as it may be—in what are proudly referred to as "restraint-free enviroments."*

The objective is to keep the highest level of function possible. With the use of well-designed lighting, proper flooring materials, level and interesting walking paths, and well-designed handrails and supports, residents are increasingly mobile. They get more exercise, which encourages physical strength and increases emotional well being. There is research, currently in progress, exploring mobility and sleep cycles to determine if more exercise in the daytime helps residents sleep better at night or results in less roaming about in the middle of the night.

Factors in the Environment Affecting Mobility

Lighting

You can't see in the dark! Insufficient lighting is one of the biggest problems in residential settings today. Older residents, particularly those with dementia, need high general illumination levels. When there is insufficient light, older people give up on activity—even walking. Glare also inhibits activity. For Alzheimer's residents a further consideration is consistent light sources to eliminate frightening shadows.

Sight

Can the residents see? Just because a resident still wears eyeglasses doesn't mean he or she can see. Are the glasses clean and when was the prescription last checked?

Seating

If appropriately designed chairs were used, and if the arms on the chairs extended beyond the seat (so that residents could just stand instead of being forced off balance as they propel themselves forward to get out of the chair), we might find more residents getting out of their chairs and walking.

Flooring

Is it safe? Carpet can make a setting seem more homelike, adding warmth, providing excellent acoustic value, and reducing glare. Carpet is available that is entirely appropriate for healthcare use. It can provide a safer walking environment and a much softer surface if a fall should occur.

A further concern for residents with cognitive impairment is that floor patterns can seem to move and be very confusing. The unsettling effects of feeling unbalanced are enough to keep the person immobile.

Contrast

Is there a clear distinction between the vertical wall plane and the horizontal floor plane? That means matching the vinyl or wood base molding to the wall, not the floor. Because of impaired depth perception, a sharp contrast between the color of the floor and the wall is necessary. Balance is adversely affected when the distinction is not clear. Again, the fear of falling makes the result predictable—residents stay put.

Handrails

Are handrails well designed for those who need to use them for support? Most are hard to use and can be particularly difficult to grip for residents with arthritic hands. A well-designed handrail allows residents to grasp the rail and permits them to glide along the rail, leaning on the forearm. An oval shape, with a broader, flat surface that can be used for arm support is much more helpful.

> *Environments can motivate mobility. They can be an invitation to "come experience me"; however, if the environment is threatening, people won't try.*

With the implementation of the Omnibus Reconciliation Act of 1987 (OBRA '87) and nursing home reform, we're coming out of the dark ages of physical and chemical restraints. For a long time we went to great lengths to minimize the mobility of demented residents, but we are beginning to see that with the use of creative interventions, allowing residents to move about has not created the horrendous problems we anticipated. Untying the elderly has not only given them freedom, but has, undoubtedly, had a positive effect on the levels of agitation and anger. Interestingly, we have not seen the dramatic increase in falls that was expected.[7]

Wheelchair Use

Nursing homes of the past never anticipated the number of people who would use wheelchairs or walkers today. Consequently, the design of many older facilities is not as kind to some residents as it could be. The lack of adequate space in bedrooms makes self-wheeling nearly impossible and forces residents to rely on staff assistance.[8] Many people in wheelchairs, for example, require more than a 5 by 5 foot turnaround space in bathrooms, and it is often necessary for designers to exceed code to meet the needs of elderly residents. Door openings are often based on clearance of the wheelchair and not the clearance of elbows of the user.[9]

Socialization

No matter how elegant and beautiful an environment, no matter how efficiently designed, no matter how safe—unless people can, in some way, participate in activities that affect their lives, the outcome is likely to be dissatisfaction, and even illness.[10]

Residents in care settings need opportunities to continue a meaningful and active life, more than just entertainment throughout the entire day. The real need is for activities and interactions that reaffirm a resident's identity as a person and restore a sense of self-worth. It is wise, whenever possible, to put opportunities for activities with meaning back into the environment and to encourage residents to maintain an active social life.

> *No matter how elegant and beautiful an environment, no matter how efficiently designed, no matter how safe—unless people can, in some way, participate in activities that affect their lives, the outcome is likely to be dissatisfaction, and even illness.*

Although many older people enjoy and benefit from socializing, there seem to be few appropriate gathering places for small groups. Many settings have a lovely lobby or other inviting social areas that are often "off limits" to frail or mentally impaired people, which makes the most interesting seating in front of the nursing station.

With more than half of residents having memory impairment, today's facility should be designed with different places for people of varying abilities to gather. Research suggests that conversation can be stimulated by activity and changing locations. When sitting at tables residents should be in appropriately designed chairs that focus attention on other people and do not recline backward.[11]

Dining

Older people can be unnecessarily hindered by dining areas that fail to accommodate their unique needs. Dining services are shaped by spaces, furnishings, equipment, and systems. For example, the majority of older people in nursing homes have some vision impairment in addition to being sensitive to glare. Most are also hearing impaired. Both of these problems cause discomfort and affect the attention span, often making conversation difficult to understand. Yet dining areas are often filled with glare and noise, and the hard surfaces used throughout, on the assumption they are safer or easier to clean, only exacerbate the problem.

Eating is often made more difficult because of the distance of the chair from the table. It can be frustrating when food on the table is out of reach. Spills may not be an indication of a resident's capability, but in fact, be the result of the chair being too far from the table.

Cognitive Impairment

Most buildings are not designed with an understanding of managing cognitive impairment. Dementia destroys a person's ability to understand events and people in his or her environment and to plan for and take care of himself or herself. Without help, such a person cannot do what most of us take for granted—the most basic activities of daily life—walking, dressing, eating, bathing or using the toilet, making a telephone call, taking prescribed medication, or cooking a meal. Many cognitively impaired residents experience diminished capacity in one or more of the following areas:

- Memory for fact: names, numbers, and sequences
- Action and motion: ability to balance, coordinate, swallow, and maneuver utensils
- Emotion: capacity to match emotions with situations (for example, a person may be expressionless or be easily agitated)
- Social behavior: ability to relate to people in conventional ways, need for smaller groups
- Judgment: ability to plan, anticipate, change behavior mid-course, override situations, and anticipate danger.[12]

As more and more healthcare settings attempt to serve a resident population that consists of large numbers of people suffering with Alzheimer's disease and other related dementias, it becomes increasingly clear that design is not just an incidental concern but integral to a well-balanced approach for this population.[13]

Physical problems are acceptable, but to most of us depression and dementia, the most significant contributors to loss of function, are not acceptable. As individual competence decreases, the environment becomes increasingly important in determining well-being. The primary focus is to maximize the capability of the environment to support residents' remaining abilities to carry out activities. Careful design planning can facilitate mental functioning, minimize some areas of confusion, and allow individuals to function more independently at whatever level they may be able.

> *Good design places the importance and focus on supporting ability and improving the quality of life.*

The number of disabled elderly is expected to grow rapidly in number, and they will be a larger percentage of the total elderly population in the future because of the changing age composition of the elderly population, particularly the higher proportion of people 85 years or older.[14]

Eighty percent of elderly people suffer from chronic limitation of mobility.[15] Forty-eight percent have arthritis, 29 percent have hearing loss, 17 percent have orthopedic impairments, and 14 percent have vision problems.[16] To that list add incontinence, sensation loss, respiration, and cardiac difficulties. Many residents have multiple problems, but environments can be designed to provide support, enhance, and simplify lives, and make them more enjoyable.

NOTES

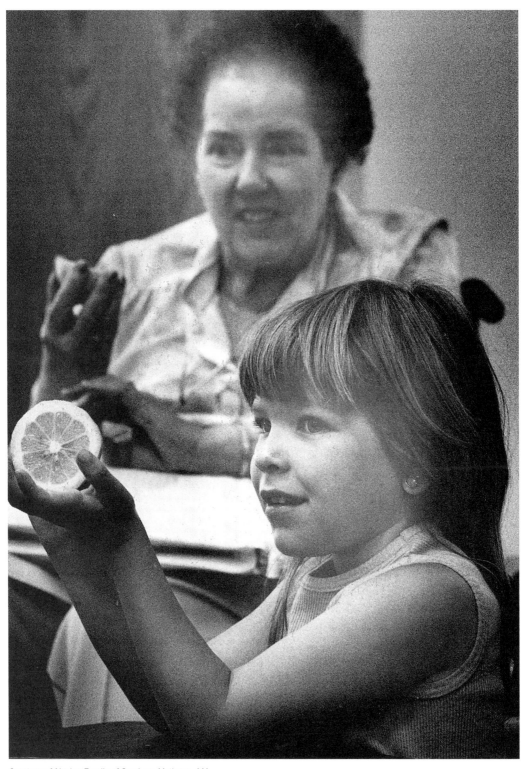

My mother died from Alzheimer's disease. My sister and I still suffer from it!

CHAPTER 4

Alzheimer's Disease: The Impact on the Family

My introduction to Alzheimer's disease came in late December 1978 when, like many other happy excited sons and daughters, I went home for the Christmas holidays. My sister and I both arrived late in the evening on Christmas Eve. Dad had been sick for several weeks, and as we walked in, we realized immediately that my father was much more seriously ill than either of us had known.

He was in a great deal of pain and my usually efficient mom, who had always been an angel of mercy with the sick, seemed neither to understand what was happening nor to have any idea what to do. After calling an ambulance and admitting my father to the hospital, I tried to find out from my mom what was wrong with Dad and why we hadn't known about it. She admitted that she hadn't told us he wasn't feeling well because she hadn't wanted to worry us, but she seemed to have no idea at all what was wrong or the seriousness of the situation. In fact, though she seemed relieved that someone else was in charge, she was uncharacteristically adamant, almost violent, in her opposition to my talking to his doctor. I'm not sure who was more confused at the time—she or I. I couldn't understand why she had no idea what was wrong with my father or why she was so strangely opposed to my attempting to find out.

When I was able to speak with his physician, I learned that my father was dying of cancer. When I questioned him further about why he had not told my mother, he seemed quite puzzled and said that he had had a lengthy conversation with both of my parents together, a conversation my mother did not remember. The doctor seemed content to accept that my mother was in denial, and that my father's illness might be more than she could deal with. He offered no advice.

I look back on this as one of the most painful times in my life. I arrived home with expectations of sharing happy times with my family, celebrating the Christmas holidays. I was full of excitement; I hadn't seen my parents for almost a year. It was so unexpected! The moment I walked in the door my life changed; it was never to be that free or that unspoiled again. I lost my father and began a long and lonely journey with my mom. Little did I know that it was only the beginning of the desperation and the frustration of trying to unravel the mysteries and cope with Alzheimer's disease.

I did not hear the words Alzheimer's disease until long after my father died, and it became increasingly apparent that my mother was suffering from something more than extended grief. It also became unavoidably clear that my mom could not continue to live alone.

In the heat and humidity of the deep South, she closed the windows, pulled the shades and draperies, and locked the doors. She lived in one of the safest small towns in America, but she was afraid. The temperature outside was 104 degrees in the shade and it's anyone's guess what it was inside the tightly closed house, with no air circulation and no air conditioning. I was afraid she would die of suffocation.

In quiet desperation, my sister, Mary, and I were confronting the undeniable truth—that though we didn't have a diagnosis or a name that would define the horror that was destroying my mother's life and ours—we had to accept that she was not getting better, despite our efforts. Her life was rapidly becoming more confusing to her and more unmanageable all the time. Finally, we could no longer avoid making inevitable and painful choices.

Day care was not an option. It didn't exist in this small town. We were trying to manage an unmanageable situation from great distances. My sister, with two very small children, lived in Atlanta, and I lived in San Francisco. We first arranged to have someone stay with mom overnight—to come in late in the afternoon, prepare an evening meal and leave after breakfast the following morning. It worked well for almost a year, until her caregiver wanted to go visit her own family for a holiday and the substitute didn't show up. Mom became hysterical and no one was able to calm her. A close friend called my sister Mary. She drove seven hours in the middle of the night, and took Mom back to her home for two weeks until her caregiver returned.

We knew time was running out, this was no longer a reliable situation and we had to make the hardest choice I have ever made. I had been through divorce and the loss of my father, and I can say, without question, that making the decision to place my mother in a nursing home was the single most painful thing I have ever lived through in my life.

Making life-altering decisions, particularly those that will forever change someone else's life, is racked with uncertainty and guilt. Mom must have said to me a hundred times in my life, if she said it once, "Please, don't ever put me in an old folks home." I have often wondered if she had as much trouble saying the words "nursing home" as I do.

As much as I know today that we made the best decision that we could have made, that during the more than nine years she lived in a nursing home, she was lovingly cared about, as well as cared for, her words are engraved in my brain as clearly today as they were then. I have never stopped feeling guilty that I couldn't have done more — that I couldn't save her from the fate she dreaded so much. Alzheimer's disease robbed my mother of her memories, her mind, and finally her life. It has been said that Alzheimer's disease is the illness that robs victims' minds and breaks families' hearts.

One of the greatest difficulties was feeling completely powerless. There seemed to be nothing I could do to change the inevitable — for once I was up against something I couldn't fix. My mother died from Alzheimer's disease. My sister and I still suffer from it!

It is important to stop Alzheimer's disease. Dr. Allen Roses, an internationally prominent researcher from Duke University, said quite accurately, "Alzheimer's is a terrible, terrible way to die...and taking care of people with Alzheimer's is a terrible way to live."

> *"Alzheimer's is a terrible, terrible way to die...and taking care of people with Alzheimer's is a terrible way to live."*

My experiences and reactions are not unlike those that many family members go through. The denial, the blame, the guilt, the fear, and the ultimate and endless sense of loss, and for some, abandonment. Placing a loved one in a long-term care setting is painful. The move is at best, a reluctant choice, and most often the decision and the selection, particularly in the case of Alzheimer's, is made by the family, not the resident. It is always a difficult and most times a painful choice. Understanding what families experience will help to provide some context for why the environmental impact is so important—for residents and for families.

The families and spouses of persons with Alzheimer's disease are usually very reluctant to give up their care-giving responsibilities. They may have promised their loved ones never to put them in a "home," and they try desperately to keep that promise. Most often it is a crisis or dramatic change in condition that pushes a family over the edge. The patient may have become incontinent, the primary caregiver may have become ill, or some other family or health changes may have occurred, and the family is suddenly making difficult choices in a time of great stress.

> *Unfortunately as Alzheimer's disease progresses, the family often bears a heavy burden. I only wish there was some way I could spare Nancy from this painful experience.*
>
> *Former President of the United States, Ronald Reagan*

This is a catastrophic time for the family who is giving their loved one to someone else for care. It is also a frightening time for the new resident, who is experiencing many changes. It is a time for care providers to be sensitive, respectful, compassionate, and very personal in their interactions. This is a time when every effort should be made to keep the family involved and informed.[1]

Most families feel that nowhere will the care be as good as they were giving at home. Finding a healthcare setting that is residential in nature is appealing, but the primary consideration is not just a pretty building. What they are looking for is a place that will treat their loved one with respect and dignity. Families want to know that their loved one will be safe and will be cared for appropriately. They are particularly concerned that the staff understand the nature of Alzheimer's disease and know how to care for their loved one. And perhaps most important, they are looking for an option that will assure that they can continue to have some level of involvement in their loved one's life. Most families want to stay involved in the care, even if they can no longer provide that care at home. They want to visit, to be involved in activities, perhaps take their loved one home for a special occasion or on short outings.[2]

Families want to know that their loved one will be safe and will be cared for appropriately.

One of the most difficult aspects of caring for a loved one with Alzheimer's is the unpredictability of the disease. The progressive deterioration is inevitable, but no one can say exactly how or when it will happen in each individual. People who live long enough with the disease can lose all ability to feed, clothe, and bathe themselves. All of this becomes even harder as the person loses understanding of what is going on around him or her, and eventually fails to recognize the loved one who is providing care. Family members continue to need reassurance of the appropriateness of their decision and that what they have done is right for them. There is no certainty about tomorrow.

A study of dementia caregivers found that, contrary to popular opinion, it was not the functional status or the extent of the individual's illness that determined a family's decision to place a loved one in a healthcare setting. It was the circumstances of the caregiver, the person with Alzheimer's disease, and the caregiving context that best predicted placement.

The Alzheimer's Association's *Guidelines for Dignity* offers care providers a framework for designing a special care program for those with Alzheimer's disease, and for families, a guide to assess and evaluate an Alzheimer's special care setting.

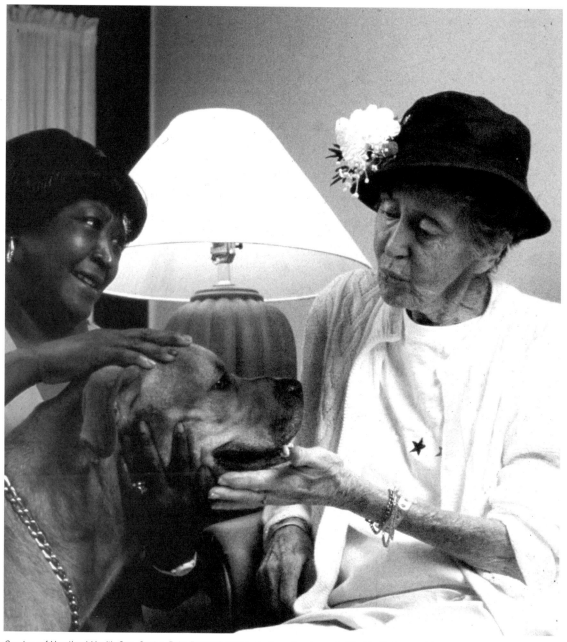

Courtesy of Heartland Health Care Center, Palm Beach Gardens, FL. Owned and operated by Health Care and Retirement Corporation, Inc.

An Alzheimer's special care unit frequently comprises the whole universe for many residents. That world can and should be a supportive environment—one that provides a sense of comfort and security. It should be as diverse as possible, not only to increase stimulation and response to surroundings for residents, but to create more interesting places for the working staff, and to support continued family involvement.

It is my hope that we provide an atmosphere of living—where residents are nurtured and find comfort and support in their environment.

CHAPTER 5

Criteria for Designing Alzheimer's Special Care Settings

It is estimated that there are now about 1.8 million people with severe dementia in the United States and an additional 1 to 5 million people with mild or moderate dementia.[1] In 1985, the National Nursing Home Survey, conducted by the National Center for Health Statistics, found that half of the residents of nursing homes with dementia were over 85, and that three-quarters of those residents with dementia were female.[2] In addition, the survey indicated that 62 percent of all nursing home residents were so disoriented or memory-impaired that their performance of the activities of daily living, mobility, and other tasks were impaired nearly every day.[3]

There are several issues that complicate the provision of long-term care for those suffering from dementia. As a cognitive disease, dementia manifests itself in behavioral and mental difficulties, but it does not necessarily lead to physical disability until the later stages. This means that the traditional medical model of nursing home care may not provide for the needs of the resident suffering from dementia.

In response to the rising numbers of residents with Alzheimer's disease in nursing homes, specialized care units are emerging as a means for managing the complex care associated with dementia. Special care units have grown from the belief that residents with Alzheimer's disease require specialized care not routinely available in nursing homes, and that people without dementia will be happier if they are separated from the more disruptive dementia patients. The intent is to encourage and support the optimum quality of life for all residents.

The first special care units for individuals with dementia in this country were established in the mid 1960s and early 1970s. Interest grew rapidly in the mid to late 1970s and the first half of the1980s, because of increasing awareness of Alzheimer's disease and the special needs of nursing home residents with dementia,[4] and SCUs in long-term care settings emerged as a care option for people with Alzheimer's disease in the 1980s. Over 60,000 people with Alzheimer's disease are being cared for in nursing homes that offer "special care units" expressly for residents with dementia — and that number is growing rapidly. Researchers estimated there would be more than 2,500 units in the year 1995, and these numbers will increase dramatically in coming years.

Residential long term care for persons with Alzheimer's disease is different from the care required for a person who has skilled nursing needs. It requires a focus on the psychosocial needs of the individual, and provides specific therapeutic activities designed to maximize remaining cognitive and physical abilities. Appropriate Alzheimer's care settings provide a specialized physical environment that enhances and supports individualized care and behavioral approaches to managing residents with dementia. Disruptive and agitated behaviors are often symptoms of the disease. Although there is diversity among special care settings, many SCUs incorporate some type of physical modification, including security measures to limit access, and most provide specialized activity programming for residents.[5]

What Makes Special Care Units Special?

What is a special care unit and how does it differ from the rest of a long-term care facility? An SCU is geographically separate, offers special activities and staff training, and is designed for people with dementia. Special care settings also have a policy or philosophy that drives all the activities and includes the resident's family as part of the care team.[6] There are five areas that make a special care unit special (Berg et al. 1991)[7]:

1. Admission of residents with dementia
2. Staff who are specially selected, and trained
3. Activities that are specifically designed for the cognitively impaired

4. Family involvement
5. A physical environment and decor designed for the safety and segregation of the residents and the common behaviors associated with dementia

The environment of an ideal SCU is designed to enhance care by creating a warm, bright, and cheerful "homelike" atmosphere,[8] and by including wandering space, special lighting designed to eliminate shadows, and wallcoverings that serve as a reminder of a more homelike setting.[9] Individual residents rooms are personalized by including many personal treasures and possessions, to make them more comforting and more comfortable .

A therapeutic milieu is a distinguishing feature of SCUs. Creating such a milieu involves meeting needs in a way that reflects compassion, patience, understanding, and creativity and providing a safe, pleasant, and clean environment.[10] In an effort to enhance the quality of life for residents, as well as to maintain consistency of staffing, it is recommended that staff receive specialized orientation and training on dementia, its manifestations, and approaches to care.[11] This is mentioned most often by providers as the single most important aspect of delivering good quality care.

Activities are emphasized as a way to provide stimulation for residents' physical, cognitive and social skills,[12] and they are provided in a manner that supports the dignity and lifestyle of the individual and assists in maintaining that lifestyle.[13] Although residents are cognitively impaired, it is assumed that they retain some ability to feel and think.[14] Privacy is respected on ideal units.

Ideal SCUs provide an outdoor area, such as a patio or courtyard, for residents to enjoy[15]—a safe physical environment that allows for some physical freedom and a sense of security.[16] Virtually all special units have some type of alarm system that alerts staff when residents leave the unit.

As Alzheimer special care settings evolve, these design elements have emerged as the basis for prototypical design. Innovative trends that raise the level of special care design involve getting away from gimmicks, to focus on designing settings that work functionally. Supported by the latest research on special care from the National Institute on Aging (NIA),[17] Sloane and Lauren Matthew have identified some of the trends. In housing, a smaller number of people in a less stimulating, and therefore less confusing, setting is definitely preferable. This cluster or pod design reduces institutional care settings in size and scale, to something that more closely resembles a home environment and allows for a variety of different groupings and activity spaces.

> *Specialized Alzheimer/dementia care is a new area. Fortunately, in the past few years, nursing care has become much more sensitive to the needs of residents, and much of what has been learned about specialized care can apply to better quality care for all residents in care settings.*

Architects are incorporating outdoor spaces in the overall design plan by adding more doors and by making the outdoor areas accessible to residents from a number of locations. Courtyards are recent innovations that provide gardening opportunities, bird feeders, outdoor seating for residents, and opportunities for other additional program activities.

Multiple special use spaces are becoming available. Private areas where a disruptive resident can be taken for one-on-one care, and separate activity spaces for groups that need special attention, are empowering to the staff. In addition, designers, working with staff members, are creating interesting opportunities for activity and stimulation such as pictures for reminiscing, wall mounted panels that attract touch, or cabinets made with various and interesting hardware, doors and drawers made for opening.

Efforts to individualize orientation to assist with effective wayfinding for residents is stimulating the discovery of more effective orientation methods or cues.[18]

Specialized Alzheimer/dementia care is a new area. Fortunately, in the past few years, nursing care has become much more sensitive to the needs of residents, and much of what has been learned about specialized care can apply to better quality care for all residents in care settings.

The options for residential care are no longer only "nursing homes." Specialized Alzheimer care residential facilities are becoming more available. Care programs for people with dementia are being influenced by architecture, facility design, technology, active appropriate programming, communication and care management techniques, environmental adaptations, and dementia-specific training. The NIA continues to study the impact of these programs on people with Alzheimer's disease, their families, and the nursing staff.[19]

Guidelines for Dignity

To meet the challenge of designing Alzheimer's special care units, guidelines were published by the Alzheimer's Association in 1992, as shown in Figure 5-1. Viewed as an effort to encourage and support innovative models to improve quality of care, these guidelines have defined the critical issues and given some structure to the process.

Philosophy of Care

The philosophy is the cornerstone of the entire program. Meeting the challenge of dementia in a long-term care residential setting is a

Guidelines for Dignity

Goal 1: Philosophy

A specialized Alzheimer/ dementia care program has a written statement of its overall philosophy and mission which reflects the needs of residents afflicted with dementia.

Goal 2: Pre Admission

There is an effective process for placement in the program, by which diagnoses are verified, the needs of the person with dementia are assessed, involvement of family is recognized (to the desired extent of the individual family), and appropriateness of the facility is confirmed.

Goal 3: Admission

The person with dementia is admitted to the program in a convenient and supportive manner, and the family is able to complete the admission requirements in a timely fashion.

Goal 4: Care Planning and Implementation

The plan of care and its implementation is resident oriented, flexible, and inclusive of family; and it is intended to promote individual dignity, optimum health and well-being and to maximize function of the person with dementia.

Care provision is the responsibility of the interdisciplinary team, committed to creating a living environment that enhances quality of life for residents and families.

Goal 5: Change in Condition

As the disease moves to late stages, the plan of care evolves and is responsive to changes in condition. A specialized program demonstrates commitment to assist families over the full course of the disease.

Goal 6: Staffing Patterns and Training

All staff, including administrators and nondirect staff (e.g. housekeeping, dietary, maintenance, volunteers), who work with residents and families in the specialized Alzheimer/dementia program receive the support of an ongoing training program.

Goal 7: Physical Environment

The physical environment and design features support the functioning of cognitively impaired adult residents, accommodate behaviors and maxzimize functional abilities, promote safety, and encourage independence of residents.

Goal 8: Success Indicators

The program is involved in efforts to evaluate the benefits of their specialized Alzheimer/dementia care.

Figure 5-1 Guidelines for Dignity: Goals of Specialized Alzheimer/Dementia Care in Residential Settings. (1992).
Reprinted by permission of the Alzheimer's Association. For more information on Alzheimer's Disease and the services provided by the Alzheimer's Association, call 1 (800) 272-3900.

process that begins with the development of a specific and sensitive philosophy of care. The philosophy recognizes the unique needs of persons with dementia who are experiencing memory loss, impairment of functional abilities and other cognitive skills, and it is a description of the distinguishing characteristics of a particular program. Examples might include "a small homelike environment," "walking paths," or "accessible, secured outdoor spaces."

Because of a resident's impairment, care providers accept an increased responsibility to be sensitive to the individual's needs and respond with a compassionate life-enriching program and environment.[20] This applies to design professionals as well. While in reality, very little research has been done to test the impact of particular physical design features on individuals with dementia, the concept that appropriate environments will improve the functioning and quality of life of individuals with dementia is one that cries for the most dedicated response.

The program philosophy describes the purpose and intent of the Alzheimer care program and defines the relationships between the philosophy and the physical environment. This is particularly important to the design process. Having a clear philosophy in place allows the program of care to determine needs that drive the design, instead of the reverse. Too often, particularly in renovation situations, the care patterns are dictated by the constraints of the budget and the environment. Good architects and designers can clear a lot of hurdles, but many renovation settings present design challenges that are much easier to address in new construction.

Many aspects of the physical and social environment affect the functioning of individuals with dementia. Providing appropriate environments will improve their functioning and quality of life.[22]

Nursing home residents with dementia are more likely than other residents to need assistance with activities of daily living (i.e., bathing, dressing, using the toilet, transferring from bed to chair, remaining continent, and eating), and behavioral symptoms are also more common. The 1987 National Medical Expenditure Survey found that 59 percent of residents with dementia had one or more of ten behavioral symptoms (wandering, physically hurting others, physically hurting oneself, dressing inappropriately, crying for long periods, hoarding, getting upset, not avoiding dangerous things, stealing, and inappropriate sexual behavior).[21]

Many aspects of the physical and social environment affect the functioning of individuals with dementia. Providing appropriate environments will improve their functioning and quality of life.[22]

The relationship between the environment and the functioning of older people has been the topic of research and theory-building for years, and it is now generally accepted that the impact of the environment is greater for individuals with low competence, including individuals with dementia, than for other people. According to Lawton[23] as individual competence decreases, the environment assumes increasing importance in determining well-being.

Lack of stimulation and exercise, as well as excessive environmental noise can cause increased disability in individuals with dementia. The literature on SCUs contains numerous examples of situations in which changing a factor that was causing excess disability resulted in dramatic improvement in an individual's functioning and quality of life. Physical design features are seen as potentially compensating for or responding to the impairments and needs of individuals with dementia in the following general ways[24]:

- Assure safety and security
- Support functional abilities
- Assist with wayfinding and orientation
- Prompt memory
- Establish links with the familiar, healthy past
- Convey expectations and elicit and reinforce appropriate behavior
- Reduce agitation
- Facilitate privacy
- Facilitate social interactions
- Stimulate interest and curiosity
- Support independence, autonomy, and control
- Facilitate the involvement of families

Characteristics of Nursing Home Residents with Dementia

To determine the priorities of special care for individuals with dementia, information about the characteristics of demented and nondemented nursing home residents is useful; see Figure 5-2. Residents with dementia are generally older than non-demented residents and are more likely to have impairments in activities of daily living, as well as psychiatric and behavioral symptoms.

The elderly have a rather broad diversity of abilities and needs that cannot be stereotyped. This is especially true in Alzheimer's care, where residents are in different stages of the disease with varying abilities and impairments, and we must continually remember that no two dementia residents are the same, and that no two days with the same resident may be the same.

Type of Nursing Home Residents

Primary diagnosis

Variable	Frequency	Limited Impaired (1)	Oldest-old Deteriorating (2)	Acute and Rehabilitative (3)	Behavioral Problem (4)	Dementia (5)	Severely Impaired (6)
Cancer	1.43	0.66	1.79	3.01	1.39	0.00	1.32
Heart disease	17.79	35.56	62.83	9.48	0.00	0.00	0.00
Stroke	10.78	0.00	0.00	18.56	0.00	19.46	20.72
Diabetes	4.05	7.77	8.57	1.10	9.47	0.00	0.00
Arthritis	5.94	8.56	14.39	11.10	0.00	0.00	0.00
Renal problems	0.64	0.00	0.00	1.74	0.00	0.06	1.44
Digestive problems	0.70	0.00	1.52	2.27	0.00	0.00	0.00
Hip fracture	1.92	0.00	0.00	9.52	0.00	0.00	0.00
Liver and gall bladder problems	0.12	0.42	0.00	0.00	0.00	0.34	0.00
Alzheimer's disease and senile dementia	15.29	12.07	0.00	0.00	22.68	42.50	20.079
Other neurological problems	10.30	0.00	0.00	24.64	0.00	0.00	27.32
Chronic respiratory problems	1.64	6.79	3.30	0.00	0.00	0.00	0.00
Other respiratory problems	0.61	0.00	1.37	0.81	0.00	0.00	1.17
Infectious disease	0.34	0.00	1.43	0.00	0.00	0.70	0.00
Other endocrine problems	0.18	0.00	0.00	0.00	1.46	0.00	0.00
Metabolic disorder	0.34	0.20	0.00	0.00	0.00	0.00	1.55
Blood disorder	0.49	0.00	3.05	0.00	0.00	0.00	0.00

Mental disorder	18.40	22.20	0.00	0.00	44.54	36.94	17.83
Atherosclerosis	2.56	0.00	0.00	0.00	20.46	0.00	0.00
Other circulatory problems	1.22	0.00	0.00	6.05	0.00	0.00	0.00
Other	5.27	5.78	1.75	11.72	0.00	0.00	8.59

Associated conditions

Cancer	3.33	4.37	14.32	2.36	4.93	0.00	0.00
Heart disease	50.60	47.13	100.00	49.95	32.83	62.03	21.23
Stroke	16.37	6.07	28.96	17.67	13.49	13.43	22.95
Diabetes	12.26	5.96	25.80	17.43	27.91	5.20	7.46
Arthritis	22.03	19.36	100.00	12.28	4.25	19.11	0.00
Renal problems	6.39	0.00	0.00	0.00	0.00	0.00	29.95
Digestive problems	7.56	4.55	55.16	0.00	0.00	0.00	0.00
Hip fracture	4.61	2.54	0.00	6.28	0.00	7.21	6.73
Liver and gall bladder disease	1.02	1.34	7.00	0.00	0.00	0.00	0.00
Alzheimer's disease and senile dementia	8.17	8.17	0.00	0.00	61.62	0.00	10.01
Other neurological problems	16.49	16.49	100.00	0.00	0.00	0.00	0.00
Chronic respiratory problems	5.16	7.59	23.40	0.00	6.82	2.61	0.00
Other respiratory problems	1.93	1.57	0.00	1.38	0.00	3.33	3.10
Urological problems	6.39	6.39	0.00	0.00	0.00	0.00	29.95
Infectious disease	75.72	75.72	0.00	100.00	100.00	100.00	100.00
Other endocrine problems	2.66	2.63	15.70	2.20	0.00	0.00	0.00

Figure 5-2 Characteristics of six types of nursing home residents, New York State. *From Special care units for people with Alzheimer's Disease and other dementias. U.S. Congress, Office of Technology Assessment. Original source: Manton, K.G., Vertrees, J.C., and Woodbury, M.A. Functionally and Medically Defined Subgroups of Nursing Home Population. Health Care Financing Review. 12(1):50-52 (1990).*

Type of Nursing Home Residents

Variable	Frequency	Limited Impaired (1)	Oldest-old Deteriorating (2)	Acute and Rehabilitative (3)	Behavioral Problem (4)	Dementia (5)	Severely Impaired (6)
Metabolic disorder	2.31	3.42	5.00	2.11	6.36	0.00	0.71
Blood disorder	6.24	0.00	51.34	0.00	0.00	0.00	0.00
Mental disorder	17.54	0.00	0.00	0.00	100.00	0.00	0.00
Eye problems	12.28	0.00	100.00	0.00	0.00	0.00	0.00
Ear problems	2.83	0.00	31.94	0.00	0.00	0.00	0.00
Atherosclerosis	5.46	0.00	27.35	0.00	0.00	7.83	3.82
Other circulatory problems	5.25	1.55	29.66	8.49	0.00	0.00	0.00
Skin problems	2.60	0.00	14.27	0.00	2.14	0.00	4.46
Fractured extremities	1.81	0.00	0.00	3.62	0.00	0.00	5.60
Comatose	1.20	0.00	0.00	0.00	0.00	0.00	6.37
Terminally ill	1.32	0.00	0.00	1.79	0.00	0.00	4.95
Alcohol abuse	3.17	4.77	0.00	0.00	26.64	0.00	0.00
Drug abuse	0.26	0.00	0.00	0.00	3.14	0.00	0.00

Limitations

Variable	Frequency	Limited Impaired (1)	Oldest-old Deteriorating (2)	Acute and Rehabilitative (3)	Behavioral Problem (4)	Dementia (5)	Severely Impaired (6)
Vision:							
No loss	74.53	100.00	0.00	100.00	100.00	91.92	54.39
Moderate loss	19.03	0.00	63.05	0.00	0.00	8.08	45.61
Severe loss	6.44	0.00	36.95	0.00	0.00	0.00	0.00
Hearing:							
No loss	80.22	100.00	0.00	100.00	100.00	100.00	100.00
Moderate loss	15.26	0.00	77.15	0.00	0.00	0.00	0.00
Severe loss	4.52	0.00	22.85	0.00	0.00	0.00	0.00
Verbal expression:							
No difficulty	66.43	100.00	100.00	91.11	83.53	51.13	0.00
With difficulty	23.72	0.00	0.00	8.89	16.65	48.87	48.31

50

Totally impaired	9.85	0.00	0.00	0.00	0.00	51.69

Reception:						
No difficulty	57.50	47.26	100.00	0.00	40.18	0.00
With difficulty	34.36	52.74	0.00	100.00	59.82	38.89
Totally impaired	8.14	0.00	0.00	0.00	0.00	61.11
Diet:						
Regular	19.56	0.00	28.35	18.81	26.83	0.19
Other	80.44	100.00	71.65	81.19	73.17	99.81
Decubiti:						
None	88.79	100.00	93.73	100.00	100.00	52.33
Single	9.57	0.00	6.27	0.00	0.00	39.88
Multiple	1.64	0.00	0.00	0.00	0.00	7.79
Discoloration	6.02	59.66	0.00	0.00	0.00	0.00
Edema	15.16	93.48	13.38	21.33	0.00	4.90
Weight loss	13.61	53.30	9.86	42.09	4.39	10.14
Severe pain	8.03	25.41	20.44	9.77	0.00	0.00
Contractures	22.49	0.00	0.00	0.00	0.00	97.90
Dyspnea	4.71	46.50	0.00	0.00	0.00	0.00
Mobility:						
No impairment	21.65	0.00	0.00	100.00	0.00	0.00
With help	24.37	0.00	62.36	0.00	38.43	0.00
Wheechairfast	38.11	100.00	37.64	0.00	61.57	36.15
Chairfast	14.74	0.00	0.00	0.00	0.00	59.27
Bedfast	1.14	0.00	0.00	0.00	021.00	4.58
Transfer:						
No impairment	29.51	0.00	0.00	100.00	0.00	0.00
With help	40.11	100.00	100.00	0.00	100.00	0.00
Bedfast	30.39	021.00	0.00	0.00	0.00	100.00

Figure 5-2 (Continued)

51

Type of Nursing Home Residents

Variable	Frequency	Limited Impaired (1)	Oldest-old Deteriorating (2)	Acute and Rehabilitative (3)	Behavioral Problem (4)	Dementia (5)	Severely Impaired (6)
Eating:							
No loss	22.12	100.00	0.00	0.00	0.00	0.00	0.00
With supervision	55.85	0.00	100.00	100.00	100.00	100.00	0.00
Totally impaired	22.03	0.00	0.00	0.00	0.00	0.00	100.00
Dressing:							
No impairment	13.22	62.72	0.00	0.00	100.00	0.00	0.00
With supervision	36.68	37.28	100.00	100.00	0.00	0.00	0.00
Totally impaired	50.10	0.00	0.00	0.00	0.00	100.00	100.00
Bathing:							
No impairment	2.25	10.12	0.00	0.00	100.00	0.00	0.00
With assistance	42.88	89.88	100.00	100.00	0.00	0.00	0.00
Totally impaired	54.87	0.00	0.00	0.00	0.00	100.00	100.00
Toileting:							
No impairment	27.37	100.00	0.00	0.00	100.00	0.00	0.00
With help	24.2	0.00	100.00	100.00	0.00	100.00	0.00
Totally impaired	48.38	0.00	0.00	0.00	0.00	0.00	100.00
Bladder control:							
Continent	39.31	100.00	0.00	100.00	0.00	0.00	0.00
Incontinent	51.59	0.00	100.00	0.00	100.00	100.00	58.92
Indwelling	7.27	0.00	0.00	0.00	0.00	0.00	32.78
External	1.64	0.00	0.00	0.00	0.00	0.00	8.29
Bowel:							
Continent	46.57	99.11	0.00	99.17	0.00	0.00	0.00
Incontinent	53.38	0.00	0.00	0.00	0.00	100.00	100.00
Colostomy	121.05	0.89	100.00	0.83	100.00	0.00	0.00

Personal hygiene:							
No impairment	12.32	54.55	0.00	0.00	0.00	0.00	0.00
with supervision	25.84	45.56	100.00	100.00	100.00	0.00	0.00
With assistance	61.84	0.00	0.00	0.00	0.00	100.00	100.00
Learning:							
No impairment	32.80	91.94	0.00	84.46	0.00	0.00	0.00
With difficulty	49.09	8.06	100.00	15.54	100.00	93.40	0.00
Totally impaired	18.11	0.00	0.00	0.00	0.00	6.60	100.00
Patient wanders	9.48	0.00	0.00	0.00	94.33	17.90	0.00
abusive	34.90	0.00	0.00	0.00	100.00	0.00	0.00
Patient physically aggressive	16.95	0.00	0.00	0.00	100.00	0.00	0.00
Severe depression	7.36	0.00	0.00	0.00	100.00	0.00	0.00
Hallucinations	6.13	0.00	0.00	0.00	100.00	0.00	0.00
Paranoia	7.65	0.00	0.00	0.00	100.00	0.00	0.00
Patient withdrawn	32.11	0.00	86.14	0.00	100.00	0.00	0.00
Delusion	4.41	0.00	0.00	0.00	82.83	0.00	0.00
Hoarding	5.66	7.25	0.00	7.81	39.77	0.00	0.00
Manipulative	11.97	0.00	0.00	36.44	78.97	0.00	0.00

Figure 5-2 (Continued)

> *Real excitement comes in understanding that when we change the way the environment functions, we can significantly change the way people function within that environment — especially people with dementia.*

Enhanced ability results in higher self-esteem and greater preservation of dignity. The difficult behaviors of the cognitively impaired are often caused by features of a poorly designed environment, which contribute to disorientation and confusion and can precipitate agitation. In response to the nature and needs of people with dementia, the goal of design should be to enable residents to function at their highest level by maximizing mobility and independence. Careful planning, well selected environmental features, and good choices can reduce agitation, wandering, and incontinence, and may well affect the most significant challenges of Alzheimer's disease.

Many problems result from a poor sensory environment, excessive stimulation, too much clutter, and no cues or orientation information in an environment that is too large. Special care units are beginning to address these issues. The more frequent use of cluster design today allows for smaller numbers of residents in these settings and smaller more residentially scaled kitchens, dining rooms, and activity spaces. The reduction of size and scale helps to make a care setting look and feel more like a home and is a more manageable for individuals who are disoriented and often confused.

Real excitement comes in understanding that when we change the way the environment functions, we can significantly change the way people function within that environment—especially people with dementia.

Challenging Behaviors

In addition to memory loss, there are a number of behavior problems, such as resistance, wandering, agitation, and incontinence, that sometimes accompany Alzheimer's disease and related illnesses. The presence or absence of these behaviors can vary greatly from one person to another throughout the progression of the disease.

There are many reasons why a difficult behavior may occur. Sometimes the behavior may be related to changes taking place in the brain; in other instances, there may be events or factors in the environment triggering the behavior. In some situations a task, such as taking a bath, may be too complex, or the person may not be feeling well.

People with dementia can also have medical problems, causes related to the person's physical and emotional health that greatly affect behavior. Impaired vision or hearing can affect a person's ability to understand what is being said. Many residents do not get enough fluids, because they no longer recognize the sensation of thirst and forget to drink, leading to dizziness and confusion—symptoms of dehydration.

People with dementia are also very vulnerable to overmedication, to reactions from combinations of drugs, and to their side effects. Sudden changes in a person's level of functioning, confusion, falling, drowsiness, or a sudden increase in agitation can all be a result of drugs.[25] Though these are not problems induced by the environment, these are situations where the results can be mitigated through environmental intervention.

Memory Loss

Memory loss with disorientation is often the first symptom of dementia, and can be frustrating and frightening for residents. Memory loss is progressive and eventually results in the inability to recognize people — including spouses and other family members. This can be painful for family members, who should be encouraged to continue to visit.[26] The needs of the physically disabled but mentally intact resident in a nursing facility are far different than those of the mentally impaired but physically active resident most often found on an Alzheimer's unit. When memory and judgment (among other abilities) become impaired, a person becomes more dependent on others to assist in everyday activities and to provide security. The demented individual may experience changes in behavior, which occasionally become management problems for the caregiver.

Agitation

Persons with Alzheimer's can be very aggressive, to the point of being a danger to themselves and to those around them. It is not always a change in personality that makes them aggressive. Often agitation is caused by confusion about the world around them, and their behavior becomes defensive, which can lead to aggression. They are defending themselves against something they simply do not understand.

Hence, sensory overload—too much stimulation—can be responsible for anger and agitation. Too many people in the environment and too much activity often produce too much movement and too much noise, which in turn invites sensory overload and agitated behavior. Sudden movements, unfamiliar sounds, startling noises, as well as glare and difficulty visually interpreting the settings, can all be contributing factors.

Distraction with a favorite food or activity and avoidance are often the most useful means of handling agitated and angry behavior. Smaller, cluster settings with several gathering or activity spaces provide opportunities for positive distraction, and the smaller settings help to reduce the number of people in the environment. Addressing vision and lighting issues, as well as noise reduction, helps to simplify the environment. Providing well designed areas for walking and access to secured outdoor areas creates an opportunity for exercise and the ability to be removed from the source of stress.[27]

Incontinence

Incontinence, which includes loss of bladder and/or bowel control and bed-wetting, is more prevalent among older people now than in the past, especially in the later stages of Alzheimer's disease. The onset of incontinence is one of the leading reasons for nursing home placement, yet too often the management of incontinence involves simply mopping up or putting residents in diapers, a practice that does little to enhance self-esteem. It is a problem of comfort, health, and dignity for individuals, as well as a costly concern for institutions in terms of staff time, supplies, and equipment.

Incontinence has many physiological causes including infections, medications, insufficient fluid intake, and changes in the brain related to dementia. Due to these changes, the urge or signal to go to the toilet may no longer be understood or received by the brain. Many times, however, the problem is caused by the resident's inability to find the bathroom or having to travel too far to reach the bathroom. Vision changes, for example, can make it difficult to see the way to the bathroom, the bathroom door, or to locate the toilet inside the bathroom.

Bathrooms should be highly visible and identifiable. Little figures of men/women or the words "men," "women" or "ladies" can be confusing to the person with Alzheimer's disease. The word "toilet" is more explicit. For more severely impaired individuals, leaving the door open, making the toilet a visible cue, is helpful.

Few elderly residents get through the night without having to use the toilet. Always have a night-light on in the bedroom and the bathroom at night.

Situation changes dramatically affect Alzheimer's residents; for example, it is not uncommon for an individual who is continent at home to become incontinent when admitted to a special care setting. These changes can often be reversed. It has been reported, in fact, that at least half of the cognitively impaired elderly with an incontinence problem could regain control.[28] By keeping the special needs of the Alzheimer resident in mind and tailoring the environment with thought and imagination, a special care setting can make using the bathroom much easier and help residents to maintain a sense of dignity and self-esteem.

Training staff to anticipate bathroom needs helps residents maintain toilet skills. Hiatt suggests that improving the bathroom configuration, hardware, and door design might enable more people to use toilet rooms independently and to spend less time negotiating the space, which, in turn, might also reduce the number of staff members required to assist one individual.[24]

Wandering

Wandering is a natural behavior and characteristic of some people with dementia. It must be considered in the design and structure of the special care setting so that the environment can be designed to support walking or wandering as meaningful activity by providing appropriate, secure, and well-defined wandering paths that allow a person to wander safely in a secure environment. Walking can be very healthy exercise, and a moderately paced walk of only five minutes helps to maintain flexibility in the joints of the lower body.

Most wandering behavior falls into three categories[30]:

1. **Goal-Directed/Searching Behavior**
   Constantly searching for something that is often unattainable such as mother, home or abstract objects. This behavior is often associated with calling out and approaching one person after another.

2. **Goal-Directed/Industrious Behavior**
   Characterized by seemingly inexhaustible drive to do things or remain busy. This habitual activity may stem from previous experience; for example, a postman delivering mail or a homemaker baking or cleaning.

3. **Apparently Nongoal Directed Behavior**
   Aimless, drawn to one thing and then another, momentarily attentive, then diverted again.

Wandering behavior can be a means for both physical and emotional release. For some people with dementia, wandering is a coping mechanism to relieve stress and tension. It may be an expression of restlessness, boredom, or the need for exercise.[31] And for some, wandering may be searching for a part of life lost to the disease or for a person, place or an object from the past. The need to recapture familiar routines may account for the wandering activity in some residents with Alzheimer's disease whose former occupations, such as a letter carrier or a farmer, involved long periods of walking.[32]

Wandering is a very common behavior seen with dementia patients and is often an expression of a need to find boundaries of

It is normal to want to walk and move about at will. In every environment, except dementia —where it is discouraged, people are encouraged to walk.

one's place. In the cases of aimless constant wandering, the need for structure and activities may be unsatisfied. For example, a resident, a woman in early to mid-stage dementia, when she is not occupied in activity, wanders aimlessly, and is distressed. If anyone says "Hello," as she passes by in the hall, she replies, "Where am I? I want to go back to England, but they wouldn't take me if they knew I'd been in a place like this....I read, but I can't remember what I read. How did I get here?"

There is also an agitated kind of pacing that occurs with some individuals. Is this an expression of need to have increased daily exercise? Is this person looking for a bathroom? Is this person troubled by unnerving delusions? The underlying purpose of the behavior should be explored for positive interventions.[33] Since trying to stop the activity may increase agitation and cause anger and frustration, a better alternative is to encourage walking by providing safe, secure, and interesting paths to walk.

Dorothy Coons, at the University of Michigan, reminds us that if we are aware of the impact of the environment, we will recognize that many so-called "difficult behaviors" are far more normal than those enforced by some care settings.[34] It is normal to want to walk and move about at will. In every environment, except dementia care settings—where it is discouraged, people are encouraged to walk. It is also normal to be angry in an environment that is unsympathetic to our needs.

Though the percentage of residents who wander may be small, the control of wandering requires a disproportionate amount of staff time. Facilities of the past were not designed to tolerate exploration and movement. Much wandering behavior may be the result of non-therapeutic environments. A study at the Corinne Dolan Alzheimer Center showed that negative aggressive behaviors were reduced when patients had an opportunity to wander freely in a protected environment,[35] and experience has shown that confinement does not necessarily stop the will to move.

The wandering associated with Alzheimer's disease is a behavior that challenges caregivers in long-term care settings and at home. Walking can be therapeutic for residents and the walking path need not be a custom design. There is sufficient experience for us to be sure that "dead end" paths lead to frustration and agitation.

The thoughtful connection of corridors that pass through common areas, and connect to other hallways or corridors, bringing them "home" again, produces an interesting and inviting walk. Aquariums, activity alcoves, a place to stop for a snack, or a place to stop and rest, provide interest along the way and ensure that the walking is more than just a meaningless activity. The continuous loop encourages a safe and secure adventure.

A continuous loop does not have to remain within the building. Walking paths can also incorporate secure, safe outdoor areas where people can explore and walk independently. Residents can walk out a door into a secure courtyard or garden, wander through the area at their own pace, and reenter either through the same door or another.

Exiting

Bells and alarms to alert staff that a resident is trying to open a door may encourage safety by preventing egress, but they disrupt the goal of a routine and orderly environment and the noise can lead to other problems such as anxiety and catastrophic reactions. The alarm system may prevent a patient from leaving while still meeting the fire code, but at the very least, it causes disruption to the unit.[36]

Although keeping the exit doors out of the wandering path is an optimal solution, it is not always possible. Camouflaging the door and the panic bar are effective solutions to controlling exiting.[37] Research at the Corinne Dolan Alzheimer's Center found the most successful way of preventing wandering Alzheimer residents from going out a door was to hide the doorknob with an 18 inch cloth barrier. Whether the fabric was the same color as the door or not, didn't seem to matter. The conclusion is that visual barriers are effective and that the inability of the Alzheimer resident to correctly interpret images prevents them from being able to recognize doors and manipulate the knobs. Visual barriers can provide cost-effective solutions, but they must be checked and approved by a fire marshal for safety.

The light and the view available through glass panels in doors attracts residents and should be omitted so it does not entice wanderers. Presenting rich views to which residents have no access is a source of frustration to the individual[38] and a form of cruel and unusual punishment. Since doors with a view encourage residents to go through the door, add mini blinds to block the view, and match the color of the blind to the door color, creating the visual illusion of a solid surface. Matching the color of doors and door handles to the surrounding walls also helps to make them visually indiscernible as exits.

There are many ways to disguise doors to discourage exiting, including covering the doorknob with a pressure-sensitive lock. Painted scenes from nature or wallpaper motifs that simulate shelves of books in a library can add interest and color, as well as effectively disguising doors, but be aware this may not be possible on all doors or allowed in every state. Taped grids on the floor not only were not effective, they often seem to encourage exiting.

In their studies researchers found that a closed blind reduced exiting by 44 percent. The cloth barrier was the most effective solution, reducing exiting by 96 percent, and the combination of the blind and the cloth barrier reduced exiting 88 percent.[39]

Persons with Alzheimer's disease or other dementias can be enrolled in Safe Return, a nationwide program that links every registrant with law enforcement agencies nationwide, and offers a 24-hour response to calls for lost or wandering Alzheimer residents. The program is available through the Alzheimer's Association and is supported by the U.S. Justice Department.

Suspiciousness

It is not uncommon for a demented resident to be suspicious, and to accuse others of stealing their possessions only to find that they have misplaced the items themselves. Other residents who display rummaging and hoarding behaviors may also actually take something, but accusations of this type are common, and staff does take precautions.

Disorientation

Disorientation is a common problem for people with Alzheimer's disease. A sense of being lost and confused is linked to brain impairments that affect short-term memory. Often a resident is searching for a familiar person, place, or possession.

After moving into a care setting, it is also not uncommon for an individual to become disoriented when waking in the middle of the night. However, careful design planning can minimize some confusion.

Name plaques, personal photographs, and other door decorations help many disoriented patients locate their rooms, though the ability to comprehend written words diminishes with the progression of the disease, making these items less useful for this population as the disease progresses.[40]

Depression

Many people who have Alzheimer's disease also suffer from depression. Medical staff has tended to over prescribe drugs, which they understand and rely on, and minimize the impact of the environment, for which there is less understanding. Currently, antidepressant drugs are prescribed, and while there is no suggestion that this practice be discontinued, I question whether even the strongest drugs can compensate for dark, dull, depressing, and uninteresting surroundings.

We can cure the chemical depression with drugs, but if we put people in depressing surroundings where they find it impossible to function, they will not be able to accomplish tasks that give them some measure of self-esteem, be more cooperative, or have a sunnier disposition.[41] We may provide the best care in the world, but if the space you're in is depressing, you're going to be depressed. Design professionals may have little understanding of the impact of Alzheimer's disease or other dementias on the individual, but they do understand very well the impact of the environment, or one's surroundings, on the individual.

Making settings warmer, more nurturing and supportive for residents can be a giant step in combating depression. There is little excuse or logic in relieving depression chemically, only to force existence in depressing surroundings.

How one feels has everything to do with one's view of self and one's life. If we're depressed, we withdraw and want to be left alone. We don't socialize or get out and move around. That is no different for the person who has dementia. Making settings warmer, more nurturing and supportive for residents can be a giant step in combating depression. There is little excuse or logic in relieving depression chemically, only to force existence in depressing surroundings.

Dementia has a strong tendency to depersonalize the victim.[42] There is no one specific design that works for all settings or all resident populations; but utilizing guidelines, the challenge becomes for architects, designers and other design professionals to team up with healthcare professionals and providers of long-term care to develop creative approaches to meet the needs of residents with Alzheimer's disease and dementia.

The success of developing well-designed special care units, in the final analysis, relies on the philosophy and dedication of staff and their relationship to the residents. The environment simply provides a context to support the program, allowing staff to be better caregivers and residents to function at the highest possible level for as long as possible—a context for living, living with dignity.

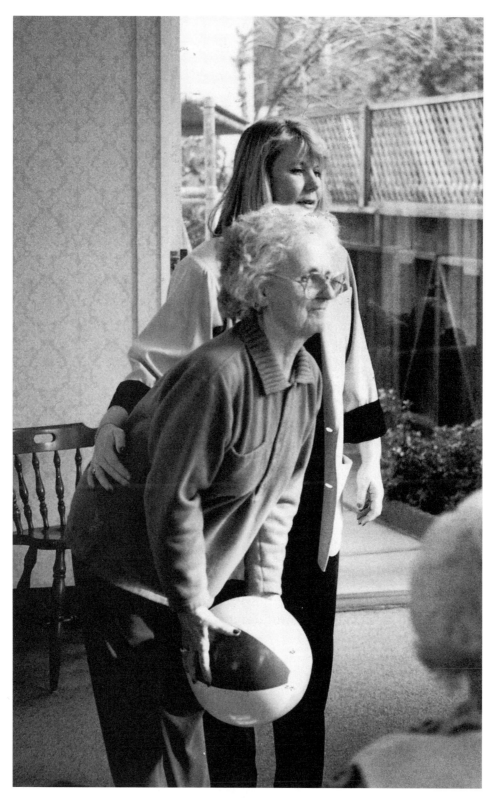

Courtesy of the Greater San Francisco Bay Area Alzheimer's Association. Photographer: Anna M. Rossi

6

Therapeutic Goals of Environmental Design

U ntil recently there has been little realization of the potential of the physical environment as a therapeutic tool in special care settings. But until such time as a cure is found and is readily available to everyone, our best hope is to concentrate our efforts on interventions to improve the quality of life for those who are attempting to live and deal with Alzheimer's disease. Providing the best quality of care possible includes in large part the environment—the surroundings, the home, the context for that care.

As early as 1985 Hiatt suggested that use of the physical environment as a therapeutic tool had been inadequately explored,[1] but until recently there has been little use of therapeutic environments, even in settings where it most likely to be beneficial.

The physical environment can play a significant role in maximizing functional independence and autonomy and should be seen as a partner or a tool in the care setting. Because of the way Alzheimer's affects the brain, each individual perceives, interprets, and responds to his or her world differently. There are no absolute answers.[2] Enhanced quality of life is still important, regardless of the eventual outcome of the disease. This is the message conveyed by a supportive physical and social environment.

Therapeutic goals are intended to provide direction in creating appropriate and supportive environments—guidelines to define the relationships between people with dementia and their environments. They should provide direction for policy, programming, and design decisions.

The following therapeutic goals are taken from Cohen and Weisman's *Holding on to Home*.[3] The authors respond directly to the needs of individuals with dementia as described by the U.S. Congress Office of Technology Assessment (OTA) in their report on Alzheimer's special care units. You may choose to add additional goals in your own planning process, but these will assist in focusing on issues most crucial to environments for people with Alzheimer's disease and other dementias.

1. **Ensure Safety and Security**

   The physical safety and emotional security of individuals with dementia is of primary concern. Those who have Alzheimer's disease, as a consequence of both the physical disabilities related to the process of aging and the cognitive impairments associated with dementing illness, are potentially vulnerable.[4] As the disease progresses the ability to reason and to make judgments diminishes, putting these individuals at risk. The design decisions for this population must be made responsibly and with care.

   Many safety regulations are addressed through various federal, state, and local codes and regulations. To insure personal safety and security for confused residents, however, we need to look beyond the things we are already doing to the things we need to do. Safety covers a range of precautions such as preventing access to toxic substances and sharp objects, providing staff to walk with residents who have an unsteady gait, and eliminating places where residents are likely to fall.

   With regard to design, the importance of security cannot be overemphasized, both to prevent residents from wandering off and to reduce the risk of injury. Providing safe, secured areas to walk and using devices to deter individuals from entering unsafe places contributes to meeting this goal. Avoid sudden loud sounds that can be startling, and evaluate the need to provide better observation of residents as they move about the unit.

2. Support Functional Ability Through Meaningful Activity

The activities in which an individual engages can contribute to a positive self-image and a sense of fulfillment. These range from helping to set the table for a meal, to baking cookies, feeding a pet, or walking in the garden. What is meaningful is determined by the resident. The environment supports the resident's experience and encourages the highest level of function by insuring that mobility needs are met through sufficient light levels, safe floor surfaces, and available handrails for support.

3. Provide Heightened Awareness and Orientation

An unpredictable or illegible environment might be confusing to anyone, but for an individual with dementia added confusion is both cruel and unnecessary. A clear path to the destination, for example, and sufficient cues and landmarks for identification, help to insure that bathrooms are located in time. Personal memorabilia placed in display cabinets adjacent to the bedroom entrance increases the ability of mildly or moderately impaired residents to locate their rooms independently (Corrine Dolan Alzheimer's Center).[5] Access to the outdoors and windows to view the outside environment help with orientation to time and season.

4. Provide Appropriate Environmental Stimulation and Challenge

Sensory deprivation can be as be as debilitating as too much stimulation. The environmental challenge in a dementia care setting is to provide sensory and social stimulation and interest without providing overstimulation. Texture, pattern, and color can be introduced through views to the outside, outdoor gardens, pets, and various textural surfaces.

5. Develop a Positive Social Milieu

Settings must provide opportunities for both passive and active social interaction. Seating can be designed to offer views to the outside, to provide opportunities for observing activities in the immediate environment, or to actively engage in conversation. Special attention must be taken to insure that views are positive and not an enticing invitation to leave. Window views of people leaving the building, getting into cars, or leaving the grounds may stimulate residents to leave themselves, especially if there is a door close by. This is not positive or the type of active participation we want to encourage. Many programs such as music and dancing can encourage active social participation.

6. **Maximize Autonomy and Control**

   Most people are much happier when they are able to make their own choices. Individuals with dementia should be allowed as much choice as possible, for as long as possible. Access to safe and secure outdoor environments insures that residents can exercise decision making skills and control over spending time inside or outside. The opportunity to bring one's own furniture and make decisions about the room decor allows the resident active participation and a chance to feel in control.

7. **Adapt to Changing Needs**

   We must be encouraged to continually remember that no two dementia residents are the same and that no two days with the same resident may be the same.[6] It is essential to respond to both the changing needs of the individuals over the course of the disease, and to differences in the needs and abilities within the residents themselves. Alzheimer's disease and related dementias are diverse and progress through definite though ill-defined stages, so the characteristics of special care residents often change over time due to "aging in place." As a consequence, environmental features appropriate for some residents may be ineffective for others.

8. **Establish Links to the Healthy and Familiar**

   People with dementia are confronted with an ongoing series of changes in themselves and their world, and it becomes increasingly important to maintain their ties to what is familiar. A comfortable and convenient environment that provides options for interaction and the routine of daily living can be as reassuringly familiar to a confused individual as using traditional elements such as fireplaces and comfortable chairs. These links to the familiar—to home and the past—will help to provide a "soft transition" into a new setting.[7]

   Familiar surroundings and the ambience of home help residents feel more comfortable and secure. If people feel uncomfortable or unsafe in their surrounding, it is likely to be reflected as adverse or inappropriate behavior.

9. Respect the Need for Privacy

Privacy is a key issue. Residents want to continue to have control of their lives, and finding the appropriate balance between socialization and privacy can be challenging. Dining rooms offer opportunities for socialization, while having one's own bedroom for privacy can offer some balance. Residents should have the same opportunity to choose from a variety of spaces where they want to spend time—just as they had previously in their own homes. The opportunity for choice may also help to reduce the sense of intrusion into personal space. Places to pursue special interests, alternative walking paths, and personalized rooms all help to increase a person's sense of control and feeling of home.

Families repeatedly ask for small private places where they can visit with loved ones. Shared bedrooms or large rooms don't offer a place to be alone with special friends, whereas a small private niche with a table and two chairs, for example, can provide intimate private space for visiting.

To these goals, I would add one additional and very important therapeutic goal:

10. Encourage Family Involvement

As residents settle into a new home experience, families need to stay involved. Regular visits and participation can be encouraged by an environment that invites family and friends in, makes room for them, makes them feel at home. This can be a setting that nurtures its residents and their families; for family members it is much easier to comfort, encourage, and nurture loved ones if they feel comfortable and nurtured themselves.

SECTION II

Sensory Environment

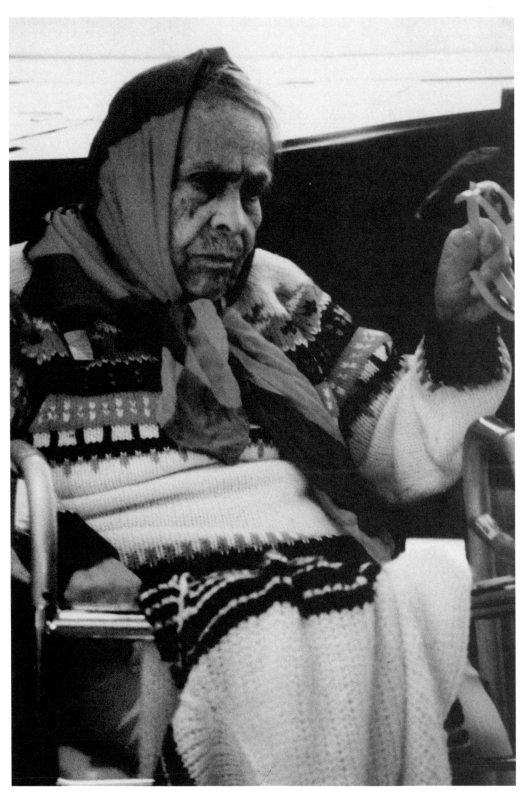

Courtesy of the Greater San Francisco Bay Area Alzheimer's Association. Photographer: Anna M. Rossi.

CHAPTER 7

Light and Aging Vision

Sunlight travels 93 million miles to reach earth where it is warmly welcomed—at least by most of us. The benefits of the full spectrum of natural light abound; however, the majority of people today spend approximately 90 percent of their time behind glass—walls and windows of closed buildings, offices, homes, and car windshields. They also wear glasses and sunglasses. All of these prevent natural light from being admitted through the eyes and coming in contact with the skin. Even plants exposed to ordinary window glass react differently to indoor sunshine than to outdoor sunshine. The reason — most ordinary glass prevents some 99 percent of the admission of ultraviolet radiation. "Sunlight starvation" may well be a condition that periodically undermines the health and well being of countless numbers of people.[1]

Without ultraviolet light, sun-loving plants will not grow properly; in fact, most plants removed from the sunlight become pale and spindly. In a similar way, sun-starved people also exhibit pallor. According to Edwin D. Babbitt, M.D., author of *The Principles of Light and Color,* published in 1878, "... put the pale, withering plant or human being into the sun, and if not too far gone, each will recover

"Sunlight starvation" may well be a condition that periodically undermines the health and well being of countless numbers of people.[1]

health and spirit."[2] Under the right conditions and length of exposure, even ultraviolet light is beneficial.

People who rarely see natural light suffer from visual deterioration as well as physical illnesses. Animals that live underground continuously may actually lose their vision. Experiments in caves have also shown that lack of sunlight causes body rhythms to become upset, and that they return to normal within three days after the subject leaves the cave. Animals whose days and nights are experimentally reversed end up with body rhythms shifted exactly 180 degrees.[3]

There are also differences in the sensitivity or resistance to ultraviolet in different people, especially in fair, light-skinned individuals compared to those with darker skin. How much exposure is beneficial depends upon the intensity of sunlight, the time of day, season of the year, and geographical location.

As beneficial, and as necessary as sunlight is for health and well-being, overexposure to sunlight would obviously be unwise, detrimental, and even dangerous. Fortunately sunscreen products are readily available and sun hats are in vogue.

Biological Effects of Light

How Does Sunlight Affect Us?

Today more than ever before, sunlight is recognized as a powerful factor in building and maintaining health. It stimulates the nervous system, improving appetite and mental attitude, and induces better sleep. Realizing the importance of natural sunlight on health, Florence Nightingale, many years ago, insisted upon allowing sunlight in the sick room.[4]

The benefits of light for the older adult come about not only in terms of vision—as a source of spatial information about the environment—but equally important in the photobiological effects necessary to maintain an older adult's health and quality of life. The benefits of sunlight on the skin, synthesizing vitamin D, are well known, but light also impacts the neuroendocrine system. Sleep disorders, depression, and reduced levels of calcium absorption result from inadequate light exposure or light deprivation.

The Sunshine Vitamin and Vitamin D Synthesis

The nutrient most associated with the sun is *vitamin D, the "sunshine" vitamin.* Most of the vitamin D we require is made in our skin under the influence of sunlight. In fact, about 10 minutes of summer sun shining on the hands and face is enough to produce 400 I.U. (international units) of vitamin D, which is twice the recommended dietary allowance (RDA) for most adults. As a result of the protective effect of the pigmentation of their skin, people with darker skin may require longer exposure.

Exposure to sunshine in the summer months allows us to make enough vitamin D to last through the winter, when vitamin D production in the skin is greatly reduced. Though it is better to avoid midday sun and use sunscreen, with a few minutes of unprotected sun exposure in the early morning or late afternoon two or three times a week, our bodies are able to make enough Vitamin D. Whether we synthesize it ourselves or get it from our diet, vitamin D is converted in the body into a hormone with many essential functions, including the regulation of calcium absorption and the maintenance of strong bones.[5]

Vitamin D synthesis also declines dramatically with decreased mobility. The elderly have a reduced capacity to produce the vitamin in their skin, and with less mobility, they quite often don't get much sun. How many nursing home residents must be severely underexposed or light-starved—particularly in the winter months?

Studies indicate that inadequate light exposure, required for calcium metabolism, results in decreased bone mass and contributes to falls and fractures. Osteoporosis is commonly associated with the aging process, and according to the National Safety council, falling down is the leading cause of accidental death in the elderly. Because many nursing home residents are often deficient in vitamin D, it is not surprising that falls are even more common in nursing homes than for the same age group living elsewhere in the community.[6]

Even people with high dietary vitamin D intake show calcium deficiencies when they don't get enough sun. Elderly people are at special risk. In one study elderly men who stayed indoors for a week began absorbing less calcium, indicating that ultraviolet radiation is necessary for adequate calcium metabolism.[7] Whether for synthesizing vitamin D or supporting calcium metabolism, there is no doubt that exposure to natural sunlight contributes to good health.

Circadian Rhythm

The term circadian means "about a day." Rhythms of the body cycling on a 24-hour period are called circadian rhythms.[8] The circadian pacemaker regulates a host of interrelated biological processes—including body temperature, hormone release, heart rate, blood pressure, and the sleep-wake cycle—that run on a roughly 24-hour schedule.

The realization of the powerful effects of the light-dark cycle on the human body clock was slow to emerge, but this viewpoint began

Three qualities of visible light are known to affect the circadian pacemaker, or body clock: intensity, wavelength and timing.

to change with three critical discoveries: that bright light could suppress melatonin secretion in humans,[9] that light could shift the timing of human circadian rhythm in core body temperature, and that circadian rhythms are often disturbed in blind individuals.[10]

In 1979, Dr. Al Lewy, then at the National Institutes of Mental Health, and Dr. Thomas Wehr began work on a hormone called melatonin, released by the pineal gland in the brain. Their studies revealed that light plays an important role in triggering and setting the biological clocks in animals. Other studies showed that exposure to light stops nighttime production of melatonin in the pineal gland. Lewy, Wehr and their colleagues found that nighttime melatonin production in humans could be stopped with high intensity light and this suggests that such brightness could be used to reset human biological rhythms.[11]

Three qualities of visible light are known to affect the circadian pacemaker, or body clock: intensity, wavelength, and timing. It appears that light intensities sufficient to almost totally suppress melatonin secretion (2000 lux) can have potent effects on the body clock. The wavelength of light that can most effectively suppress melatonin, and presumably affect human circadian rhythms, is in the blue-green range of the visible spectrum. The timing of light exposure is the third critical factor.[12]

Circadian rhythm affects our hormonal systems and sets our body rhythms. The biological clock triggers many daily activities, each at about the same time every day—hunger, going to sleep, and getting up, among others. Generally the biological clock lags behind real time, and with no cues from daylight, traffic noises, or temperature changes, one could feel sleepy later and later each day.

The use of bright light to reset biological rhythms is one of several innovations to follow recent findings on the effect of light on humans. We now know that the light-dark cycle synchronizes human rhythms to the 24-hour day.[13] Light rays strike the retina, triggering nerve impulses that travel to the brain along pathways that have nothing to do with vision in the sense of image processing; they function strictly as light meters.[14] The pineal gland converts light into nerve impulses, which cause the gland to secrete melatonin,[15] which then acts on a biological clock within the hypothalamus. "The result is that fundamental biochemical and hormonal rhythms of the body are synchronized, directly or indirectly, by the daily cycle of light and dark."[16]

Circadian rhythm takes on increasing importance when we consider that chronic illnesses tend to be *rhythmic disorders* characterized by chemical processes whose cyclings and pulsings have gotten out of sync. This is evidenced in Alzheimer's disease, depression, epilepsy, hypertension, schizophrenia, and others.[17]

In addition to setting our body rhythms, sunlight bolsters the immune system. It can double the ability of certain cells to engulf bacteria, and it affects the rise and fall of cortisol, which influences immunity. In laboratory rats, for example, a single exposure to ultraviolet light boosts the number of infection-fighting cells for up to three weeks.

The elderly, especially those with dementia, may receive levels of light exposure that are insufficient to provide for optimum circadian rhythm. Investigators have measured light exposure in a number of elderly subjects, healthy and active, as well as demented and institutionalized, and found extraordinarily low levels of light exposure.[18] In experiments with elderly rats, increasing levels of light exposure can improve the rest/activity rhythm, causing it to resemble the rhythm of young rats.[19]

Relevance of Natural Light to Aging

Melatonin is the chemical that relays information in the body regarding the light-dark cycle. High levels of circulating melatonin signal the body that it is nighttime, but the pineal gland secrets the hormone melatonin at night in decreasing amounts as people age. With less circulating melatonin to provide internal stability, it is conceivable that the elderly are even more dependent on daily light exposure.

Elderly persons retain their sensitivity to the chronobiologic effects of bright light, and they retain the capacity to regulate core body temperature rhythm with appropriately timed bright light exposure.[20] Sunlight has an effect on other diseases as well—all with significant impact on the elderly. Sleep disorders and seasonal depression (SAD) are the two disorders with the most clear response to bright light. There is also some data to support benefits of bright light exposure in other forms of insomnia, nonseasonal major depression, and agitated behaviors in the demented elderly.

Sleep Disorders

Sleep is controlled by both voluntary and involuntary factors. The involuntary factor is the circadian rhythm for sleepiness and alertness, which is timed by the circadian pacemaker, the setting of which is influenced by daily exposure to bright light and melatonin. In old age, it is more common for a person to get sleepy early in the evening and to have middle of the night awakenings. Many elderly people suffer at least mild symptoms of the chronic insomnia of old age. Evening light exposure has been remarkably effective in improving sleep quality.[21] Given the potential hazards of sleeping pills (confusion, falls, nighttime breathing problems, lack of efficiency), studies of the effects of brighter lighting on sleep in the elderly should be a health priority.

Seasonal Affective Disorder (SAD)

Light is also being enlisted to fight emotional disorders. Growing evidence suggests that seasonal variations in light levels can have a profound impact on mental health. This is dramatically evident in people suffering from seasonal affective disorder (SAD), an affliction that strikes an estimated five million Americans. This recurring annual ailment is marked by abnormal sleep patterns, fatigue, weight gain, withdrawal from friends and family, and depression of clinical depths. SAD strikes the majority of sufferers as days shorten in late October or November, holding them in its grip for three to four months each year. Though they may be outgoing and vivacious in the summer, people with SAD find themselves increasingly despondent and anxious as winter approaches. Then as spring arrives and the days lengthen, their depression lifts.

It was not until 1987 that the American Psychiatric Association recognized SAD as a true affective (mood) disorder, listing it in the Diagnostic and Statistical Manual of Mental Disorders, third edition, revised. But this is one case where recognition of an illness has been nearly simultaneous with the discovery of a treatment: light therapy.[22] Psychiatrists still don't know what causes SAD, though there seems to be a genetic predisposition and, like other types of depression, it strikes women more often than men. It seems clear that the decreased amount of winter daylight, however, is important. Researchers working on that assumption began artificially extending patients' daylight hours. They exposed them to fluorescent lights of an intensity of 2,500 lux—far brighter than ordinary room light, which is about 500 lux or less—for a total of two hours daily. The results were astonishing. Severely depressed patients who'd resisted antidepressant drugs showed dramatic improvement in a week or less.[23]

> *Though it remains unclear exactly how light fights depression, as in SAD, it is thought that it may work through the body clock or by affecting melatonin levels.[24]*

Seasonal affective disorder, or winter depression, is the mood disorder that is most responsive to bright light therapy, but since no systematic studies of SAD in the elderly have been done, we can only guess as to how common winter depression is in old age

Nonseasonal Depression

Nonseasonal major depression is common in old age and more complex than SAD. Results are preliminary, but evidence suggests that if light can combat winter depression, it might also work against the nonseasonal kind. Dr. Daniel Kripke, professor of psychiatry at the University of California at San Diego, has been using light therapy since 1981 on patients hospitalized for depression. "The benefit we're seeing is actually more than you would expect to see with antidepressant drugs in a comparable time period," he reports. Though it remains unclear exactly how light fights depression, as in SAD, it is thought that it may work through the body clock or by affecting melatonin levels.[24] The effectiveness of bright light exposure in treating the elderly for nonseasonal major depression is unknown; while some patients have responded, others have not.

Agitation in Dementia

Degenerative brain diseases such as Alzheimer's disease are prevalent in old age. Dementing illnesses not only affect memory and intellectual function, but can also cause severe behavioral symptoms that are disruptive and that can be dangerous. Increased agitation has been attributed to decreased light levels. Several investigators have shown that bright light exposure can reduce agitated behaviors and improve the sleep/wake cycle in persons with advanced Alzheimer's disease.[25]

For many of those with dementia, bright light exposure often proves too stimulating. Glancing at light fixtures for a period of time is difficult, and the glare from bright light fixtures can be uncomfortable. If bright light exposure is shown to benefit those with dementia, better methods of delivering light should be explored. Singer and Hughes at the Oregon Health Sciences University in Portland, Oregon, have indicated that issues such as proper timing, intensity, and methods of light exposure in restless, confused elderly people who may be sensitive to the effects of glare or stimulation from bright light need to be addressed. Already, some investigators are experimenting with illuminating entire rooms at a lower intensity, as opposed to using a light box.[26]

Since well over 50 percent of nursing home residents suffer from Alzheimer's disease or some type of dementia, it seems particularly important to note that there is some evidence that light relieves the symptom in Alzheimer's disease called "sundowning." Residents become confused and agitated around sunset. People with

"We now know that the powerful hold that light has on us is less magical than it is biological."

Alzheimer's disease also show a degeneration of the eyes that could be light-related.

According to a 1992 article in *The New York Times Good Health Magazine*, in 1991 over $15.5 million was spent by the U. S. National Institute of Mental Health on light and light therapy experiments.[27] "We now know that the powerful hold that light has on us is less magical than it is biological." It is encouraging to note the increased interest on the part of researchers in investigating the possible effects of light, relative to the elderly and Alzheimer's disease.

Aging Vision

Of all our senses, vision is arguably the most precious. Most of us experience normal changes in vision as we age, and these changes, typically, can be corrected with standard prescriptive glasses or contact lenses. Vision impairments, vision that cannot be corrected by medical or surgical intervention or regular glasses, however, may mean unnecessary loss of independence and diminished quality of life for far too many people. Vision impairment results primarily from age-related eye diseases such as cataracts, macular degeneration, diabetes or glaucoma, and spans a continuum, from blindness at one extreme to partial sight at the other.[28] Surveys have shown that most older Americans fear severe vision loss more than any other physical disablilty.[29]

It is conservatively estimated that as many as 2.7 million older people currently experience severe vision impairment, and with the aging of America, these numbers are expected to increase to 6 million by the year 2030.[30] In the United States the 85 and over population is currently the fastest growing age group, and 27 percent have severe vision impairment.[31] The number of people 65 years and older is also experiencing a sharp increase of 90 percent.[32]

The vision problems of older adults tend to be both overlooked and undertreated, and all too often, this leads many older people to needlessly experience functional disability and a decreased quality of life.

The vision problems of older adults tend to be both overlooked and undertreated, and all too often, this leads many older people to needlessly experience functional disability and a decreased quality of life. Vision loss is one of the most common and potentially disabling conditions of later life.[33] It is highly disruptive to the everyday activities for older persons, yet there is a tendency to accept it as a "normal" part of the aging process.

Since increasing incidence of vision impairment with advancing age is undeniable, our homes, places of business, and particularly, healthcare settings should be designed to enable people of all ages to carry out their activities with relative ease, safety, and comfort. Unfortunately, we know that the special needs of older eyes are not always met.

Just as the body ages, so does the eye age.[34] These changes to the healthy aging eye differ from loss of visual function due to specific eye diseases.[35] Presbyopia, or loss of focusing power, is a natural part of the aging process and one of the changes that can be corrected with glasses. Though the eye stops growing in the early teen years, the lens continues to grow. Eventually as the elasticity diminishes, some of its focusing ability is lost, resulting in presbyopia.[36]

The pupil becomes smaller as the eye ages, and the lens more dense. This combines to reduce the quality of images and leads aging eyes to need more light and more contrast on task activity. Many older adults experience increased difficulty perceiving patterns, requiring greater contrast for recognition. Color perception may be affected: white may be indistinguishable from yellow and blue may appear as gray.

The normal aging eye adjusts more slowly than a young eye, causing difficulty in adjusting to changes in levels of illumination. When moving from a normally illuminated room into bright sunlight, for example, or entering a dimly lighted entryway from bright sunlight, the dramatic change in illumination often results in temporary blindness until the eyes adjust.

Changes to the Healthy Aging Eye

The changes in visual function from age-related vision loss are not correctable by ordinary glasses, contact lenses, medical treatment, or surgery. This condition, known as low vision, typically results from cataracts, glaucoma, diabetic retinopathy, macular degeneration, or stroke. It is particularly important that designers be aware of the effects of functional vision loss so that they can effectively address the resulting needs of residents who deal with these problems. The three most common types of functional vision loss are:

1. Overall blurred vision
2. Central vision loss
3. Peripheral (side) vision loss

Figure 7.1 shows how such losses affect what a person sees.

Age-Related Vision Loss

Overall Blur

Overall blur can be caused by cataracts, corneal scars, or diabetes. Cataracts cause cloudy images and increased sensitivity to glare; images may appear hazy, making it difficult to recognize facial features and other details without the right contrast.

Three Types of Functional Vision Loss

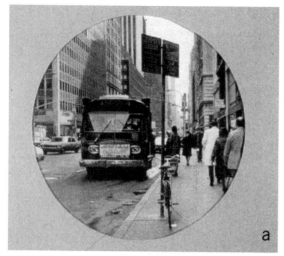

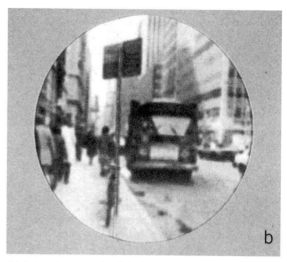

(a) Normal vision: a person with normal vision or vision corrected to 20/20 with glasses sees this street scene. The area of the photograph is the field of vision for the right eye.

(b) Cataract: an opacity of the lens results in diminished acuity but does not affect the field of vision. There is no distorted empty or dark area, but the person's vision is hazy overall, particularly in glaring light.

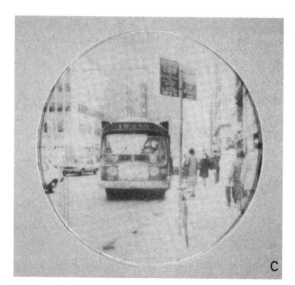

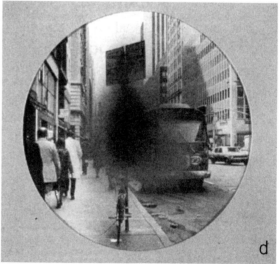

(c) Corneal pathology: an injury or damage to the cells of the cornea results in a distorted or cloudy image and increased glare sensitivity. Clear detail is no longer discernible, but the field of vision is normal.

(d) Macular degeneration: the deterioration of the macula, the central area of the retina, is the most prevalent eye disease. This picture shows the area of decreased central vision called a central scotoma. The peripheral, or side, vision remains unaffected so mobility need not be impaired.

Figure 7-1 A photographic essay on partial sight. *Courtesy of The Lighthouse, Inc.*

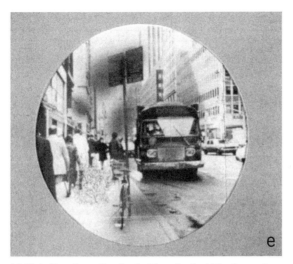

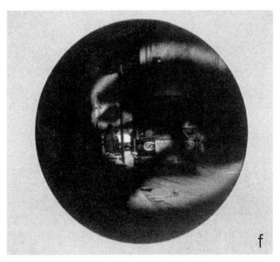

(e) Diabetic retinopathy: the leaking of retinal blood vessels may occur in advanced or long-term diabetes and affect the macula or the entire retina and vitreous. Not all diabetics develop retinal changes, but the likelihood of retinopathy and cataracts increases with the length of time a person has diabetes.

(f) Glaucoma: chronic elevated eye pressure in susceptible individuals may cause optic nerve atrophy and loss of peripheral vision. Early detection and close medical monitoring can help reduce complications.

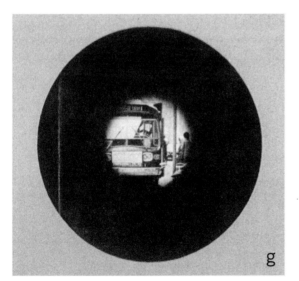

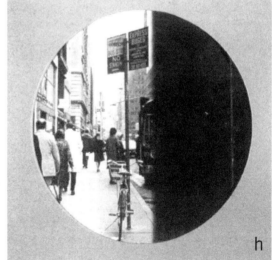

(g) Retinitis pigmentosa: A congenital degeneration of the pigmented layer of the retina that leads to a severe loss of peripheral vision. Even though central vision may remain clear, traveling is difficult, because of side vision loss.

(h) Hemianopia: A defect in the optic pathways in the brain can result in vision loss in half of the field of vision. The most common defect, right homonymous hemianopia, occurs in corresponding halves of the right field of vision, causing reading impairment. It can also happen in the left field of vision, in the upper half or the lower half.

Figure 7-1 *Continued.*

Persons with overall blurred vision may experience increased sensitivity to light, a marked decrease in the intensity of color, and due to lack of contrast they may experience particular difficulty out of doors.

To assist persons with blurred vision who may have difficulty recognizing faces, always introduce yourself when you enter a room and say good-bye when you leave. It is important to remember also, when talking, not to stand in front of a window.[37]

Central Vision Loss

This type of vision loss is most often caused by macular degeneration. For those who have central vision loss, type and images appear distorted and segments of words may be missing. There is increased sensitivity to light, altered color vision, and faces may be hard to recognize.[38] Residents can see you but cannot make out details such as facial features or name tags.[39]

Again, always introduce yourself when you enter a room and say good-bye when leaving. This may seem an oversimplification, but it is especially important for those who have cognitive impairment in addition to vision loss.

Again, always introduce yourself when you enter a room and say good-bye when leaving. This may seem an oversimplification, but it is especially important for those who have cognitive impairment in addition to vision loss. Window coverings and lighting can be adjusted as necessary to reduce harsh sunlight.

Peripheral Vision Loss

Peripheral (or side) vision loss is most often caused by glaucoma or stroke. It commonly causes loss of half of the visual field and is particularly serious because of the resulting loss of independence.

Persons with loss of peripheral vision have the capacity to see only straight ahead. They are hesitant when moving about and need to move their heads from side to side to scan their surroundings. It is important not to rearrange furniture.

Vision in Alzheimer's Disease

Relative to their healthy elderly counterparts, individuals with Alzheimer's disease show significant impairments in at least one visual function, though they often have multiple deficits. These impairments occur in such basic visual capacities as color discrimination, depth perception, contrast sensitivity, and their ability to resist or ignore visual distractions.[40]

The status of vision in Alzheimer's disease is not merely an exaggeration of the normal aging process. Persons with Alzheimer's disease, relative to healthy elderly persons, show significant, selective losses in color discrimination and contrast sensitivity. There is a disproportionate impairment in the discrimination of the blue color axis (short wavelength), and they have particular difficulty in distinguishing between blue and green hues and between blue and violet hues. There seems to be little difference in discriminating between yellow and orange hues.[41] As we learn more about the effects of Alzheimer's disease on color sensitivity, we may need to rethink our color selections for special care settings. While blue, green, and violet in their various shades and tints may be very restful for many, the indications are that copious use of these colors may not be the best choices for dementia settings.

With a better understanding of vision loss it is easier to understand the importance of adapting the environment to accommodate for changing abilities.

Besides the changes in color vision, persons with Alzheimer's also experience depressed contrast sensitivity at all spatial frequencies. High but not low frequency loss is characteristic of normal aging.[42] Added to these changes, impaired depth perception and a decreasing ability to focus or shut out distraction make the normal activities of every day life increasingly more difficult.

Sensory losses can masquerade as cognitive losses. Many individuals with Alzheimer's disease have selective deficits in vision as well as cognition, which raises interesting questions about the impact of visual dysfunction on cognition. In many cases, visual deficits can predict cognitive problems.[43] It can be extremely useful in the care and understanding of individual residents to be aware of the possibility they may experience difficulties in activities of daily living that are attributable to specific visual dysfunction. For example, problems in spatial orientation and mobility may be related to deficient depth perception, and losses in central acuity have been associated with functional disability in nursing home residents.[44]

With a better understanding of vision loss it is easier to understand the importance of adapting the environment to accommodate for changing abilities. We may find also that interventions designed to cope with vision loss can help to ease the agitation and confusion of the cognitively impaired who also experience some of the same losses. One can only imagine how frightening it must be, trying to make sense out of blurred and undefined images and missing parts.

Elderly vision should be checked regularly. When admission intakes are done, vision should be evaluated and the vision status should be included in the medical information used to create the resident's care plan. The presence of a vision problem, the diagnosis, medications prescribed, and the resident's sensitivity to light should be documented.[45] For the resident with Alzheimer's disease, records of past eye exams and the insight of family members can provide useful information. Having more knowledge available about the integrity of a resident's basic visual capacities can only be helpful in the evaluation of adaptive functioning, and in understanding the resident's world.[46]

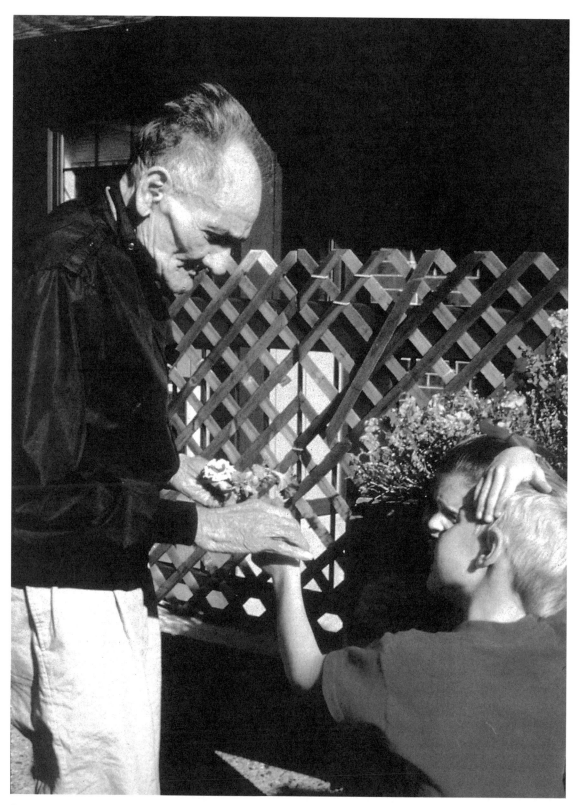

Courtesy of Foxwood Springs Living Centers, Raymore, MO.

CHAPTER 8

The Dramatic Effect of Lighting

Scientific research on the effect that light has on the body is raising consciousness levels, giving us a new awareness of the importance of light in the indoor environment and of how important natural sunlight is to our health and well-being. It is interesting that, whether by intention or not, we have all but eliminated natural light from most of our elderly housing environments.

Lighting needs for the elderly are quite different from those of a younger person, and design professionals have a big challenge ahead of them to understand appropriate lighting for long-term care. Judgments about lighting are too often based on personal perception; however, architects and designers are becoming more aware of the importance of how a building's design and orientation to light affect the general health and well-being of its residents. It is important for all designed spaces, particularly those in long-term care settings, to incorporate as much natural sunlight as possible within the built environment, balanced with artificial light. We need to provide patios, porches, and balconies to encourage residents to spend time out of doors.

A first step in that process would be to have the lighting for long-term care settings evaluated by an 80-year-old.

Lighting is not a subject that is easily understood, and until recently it has been a low priority in the environment. Designing good lighting systems for the elderly has proved especially challenging, due to the absence of postoccupancy studies and a lack of established guidelines. The greater challenge, however, to understanding appropriate lighting for long-term care involves a willingness to "see" things differently.

A first step in that process would be to have the lighting for long-term care settings evaluated by an 80-year-old. Who better to assess light levels, the presence or absence of glare, even light distribution, and how much illumination is actually needed for visual acuity? Such an evaluation would lead to significant changes in lighting systems, most probably resulting in increased mobility, socialization, and greater participation in activity programs by residents.

Vision begins to decline as early as age 40. The changes in visual acuity that affect depth perception and the ability to distinguish details, and that cause difficulty in focusing, necessitate much higher levels of illumination. A 60-year-old person may require two to three times as much light as a 20-year-old,[1] and the amount of light required doubles for each 13 years after the age of 20.[2]

As the eye ages, the visual field narrows and the pupil gets smaller, decreasing the amount of light that enters the eye. The pupil size of the average 5-year-old, for example, is 7 mm, whereas the pupil size of the average 65-year-old is 2.5 mm. In addition, the lens of the eye thickens with age, loses transparency, and turns a yellow-brown in color, and the sensitivity of the retina diminishes. The combined effect of the reduction in size of the pupil and the thickening of the lens results in two-thirds less light reaching the retina by age 65.[3]

Lighting in Healthcare Settings

As healthcare settings take on a decidedly more residential and homelike feeling, one of the most influential and important design details is lighting. Warmer, more residential lighting helps to create a facility's image, but in more practical terms, lighting is being designed to increase function, minimize the discomfort and hazards associated with glare, and improve the poor color rendition of low quality fluorescent light.

Long-term care settings and Alzheimer special care units can accommodate aging residents experiencing cognitive difficulties and diminishing physical dexterity, and still have a residential atmosphere. It's important, however, to remember that residents in long-term care settings, particularly those in dementia SCUs, are not able to physically modify their environment to avoid glare or to improve lighting conditions to meet their needs. If they have difficulty seeing or are unable to avoid problem areas, such as a poorly lighted dining room, residents may endure daily torment that may lead to additional serious problems such as anxiety, confusion, and anger.

New technologies and changing attitudes toward healthcare are stimulating fresh approaches to lighting design for these settings. Compact fluorescent and T-8 lamps, for example, are now regarded as important design tools, and contribute to more varied approaches in lighting.

Well-designed lighting plans, using more indirect ambient lighting, make safer and less stressful environments where residents feel more comfortable. Decorative fixtures sensitively integrated with the architecture, and not merely fixtures applied to the wall or ceilings, make the setting more homelike.

Primary areas of concern in lighting design for long term care and Alzheimer's special care settings are:

Criteria for Lighting

- *Raise the level of illumination.*

    Lighting levels need to be increased to counteract the loss of sight and visual acuity that occurs throughout the aging process.

- *Provide consistent, even light levels.*

    Uneven brightness patterns can produce frightening shadows and/or create the illusion of steps or edges where light and shadows meet. This can produce increased levels of agitation and confusion.

- *Eliminate glare.*

    Glare reduction not only contributes to comfort, it also helps to minimize falls and maximize attention span. The behavioral implications of glare serve to produce confusion, agitation, and anger.

- *Provide access to natural daylight.*

    Sunlight stimulates the circadian and neuroendocrine systems that regulate the body's entire homeostasis.

- *Provide gradual changes in light levels.*

    Transition spaces between outside daylight areas and indoor spaces should provide gradual changes in light levels.

- *Provide focused task lighting.*

    Attention to the special needs of task lighting assists residents in seeing and in task performance.

- *Improve color rendition from lamps or light sources.*

Raise the Level of Illumination

Insufficient lighting is one of the most obvious problems and one of the deficiencies most often cited in the Omnibus Reconciliation Act of 1987 (OBRA). Lighting levels need to be increased to counteract the loss of sight and visual acuity that occurs throughout the aging process.

Most light level requirements are based on the Illuminating Engineering Society's (IES's) schedule, which was originally developed from data using subjects with an *average* age of 23 years old. The schedule has since been adjusted to a three level range partially based on the age of the users (see Figure 8-1); however, the oldest group considered was only 50 years old. In addition, the medical and hospital schedule that is most commonly applied to long-term care was developed based on the needs of the medical practitioner—not the elderly resident.

Many facilities do not provide adequate environments to support abilities of older adults or the cognitively impaired. Only skilled nursing facilities have regulations for lighting, and those vary from state to state. There are currently no nationally recognized regulations for lighting. Since the average age of nursing home residents is 86, and 83.5 years for assisted living, we can only wonder how many residents are unable to manage on their own due to inadequate light.

Fortunately, proper lighting can help compensate in many ways for poor vision. Improved lighting and an enhanced visual environment often result in renewed interest and optimism, and in older people regaining mobility and remaining active.

General ambient illumination should be provided in every room, the best sources being natural daylight and dimmable fluorescent lamps. Manufacturers now make lamps, both fluorescent and incandescent, that mimic the light of the sun, as well as window glazing and eyeglass lenses that pass a more complete range of light. Energy efficiency and the availability of full spectrum lamps now make fluorescent a viable source.

A combination of low-brightness, direct fixtures and properly applied indirect fixtures is another reliable approach for general illumination. To make this combination successful requires use of indirect fixtures that provide a uniform ceiling brightness and down lighting with the same luminance as the ceiling. The Illuminating Engineering Society defines a uniformly bright ceiling as one that includes no areas four times brighter than the area between fixtures.[4] However, because of the extreme sensitivity to glare for older adults, a 3:1 ratio is preferred.

Minimum Illumination Levels

Areas	Ambient Light	Task Light
Administration (Active)	30	50
Activity Areas (Day only)	30	50
Visitor Waiting (Day)	30	
Visitor Waiting (Night)	10	
Barber/Beautician (Day)	50	
Chapel or Quiet Area (Active)	30	
Hallways (Active Hrs)	30	
Hallways (Sleeping Hrs)	10	
Dining (Active Hrs)	50	
Exterior Entrance (Night)	10	
Interior Entry (Day)	100[a]	
Interior Entry (Night)	10	
Exit Stairway & Landings	30	
Elevator Interiors	30	
Medicine Prep	30	100
Nurses Station (Day)	30	50
Nurses Station (Night)	10	50
Physical Therapy Area (Active Hrs)	30	50
Occupational Therapy (Active Hrs)	30	50
Examination Room (Dedicated)	30	100
Janitors Closet	30	
Laundry (Active Hrs)	30	50
Clean/Soiled Utility	30	
Commercial Kitchen	50	100
Food Storage (Non-Refrig.)	30	
Staff Toilet Area	20	60
Resident Room	30	75
Wardrobe	30	
Bathroom entry	30	
Bathroom	30	
Make-up/Shaving area	30	60
Shower/Bathing Rooms	30	

[a] Utilization of daylight is encouraged in entryways to provide a transition between outside and interior illumination levels.

Note: Ambient light levels are minimum averages measured at 30 inches above the floor in a horizontal plane. Task light levels are absolute minimums taken on the visual task. For make-up/shaving the measurement is to be taken on the face in a vertical position.

Lamp color: The lamp shall have a color rendering index (CRI) of 80 or higher. Exam rooms lighting shall be 90 CRI or higher.

It should be understood that the values listed are minimums. The optimum solution for task lighting is to give the user control over the intensity and positioning of the light source to meet his or her individual needs.

Figure 8-1 Minimum illumination levels, using daylight and/or electric lamps with a CRI of 80 or greater. *Courtesy of Illuminating Engineering Society of North America. From RP-28-96 Recommended Practice for Lighting and the Visual Environment for Senior Living.*

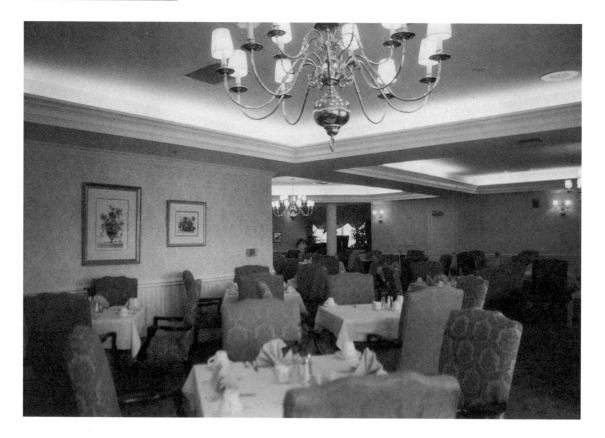

Provide Consistent, Even Lighting Levels

It can be a tricky feat to insure consistent and even illumination of wall and floor surfaces. Pendent indirect lighting and cove lighting provide the most even illumination of a space and an excellent solution to the challenge of providing high levels of ambient light without glare in large spaces.

To achieve high levels of even illumination and still maintain a more homelike feeling, combine indirect cove lighting for general illumination, with floor and table lamps, sconces, and chandeliers. See, for example, the dining room shown in Figure 8-2. When chandeliers are used, filament wrapped or frosted bulbs should be specified to control glare. Translucent shades can also be used.

Chandeliers and sconces are wonderful tools for creating an ambiance of home. They are an important part of the design equation, but they can never supply enough light to fill a room and meet the visual needs of aging eyes. Use them and use them often, but they should not be considered light sources. Also, in the absence of general illumination there is a risk of inadvertently producing scalloping effects of light and dark contrasting areas.

Recessed down light fixtures are not particularly successful in residential settings for the elderly primarily because of poor light distribution. In addition, they add little to a "homelike warmth" and produce both direct and reflective glare, as well as shadows. Whether a ceiling down light is successful depends on the type of fixture, the height of the ceiling (the higher the ceiling, the greater the chance of success), and the amount of glare it produces.[5] Pools of light, also, can distort perception of height and depth, causing stumbling or tripping.

Eliminate Glare

As we age, increased sensitivity to glare is a major problem. It affects both vision and balance for the elderly, and is frequently responsible for limiting mobility and activity—even walking. Reflective glare and lighting that is either too bright or too low can add up to eye strain, headache, and lowered ability to accomplish tasks. It is critical to understand what causes glare, in order to eliminate or control it. There are two types of glare: (1) direct glare, and (2) reflected glare.

Direct glare, which comes from inappropriately shielded light sources, must be avoided. Glare can result from natural daylight streaming in from windows or skylights. If the ambient light level (general illumination) of the room is too dim, compared to the daylight coming in the window, glare will result. Daylight should be balanced and controlled, but should definitely be utilized. Dirty or smudged windows are not a method of controlling glare; to the contrary they only makes the problem worse.

Looking directly into bright lights or unshielded bulbs is not visually healthy for persons of any age, but the damage may be more noticeable in the elderly. When lighting is exposed, without proper reflectors and diffusers, it can be harsh and irritating. The eyes don't adjust quickly and it can be painful and hasten the deterioration of the retina. The response to glare is categorized as either discomfort glare or disability glare. Discomfort glare is annoying; disability glare is severe enough to inhibit an individual from performing visual tasks. *Reflected glare* is created by strong light bouncing off a smooth reflective surface. The camera is one of the best means of highlighting the problem; photographs dramatically illustrate how light directed down from the ceiling or through a window, reflecting off highly polished vinyl floors, appear as "hot spots" that can be blinding.

An 89-year-old resident in a Personal Care unit who visits her sister in the Nursing Care section was quoted as saying: "The glare off the floor just throws me! Going down the hall is the worst part of the journey."[6] Because light and glare are often confused, frequently it is mistakenly assumed that the elderly avoid light, when in reality, they are avoiding glare.

Reflected glare can be controlled by carefully selecting paint, wallcoverings, countertops, and other surface materials with matte finishes. Highly polished, reflective floor surfaces are not acceptable; in today's world better choices are available. The same is true for furniture finishes, as well as accessories, artwork, and signage.

Provide Access to Natural Daylight

Most residents seem to seek out natural sunlight. There are many benefits to providing access to safe outside spaces, not the least of which is that it requires little effort to appreciate the joys of nature. Access to interior courtyards near residents' rooms and shared porch spaces offer opportunities for exercise, fresh air, and sunshine. Skylights, as well as indoor atriums and greenhouse windows, are designs that offer greater access for exposure to natural daylight, and are increasingly popular ways of maximizing natural light. Figure 8-3 shows one attractive example.

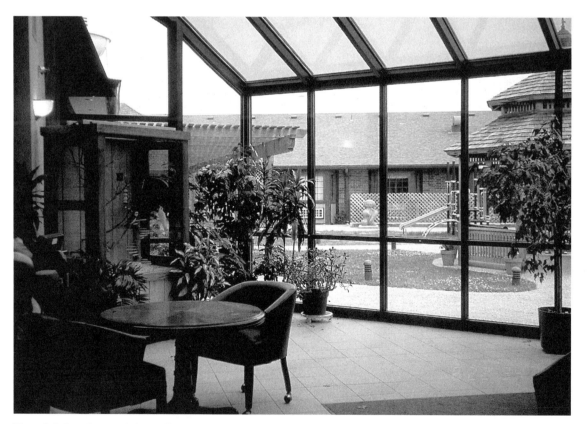

Figure 8-3 Greenhouse windows offer greater access for exposure to natural daylight. *Courtesy of Foxwood Springs Living Center, Raymore, MO.*

Provide Gradual Changes in Light Levels

Older eyes adapt much more slowly to changes in light level. Transition areas should be provided so that sensitive eyes have time to adjust from bright daylight to lower ambient interior light levels. Moving from a dim corridor into a bright room, or from daylight into a dark lobby can cause momentary blindness, and this temporary loss of vision may cause the edge of a rug or a step to be obscured.

Changes in the floor level should not be made until the eyes have sufficient time to adjust. A seating area in an entry vestibule, for example, gives the older person a place to rest while his or her eyes adjust.

Provide Focused Task Lighting

Behavior and attention can be directed by reducing the brightness of the environment as a source of distraction.[7] Task lighting is often provided by adjustable lamps that allow considerable variation in the distance separating the light source from the task. Lamps in the 3,500 to 4,000 degree Kelvin range are best for task lighting. Care should be taken to avoid direct glare from the light source. Local task lighting can be useful even when there is good general lighting, but if no local task light is available, the general lighting should provide illumination of about 300 lux (30 fc) to 750 lux (75 fc) at the work surface.

Undercabinet incandescent strips or low-voltage lights are excellent ways to balance lighting in task areas. The placement of undercabinet task lighting may cause some veiling reflection, however, which can be eliminated by special lenses that block downward light.[8]

Incandescent lamps create heat that can cause problems. Because of the intense heat they generate and the high concentration of ultraviolet light, which contributes to deterioration of the eye and can cause skin cancer, halogen lamps are poor choices for task lighting. An ultraviolet blocking lens must be used with halogen lamps.

Improve Color Rendition from Lamps or Light Sources

Lamp color should not distort the true colors of the environment or the people who live in that environment. Cool-white fluorescent lamps are known by designers as "cruel white," but until recently they were the most frequently used fluorescent lamp. Because their light is deficient in both the red and blue-violet areas of the spectrum, color lost its warmth and aliveness, and skin took on a lifeless pallor. Knowing the effect of the "cruel white" lamps raises the question of why they were used in healthcare settings. Fortunately, today the cool-white fluorescent is being replaced in many healthcare settings with the much kinder full-spectrum fluorescents, the triphospher T-8, and compact fluorescents.

The full-spectrum fluorescent light reflects more accurately the true color of people and objects and is the closest match to sunlight in commercially available lighting. It also helps to reduce eye fatigue. Compact fluorescents, using rare-earth technology with good color quality, are also an ideal source to make fluorescent lighting look like incandescent. For indirect ambient light in areas without natural daylight, the color rendering index (CRI) should be 80 or above; full spectrum fluorescent light 91 CRI.

Using Natural Light

In the days before artificial lights, an architect's number one task was to fill the interior space of a building with an abundance of natural light. Perhaps it's time to go back to that.

Richard Wurtman, a photobiologist at the Massachusetts Institute of Technology, says the change in lighting over the past 100 years is like an experiment in which we've all been testing an unknown new drug. "The findings already in hand suggest that light has an important influence on human health, and that exposure to artificial light may have harmful effects of which we are not aware."[9]

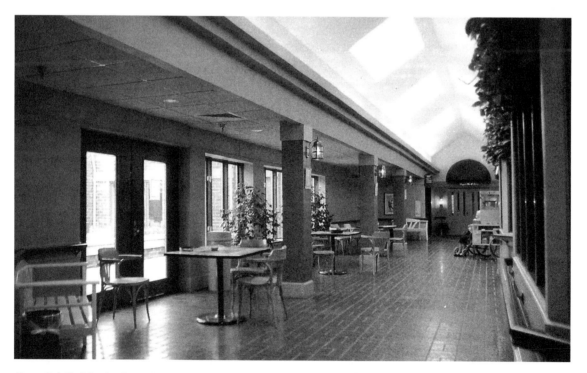

Figure 8-4 Skylights by day and cove lighting by night provide interior lighting needs. Decorative fixtures add to the outdoor look. *Courtesy of Peachwood Inn/Borden Court, Rochester Hills, MI. Architect: Hobbs & Black, Associates Inc. Designer/Assistant Professor: Jeanne Halloin, Michigan State University.*

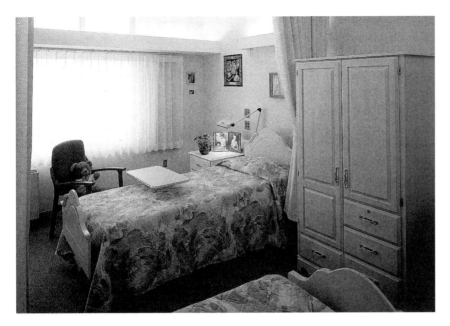

Figure 8-5 Light shelves, set above standing eye level, reflect light into a space and onto the ceiling, while allowing the lower portion of the window to be treated in a traditional manner. *Courtesy of Holladay Park Plaza, Portland, OR. Architect: WEGroup Architects/Interior. Design: Center of Design for an Aging Society. Lighting Design: Center of Design for an Aging Society & Interface Engineering. Photographer: Charlie Borland.*

We need to be concerned about the missing ingredients of light that neither incandescent nor fluorescent light gives us.

We are only beginning to understand the deficiencies caused by and the impact of light starvation on the large elderly populations, who tend to spend significant amounts of time indoors. According to Dr. Robert E. Jenkins, Director of the Clymer Health Clinic in Pennsylvania, "A room lighted with fluorescent lighting is less than one-tenth as bright as the area under a tree on a bright sunny day."[10]

It is being documented with greater frequency that the illumination level for indoor lighting is typically equivalent to that of twilight (Luke Thornton, Duro-Test Corp.) and the equivalent of biological darkness. These light levels are barely adequate to see, and, without question they are not sufficient to send an effective signal to the biological clock for the regulation of hormones and rhythms.[11]

Daylighting design refers to architectural design solutions that gather, direct, and reflect natural light deep into single or multistory buildings. Most long-term care settings designed to shelter the elderly have little natural light penetrating inside. The buildings themselves have become the barriers between natural light, the frail elderly person, and ultimately, that person's health and well-being.

High ceilings, large windows, and north-facing skylights to maximize natural lighting, while minimizing direct light, were all typical characteristics of building construction over 80 years ago. Houses were sited to take advantage of natural daylighting. These strategies can still work; see Figure 8-4.

Daylighting

Sunlight is a source of well being and provides residents with a sense of orientation, a subconscious reference to time—both the hour of the day and the changing of the seasons.

In designing long-term care settings, daylighting is important for a number of reasons. Sunlight is a continually available source of light, warmth, and energy, yet we consistently ignore it, minimize its potential, and replace its free energy with mechanically engineered lighting, heating, and cooling. With so much interest in technology and the development of sophisticated "state of the art" mechanical/electrical systems, we seem to have forgotten this source of energy known as daylight—abundant, economical, and an effective source of energy that can dramatically reduce lighting costs.[12]

Architects have used effective daylighting methods to bathe interiors with warm, indirect sunlight, raising illuminance levels to as much as 3,500 lux (350 fc). Interestingly, in facilities where luminance levels were substantially elevated, sleep disorder problems were reduced.[13] Clerestories, large windows, and high ceilings all help the designer to maximize daylighting. If ceilings are dropped or suspended, they should be designed well back from the window wall to avoid reducing the daylighting impact.

Light shelves, like the one in Figure 8-5, are set above standing eye level, and reflect light into a space and onto the ceiling, while allowing the lower portion or viewing window to be treated in a more conventional manner with some type of sun control or window treatment, such as sheer draperies.

Sunlight is a source of well being and provides residents with a sense of orientation, a subconscious reference to time—both the hour of the day and the changing of the seasons. Curiously, skylights are as effective in providing this sense of well-being as are windows, confirming that it is daylight, and daylight alone that achieves this positive response. 3M and Andersen Windows are working jointly on a glazing material for skylights that would diffuse the natural daylight and yet allow a view of the sky.[14] Designing in light color palettes, using finishes with a high reflective value, and keeping furniture as low as possible near windows, all help to optimize daylighting.

New technology is now available, using photocells, which allows linking ambient artificial light sources to available daylight to provide a constant preset illumination level. Through the integration of natural and artificial lighting systems, a predetermined foot-candle level can be maintained.[15]

Not only is daylighting a cost-effective strategy, it is a strategy for human health and well being. Any interior space is enhanced by the maximum use of daylighting; it contributes an element of quality unrivaled by any artificial light. Perhaps the greatest benefit is seen in naturally lit space where human beings feel the warmth of the sun and sense they are connected visually to the greater environment.

Eunice Noell, of the Center of Design for an Aging Society, suggests, "If the intensity of daylight can penetrate into the now 'twilight' environments, perhaps some of the elderly residents' problems may be reduced, be less debilitating, or never develop." This is certainly incentive enough for putting more natural light into the living environments we design.

Lighting Technologies for Health Care

The *fluorescent lamp,* now the world's most frequently used light source, is the prevalent form of light used in schools, businesses, healthcare facilities and industry, largely due to both the energy efficiency and reasonable cost. In most healthcare settings the lamps are likely to be full-size or T-12 straight tubes or U-bent fluorescent.

Fluorescent lamps are efficient sources, by themselves, but coupled with the technology of trichromatic phosphors, reduced diameters, and electronic ballasting, even better efficiencies can be realized. Two options are available using this added efficiency, either more light for the same wattage or original light levels at reduced wattage levels. In the case of T-8 trichromatic lamps, the same high level (3,050 lumens) of a T-12 40-watt cool white lamp is provided at a reduced 32 watts.

Because of its poor color rendering, cool-white fluorescent, the most frequently used light tube, deficient in the red and blue-violet spectrum, is no longer available. It is being replaced by the T-8 lamp with rare-earth technology. Warmer colors are available with other lamps, like deluxe warm white, but these are more expensive.

Full-spectrum fluorescent light reflects the true color of people and objects more accurately and is the closest solar match in commercially available lighting. They are used in art museums, photographic studios, and dental labs where seeing true color is crucial, because they have the total range of colors found in natural light.[16] A 4 foot, 40-watt full-spectrum tube costs about two to three times as much as other fluorescent tubes. Considering the benefits, however, that doesn't seem a lot of money.

> *Two options are available using this added efficiency, either more light for the same wattage or original light levels at reduced wattage levels.*

Full-spectrum lighting also helps to reduce eye fatigue. In 1974 Maas, Jayson, and Kleiber at Cornell University found that students in a study group working under full-spectrum lighting showed significant increases in visual acuity (perception) and were much less fatigued than those in a second group studying under conventional cool-white fluorescents.[17]

Incandescent Lamp Wattage (watts)	Suggested CFL Substitute (watts)
25	5 — 9
40	7 — 11
60	13 — 17
75	13 — 20
90	23 — 26
100	25 and above

Philips Energy-Saving Lamp Substitution Guide

Figure 8-6. Compact fluorescent lamp substitutes for incandescent lamps. *Used with permission of Philips Lighting Company.*

T-8 lamps

The T-8 lamps are replacing most common T-12 fluorescent linear lamps. They are inherently more energy efficient and provide lower operating cost. The higher color rendering indexes provided by trichromatic lamps allow for enhanced color rendering; therefore, clearer color differentiation and visually more vibrant color, as in flesh tones, for example, will result.

Selection should be made according to color temperature and color quality. The recommended color temperature for residential healthcare settings would be 3,000 to 3,500 degrees Kelvin. Since the aged eye has reduced sensitivity to the shorter wavelengths, a CRI (color rendition index) of 80 or above is recommended.

compact fluorescent (CFL)

The compact fluorescent (CFL) lamp is the ideal source for table lamps and wall sconces to make fluorescent lighting look like incandescent (see, e.g., Figure 8-6). The smaller and low-wattage lamps called "PL" lamps range from 5 to 26 watts. All compacts are rare-earth technology and offer good color quality. Choose 2,700 or 3,000 degrees Kelvin to match incandescent or choose 3,500 degrees Kelvin to match T-8 or other full size or U-bent lamps.

There are two primary types of compact fluorescent lamps: integral and modular. Integral CFLs are screw-in types that have a ballast integrated into the system. Integrals are common in retrofit applications where they are replacing incandescent lamps. Modular CFLs use either adapters for conversion or are directly hard-wired and will be more common in new construction applications where the conversion to a CFL is ensured. Figure 8-7 gives some guidance on what lamp to use where.

Figure 8-7 Quick reference table/lamp energy-saving substitutions. *Used with permission of Philips Lighting Company.*

QUICK REFERENCE TABLE   ENERGY-SAVING SUBSTITUTIONS

Present Lamp	Suggested Substitute Energy-Saving Lamps	Approximate Light Levels[a]	Watts Saved per Socket	Annual Energy Cost Savings per Socket[b]
Tungsten Halogen Lamps				
500T3Q/CL	$$$ 400T3Q/CL	88%	100	$40.00
Compact Fluorescent Lamps				
25 Watt Incandescent	$$$ Earth Light Specialty SLS 9	179%	16	$6.40
	$$$ PL-S 5/27/SYS	104%	18	7.20
40 Watt Incandescent	$$$ Earth Lightght Specialty SLS 9	86%	31	12.40
	$$$ PL-S7/27/SYS	80%	31	12.40
	$$$ Earth Light Specialty SLS 11	120%	29	11.60
	$$$ PL-S9/27/SYS	110%	29	11.60
60 Watt Incandescent	$$$ PL-C 13/27/USA/SYS	100%	46	18.40
	$$$ Earth Light Universal SLS 15	105%	45	18.00
	$$$ Earth Light Table Lamp SL/T 16	105%	44	17.60
	$$$ Earth Light Outdoor SL/O 17	101%	43	17.20
75 Watt Incandescent	$$$ Earth Light Outdoor SL/O 18	93%	57	22.80
	$$$ Earth Light Universal SLS 20	102%	55	22.00
	$$$ Earth Light Table Lamp SL/T 20	102%	55	22.00
100 Watt Incandescent	$$$ Earth Light Universal SLS 25	102%	75	30.00
65 BR30 Flood	$$$ Earth Light Flood 5LSSl30 15	88%	50	20.00
	$$$ Earth Light Flood SLS/R30 20	99%	45	18.00
65 BR$0 Flood	$$$ Earth Light Flood SLS/R40 15	99%	50	20.00
	$$$ Earth Light Flood SL/R40 18	117%	47	18.80
	$$$ Earth Light Flood SLS/R40 20	128%	45	18.00
85 BR$0 Flood	$$$ Earth Light Flood SL/R40 18	86%	67	26.80
	$$$ Earth Light Flood SLS/R40 20	95%	65	26.00
60 G30 Globe	$$$ Earth Light Decor Globe SL/G 18	112%	43	17.20
Fluorescent Lamps				
F30T12/CW/RS	$$$ F30T12/CW/RS/EW	87%	5	$2.00
F30T12/WW/RS	$$$ F30T12/WW/RS/EW	85%	5	2.00
F40CW	$$$ F40SPEC$1/RS/EW	85%	6	2.40
F40CWX	$$$ F40/$1U/RS/EW	122%	6	2.40
F40D	$$$ F40DX/RS/EW	72%	6	2.40
F$0SPEC30	$$$ F40SPEC30/RS/EW	81%	6	2.40
F$0SPEC3S	$$$ F405PEC3S/RS/EW	81%	6	2.40
F40SPEC41	$$$ F40SPEC41/RS/EW	81%	6	2.40
F40WW	$$$ F40SPEC30/RS/EW	84%	6	2.40
F40WWX	$$$ F$0/30U/RS/EW	122%	6	2.40
F40/30U	$$$ F40/30U/RS/EW	81%	6	2.40
F40/35U	$$$ F40/35U/RS/EW	81%	6	2.40
F40/41 U	$$$ F40/$1 U/RS/EW	81%	6	2.40
F40/50U	$$$ F40/50U/RS/EW	81%	6	2.40
F96T12/CW/HO	$$$ F96T12/CW/HO/EW	84%	15	6.00
F96T12/D/HO	$$$ F96T12/DX/HO/EW	69%	15	6.00
F96T12/SPEC30/HO	$$$ F96T12/SPEC30/HO/EW	84%	15	6.00
F96T12/SPEC35/HO	$$$ F96T12/SPEC3S/HO/EW	84%	15	6.00
F96T12/SPEC41/HO	$$$ F96T12/SPEC41/HO/EW	84%	15	6.00
F96T12/WW/HO	$$$ F96T12/30U/HO/EW	90%	15	6.00
F96T12/30U/HO	$$$ F96T12/30U/HO/EW	85%	15	6.00
F96T12/41U/HO	$$$ F96T12/41U/HO/EW	85%	15	6.00
F96T12/CW/VHO	$$$ F96T12/CW///HO/EW	87%	30	12.00
F48T12/CW	$$$ F48T12/SPEC41/EW	82%	8.5	3.40

[a] For compact fluorescent lamps: Light levels based on comparison to A-19 SoftWhite bulbs or BR floods.
  For standard fluorescent lamps: Ballast factor of .95 for standard lamps and ballast factor of .88 for EW lamps was applied to achieve light output levels.
[b] Based on 4,000 operating hours/year and $0.10/KWH

CFLs typically are four to five times more efficient than incandescent lamps, supplying 50 to 80 lumens per watt (LPW), compared to 10 to 19 LPW. They are an excellent replacement for incandescent lamps, which consume four to five times more electricity for the same light levels as CFLs. An added benefit to CFL is their rated life of 10,000 hours —10 to 13 times longer life than for incandescent lamps.[18]

The larger high-powered CFLs, such as Biax, come in wattages ranging from 18 to 55 watts. These compact fluorescent lamps used with electronic ballasts, provide excellent lighting and value. Depending on the fixture design, these high-wattage CFLs can be used in place of T-8s for indirect lighting systems, such as pendent indirect fixtures. Use 2700K or 3000K to match incandescent or choose 3500K to match the T-8 or other full size lamps.

Incandescent bulbs

Incandescent bulbs are most commonly used in today's homes. Although they emit a fairly complete range of the visible color spectrum, they are deficient in the blue end of the spectrum. Typically, incandescent lamps are yellow and give off a warm glow. However, incandescent bulbs generate more heat, a potential burn and fire hazard, and less light per watt than fluorescent tubes. A 150-watt incandescent bulb, for instance, throws off about the same amount of light as a 40-watt fluorescent light, which last about 10 times longer.

Electronic ballasts

Electronic ballasts for fluorescent light sources eliminate flicker, are energy efficient, and allow for dimming. Dimming can be particularly important for nighttime corridor illumination. Flicker associated with the old magnetic ballasts can trigger seizures in epilepsy patients and cause agitation and confusion, creating behavioral problems in residents with dementia. In addition, the eye is affected by flicker, causing eye fatigue.[19]

Electronic ballasts eliminate perceptible flicker and most audible hum. Healthcare interior designer Pat Hennings uses the assistance of hard-of-hearing residents who use hearing aids to help identify standard magnetic ballasts that need to be replaced. The humming noise generated by the old magnetic ballast is annoyingly identifiable to someone using a hearing aid.

Dimming and Control Issues

The ability to control all lighting, to brighten or soften light levels, is essential; therefore step level switching or dimmers are quite necessary. Step level switching requires that part of the lamps be wired to a separate ballast and circuit, to be controlled by a switch. For example, one popular pendent indirect fixture has six CFLs on top and one 18-watt CFL below. Two switches control the up lighting and one switch controls the down light, giving flexibility.

All light fixtures specified must carry a UL label. UL stands for Underwriters Laboratories, whose standards are the basis of national (ANSI) and regional electrical codes. Every light fixture, including table lamps, must carry a UL sticker. Using non-UL approved fixtures may void the building owner's fire insurance. It's always better to be safe than sorry.[20]

The ADA Approved label found on some fixtures refers only to size (ADA refers to the Americans with Disabilities Act). This compliance has nothing to do with the light the fixture produces; it simply means that the fixture does not project more than 4 inches out from the wall.

Maintenance

Specifying an interior lighting system is only part of the job; the other part is ensuring that the system continues to function to the performance standards to which it was designed. Even though most lighting designers provide detailed fixture schedules, it seems that all too often the specs are rarely looked at, and even more rarely adhered to.

Fixture schedules detail the exact fixture location, fixture description, manufacturer's name and catalog number, and lamp type used. In order to make the odds more favorable that the lighting system will be maintained, owners and operators must be convinced it is worth maintaining. Maintenance schedules for all lighting systems are important. When lamps are replaced, they should be replaced with those that were initially specified. Design professionals can help insure that required maintenance is performed by providing the maintenance staff with a notebook of the original specifications, accompanied by supplier's names and telephone numbers.

Fluorescent lamps will dim over time and need to be replaced when they start to flicker. This flicker is especially agitating to older residents whose eyes are sensitive to light changes and unable to make adjustments quickly. It can also provoke agitation and confusion in residents with dementia, and be a source of eye fatigue and "office headache" for staff. Ballasts will also have to be replaced periodically.

Other factors that can influence how well a lighting system is maintained, once the designer is gone, are simply factors affecting the ease of maintenance[21]:

- Minimize the number of different lamps on a job.
- List fixtures and which lamps go with which fixture.
- Take time to educate the building owner or administrator as to why certain lamps were selected over others, and how to replace lamps as needed so that the integrity of the plan is maintained.
- Specify light sources that are easily available.
- Provide training to educate the staff.

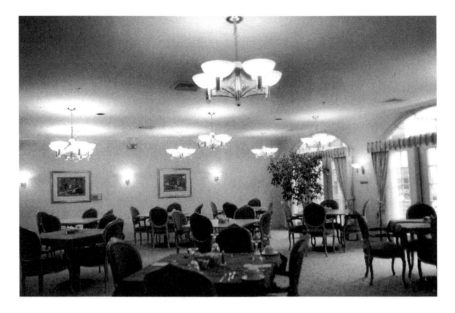

Figure 8-8 Pendant fixtures with both direct and indirect capabilities light the ceiling, reflecting light throughout this dining room, as well as lighting the tables below. *Courtesy of Waltonwood, Rochester Hills, MI. Designer/Assistant Professor: Jeanne Halloin, Michigan State University.*

Lighting Solutions for Dementia

In providing successful lighting solutions for dementia settings, more familiar residential appearance should be encouraged. Older residents, particularly those with dementia, need lighting design that provides high general illumination levels and consistent light sources that eliminate frightening shadows and that avoid distraction and glare.

It is not uncommon for adults with Alzheimer's disease to hallucinate or experience delusions, seeing, hearing, or experiencing things that aren't really there. Dim shadows and glare can distort images even further, contributing to a resident's hallucination. Special care must be exercised to avoid triggering any of these behaviors.

> *Older residents, particularly those with dementia, need lighting design that provides high general illumination levels and consistent light sources that eliminate frightening shadows and that avoid distraction and glare.*

Problems arise, however, when trying to provide the necessary or desired amount of light. Using only chandeliers and wall sconces provides insufficient ambient light. The high ambient light levels can be achieved by using pendent indirect fixtures or light valances mounted to walls and ceiling coffers. These enhance the residential quality without producing glare and shadows, as shown in Figure 8-8.

Balancing Natural and Artificial Light

Today's assisted living and skilled healthcare facilities are designed with a residential and more homelike look, and light fixture selection is important in carrying out the design theme. It is important to obtain the required illumination levels with ambient (general) lighting without sacrificing the residential character. Fixtures with residential design appeal can still be used, in combination with the indirect light systems mentioned above, to provide both a homelike feeling and adequate light in the space. Residential fixtures such as chandeliers, lamps, and wall sconces can be successfully used for ambience, but they do not provide consistent and even distribution of light on room surfaces. The secret to success lies in the skilled use of combinations.

Table Lamps

Table lamps provide a warmth and intimacy unmatched by overhead fixtures. An average table lamp will light 40 to 50 square feet. Although table lamps on either side of a sofa need not be identical they should have the same visual weight and height.

The correct height for a table lamp is determined by the seating and the height of the table beside it. To avoid glare, the lamp should be tall enough for the bottom of the lampshade to fall at the eye level of the person seated next to it. Shades should be selected for the required wattage as well as the ambience they provide. Translucent white and ivory shades, for example, give off a gentle overall light, while opaque shades focus light down for reading or for illuminating objects on a table. White lamp shade linings are the best choice for reading or specific tasks.

Sconces

Wall sconces are an often overlooked solution for brightening dark spaces. Compact but decorative, they add just enough extra light to complement other lighting sources in the room. They are a natural choice for the living room, dining room, and bedroom. They add decorative interest as well as lighting artwork and details at eye level. Wall sconces can also be used to light a hallway or any dark area where there is no space for a table lamp. They are appropriately mounted at eye level for home use, however, in residential settings for the elderly, they should be raised to avoid becoming a source of disabling glare. If the light bulbs are exposed, use small chandelier shades to avoid glare and soften the lighting effect.[22]

Chandeliers

Available in many decorative styles, chandeliers add both presence and weight to a room. Whether hung above a dining room or kitchen table, or used as general lighting in foyers, they bring the glow of candlelight to any setting. The light intensity of a chandelier can be controlled by dimmers to accommodate lighting for diverse activities. Chandelier shades allow for higher wattage without glare and help to direct light down where it is needed.

To determine the size of a chandelier for a dining room, add the two dimensions of the room in feet and convert the total to inches. This should appropriately equal the width of an appropriate chandelier. A 10 by 13-foot dining room, for example, would take a 23-inch wide fixture. Chandeliers should also be at least 12 inches smaller in width than the width of the dining table.[23] Shades add 2 to 4 inches to the total width of the chandelier. In dining rooms with 8-foot ceilings, hang chandeliers about 30 inches above the table. Add 3 inches for each foot of ceiling height over 8 feet, and remember to order extra chain for higher ceilings.

Cost Efficiency

There are both environmental and economic reasons to design more energy efficient lighting systems. Most U.S. utilities (but not all) offer rebates to install energy efficient lighting in new or existing buildings. The average rebate is about $0.25 per square foot for a complete program costing about $1.00 per square foot, and saving about $0.33 per square foot. Simple payback is achieved in slightly over 2 years.[24]

> *There are both environmental and economic reasons to design more energy efficient lighting systems.*

Energy, however, is not the only component of lighting that is increasing in cost. Lighting fixtures or luminaires that are energy efficient and provide good light quality are not inexpensive. Everyone is looking for ways to save money, and often life cycle and less tangible costs, such as discomfort and disability glare, are not considered.

"The cheapest possible solution is not always the best value" (E. Noell). The Center of Design for an Aging Society specified indirect fluorescent lighting producing 6,100 lumens and using only 64 watts of energy on a recent project. The specification was changed by the owner to incandescent down light fixtures producing only 1,090 lumens and consuming 120 watts. The results: one-sixth the light for twice the energy cost and the owner saved only a few dollars on the initial purchase of the fixture, a graphic illustration of costly, long-term false economy.[25] Careful planning and balancing initial costs against true life cycle costs can avoid short-sighted and wasteful investment in inadequate and/or poor quality lighting.

> *The physical surroundings contribute to the residents' comfort and ability to function safely and support their function, adding to the quality of living, rather than rendering daily tasks more difficult, hazardous, or impossible.*

As we learn more from research about the needs of aging eyes, we must use the information to design spaces that allow the elderly, particularly those with cognitive impairments, to continue to function with as much ease and confidence as possible. The physical surroundings contribute to the residents' comfort and ability to function safely and support their function, adding to the quality of living, rather than rendering daily tasks more difficult, hazardous, or impossible.

Guidelines can be developed based on the visual tasks to be performed in given spaces and our knowledge of the vision changes that take place in aging eyes. A complete analysis of the kinds of visual tasks that are likely to occur helps to prepare the lighting designer to provide flexible lighting applications to solve unique lighting needs.

Environmental improvements, particularly in lighting, energy, and building design, are necessary. We must support the visual tasks performed by aging eyes.

Checklist for Lighting

❏ Provide transition areas to make adjustment between spaces with differing levels of brightness.

❏ Provide even light distribution that does not create shadows

❏ Use ambient indirect lighting systems to produce sufficient light levels and prevent glare.

❏ Supplement with "residential style" fixtures for decorative effect.

❏ Use task lighting for specific activities requiring close proximity. Fixtures should allow for flexible positioning, directional control, and easy lamp replacement.

❏ Consider using compact fluorescent lamps for task light, as they alleviate burn hazards produced by incandescent lamps.

❏ Use appropriate carpet to prevent glare on the floor.

❏ Use nongloss wax on floor tile; high gloss finishes create glare.

❏ Use semigloss or eggshell enamel paint; high gloss finishes create glare.

❏ Provide adjustable window coverings to control sunlight.

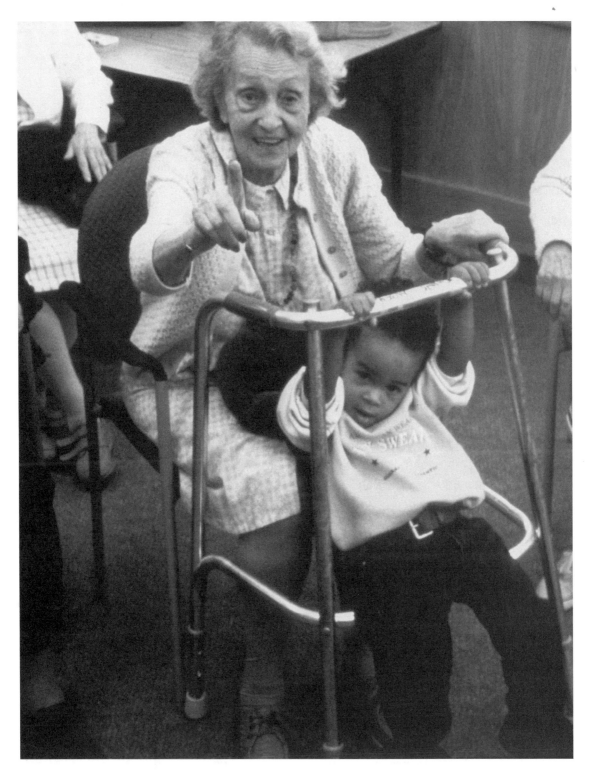

Courtesy of the Norma and Joseph Saul Alzheimer's Disease Special Care Unit of the Jewish Home and Hospital for Aged, Bronx, NY.

CHAPTER 9

The Impact of Color in Environmental Design

The average person doesn't give much thought to light or color, but then we have not been conditioned to think of light as having an effect on our quality of life or to think of color impacting our lives. Earlier civilizations, however, recognized the importance of color and understood that the light that comes from the sun is the foundation for color.

There is increasing evidence that light and color relate to more than just illumination or aesthetic value in shaping our lives. They influence our sleeping, wakefulness, emotions, and health, playing a major role in our everyday living. How people feel directly affects their quality of life, which can be enhanced with a better understanding of the correct use of light and color.

For the last 100 years the visible spectrum has been virtually ignored by physicians. Until recently, the modern medical profession disdained color as a therapeutic agent, but today the long held fascination with the magical properties of light and color is working its way back into the medical field. Both the emotional and physical aspects of color are now being acknowledged as having therapeutic potential.[1]

Architects and designers throughout the world share a renewed interest in the role of color in the built environment. Visible light, as well as ultraviolet (UV) or infrared radiation, has measurable biological effects (Thomas R. C. Sisson).[2] Visible blue light, for instance, is used by doctors and hospitals throughout the world to treat newborn infants with jaundice.[3]

Scientists in the fields of psychology and medicine indicate that both light and color influence the emotions and affect the autonomic nervous system, as evidenced by changes in heart rate, blood pressure, respiration, cortical activation, muscular tension, and other changes in internal organs stimulated by nerve endings in the skin.[4] However, despite our scientific understanding of so many other subjects, we are just discovering the significance of color, its role in our lives, and its importance in our environment. This renewed interest in light and color has encouraged many of us, especially designers, to become more educated as to their use and effect.

From a biological point of view, color is an optical illusion; using spectral light as its palette, the human brain perceives an estimated seven million different hues.[5] Though researchers and theorists have shown that color doesn't have to be noticeable to have a noticeable effect on patients and medical staff alike, color has the ability to stimulate the brain and the autonomic nervous system. Hospitals now use it to help reduce anxiety and speed recovery. Since how we feel and the way we behave are so strongly impacted by light and color, color is a logical tool to use in healthcare settings.

Since how we feel and the way we behave are so strongly impacted by light and color, color is a logical tool to use in healthcare settings.

Designers have long understood the existence of a relationship between color and how people feel and respond. Only a few years ago the popular trend was to have "our colors done" to determine the color tones that make us look our best. It was a conscious effort to surround ourselves with appropriate colors in our homes and to look our best in our clothing. Most of us have at some time worn an unflattering color, only to be asked by friends, "Do you feel O.K.? You look a little pale" or told "You don't look well"—graphic results of how the wrong color reflecting on the skin can change the look of skin tones.

In recent years, the colors used in healthcare have changed dramatically. Instead of white, yellow, beige, and "hospital green," we are seeing more stimulating and pleasing colors like soft apricot and peach tones. This is no accident. As the healthcare community becomes more familiar with the effects of color, it will be used to much greater benefit.

Carefully adjusting the brightness to softer colors of the same hues helps avoid monotony, and in addition keeps the eyes from being distracted, causing them to work overtime and produce fatigue. Yellow-based pinks, such as salmon, coral, peach, or a soft yellow-orange will provide residents with pleasant surroundings. The pale tints, soft apricot and peach, accent the skin's own natural pigmentation, and of all the colors, are the most flattering to human skin tones. Turquoise and aquamarine, considered "universal" colors, also compliment most people's skin tones. When people look better, they feel better!

The importance of projecting a positive message in health care setting cannot be overestimated. Color communicates value and image. While clean, fresh, updated colors send the message, "we care about our residents" and help to reinforce a sense of confidence in family members, out-of-date color schemes and a rundown appearance send an altogether different message of lack of attention and possible neglect.

Before selecting color schemes, lighting, or wayfinding and cueing strategies, it is crucial to understand the physical effects of aging on residents' eyes, along with the resulting behavioral and psychological changes.

Age-Related Changes

Without the help of feedback from the eyes and the brain, which helps us to experience light and color, we would not be able to see color or attach perceptions to it. It is the upper two-thirds of the brain where ideas take shape and become perceptions.[6] This may help to explain why color cueing is often not particularly effective for people with Alzheimer's disease.

The majority of the individuals being cared for in long-term care settings are elderly, and can be expected to have visual impairments; many may also be cognitively impaired. Together, these visual and cognitive deficits make it difficult for the individual to interpret and understand the environment. The challenge becomes adjusting the environment to help compensate for these changes.

The issue of color in residential settings for Alzheimer's and its effect on resident behavior is an area that is frequently debated among the experts. Some people with dementia retain the ability to recognize and attach importance to colors long into the course of the disease, though evidence suggests that most Alzheimer's and other dementia victims will eventually lose this ability.[7]

Age has a negative effect on human vision and the ability to see. This is primarily due to inevitable changes in the lens of the eye (which after age 60 becomes noticeably harder, thicker, and more yellow), and to a reduction in the size of the pupil. The hardening of the lens reduces its ability to change shape, and therefore, to accommodate for variations in distance.[8] In addition, the altered composition of the aging lens and the presence of intraocular particles, which cause light to scatter instead of focus on the retina, are mainly responsible for the phenomenon known as glare.[9] The end result of all these changes is that both the quality and the amount of light entering the eye are negatively affected, altering the image received.[10]

Decreases in depth perception and color differentiation are common in normal aging; visual memory is also reduced.[11] Together, these changes alter visual perception, causing a negative impact. For example, impaired depth perception may cause a person to perceive a shadow on the floor as a step or a hole, and this visual misinterpretation, based on visual misinformation, can severely impair an individual's ability to function safely.[12]

The yellowing of the thickened lens filters out the short wavelengths and distorts color perception, causing *older people to perceive colors and color combinations differently from younger people.* These age-related changes in color vision manifest themselves by a loss in color discrimination, especially along the blue-yellow axis. What the older person recalls may not match the "real" color.[13] Other changes make it more difficult for the older person to adjust to sudden changes in light level.

Cooper, Ward, Gowland, and McIntosh[14] studied color vision in a well elderly population. Their study confirmed the earlier findings of loss in the ability to discriminate color, and found selective decrease in the ability to discriminate among unsaturated colors, which was more pronounced for "cool" hues and more noticeable after age 60. The ability to discriminate red (hue) and the brightness factor of color persists longest.[15]

These findings indicate that elderly people are best able to discriminate highly saturated colors at the "warm" end of the spectrum, and that colors with a high degree of brightness (e.g., yellow) are particularly visible. Conversely, pastel tones, especially those at the "cool" end of the spectrum, are less easy to see. Pastel blues, lavenders, and pinks may appear so similar that it is difficult to distinguish one room's color from that of a neighboring room. Cooper found blue/purple at Munsell chroma two was the most difficult color for older people to see; it appeared gray to many individuals after age 70.[16]

There are a variety of visual impairments that affect the elderly population, including cataracts (which produce overall haziness), macular degeneration, and glaucoma; these impairments result in varying degrees of loss of central and peripheral vision (as discussed in Chapter 7), and a wide range of color vision defects.[17] In addition, many of the elderly, particularly men, are affected by varying degrees of color blindness.

It is important to remember that not only do elderly individuals vary considerably in their capacity to see, but they are affected at dif-

It is important to remember that not only do elderly individuals vary considerably in their capacity to see, but they are affected at different rates by the aging process.[18]

ferent rates by the aging process.[18] For example, while acuity begins to fail sometime after age 40, losses in the ability to discriminate color usually are not noted until after age 60.[19]

Color is important. It greatly enhances the ambience of the environment for residents, families, visitors, and staff, but with little research available on how to make environments visually accessible, the design team needs to be aware of the special needs of the older population. To put this in perspective, color is an important element in the overall design, but for aging vision, clearly, contrast takes on even more importance than color alone.

> *Color is an important element in the overall design, but for aging vision, clearly, contrast takes on even more importance than color alone.*

Contrast

More than 10 million Americans have significant vision problems, and over 3 million have partial sight. Most of these individuals have deficits in color perception that accompany their eye diseases, and reduce the effectiveness of certain color combinations. Between congenital color deficiencies and those acquired with eye diseases, there are some 35 million people in the United States alone with reduced ability to distinguish colors.[20]

Nothing is more effective in enhancing residents' visual function than high contrast. The two factors primarily responsible for impeding older people in the performance of activities of daily living are the presence of glare and the difficulty encountered in seeing the edges of pale colored objects.[21] In designing for elderly persons, color should be thought of in terms of relationships to establish contrast between light and dark. Light entryways and dark door jambs, for example, help people differentiate between a door and its frame; light walls and darker floors, or lighter floor and dark furniture are also helpful.[22]

Tabletops and countertops should stand out strongly from floors. Often an edge band of contrasting color on a table top or other raised surface can help residents to see it more easily. Contrasting countertops, for instance, help to define a sink from the surrounding counter surface, as shown in Figure 9-1.

The same principle also applies in the bathroom. Using the toilet may depend on being able to locate it. Distinguishing the toilet from the wall or floor in, for example, a totally white bathroom is at best confusing

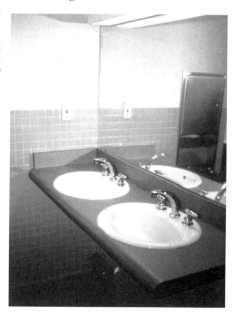

Figure 9-1 Contrasting countertops help to define a sink from the surrounding surface. *Courtesy of On Lok Senior Health Services, San Francisco, CA. Architect: Barker Associates. Interior design: Elizabeth Brawley, IIDA Design Concepts Unlimited.*

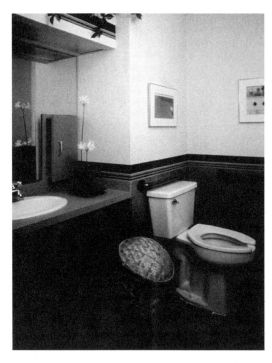

Figure 9-2 Contrast between the vanity surface and the lavatory bowl increases visibility. People in wheelchairs need one side of the toilet clear for access. *Morton Plant Family Center, Clearwater, FL. Interior design by and courtesy of Susan Behar, ASID/Universal Design. Photographer: George Cott.*

and perhaps altogether impossible for some. A colored wall can provide visual contrast with a white toilet, making it easier to see and more likely to be used, while colored toilet seats give added definition. See the example shown in Figure 9-2.

The best color contrast for ease of vision, to accommodate persons experiencing difficulty with depth perception, is provided by black against white. While it might provide excellent contrast, however, an environment created totally in black and white would be cold and would become very boring. However, many pleasing and highly effective contrasting color combinations can be devised by designers skilled in using color.

It can be difficult to accommodate varying impairments, because color choices that "read" well for a person with one visual deficit may be indiscernible to another person with a different impairment. Knowledgeable choices, implemented with skill, can help substantially to increase function. These details are especially meaningful in an Alzheimer special care setting, since the cognitive deficit in persons with Alzheimer's is often compounded by visual deficits. Design professionals should be aware that the deficits that prevent residents from interpreting the environment accurately impede function.

The Alzheimer's Association's "Guidelines for Dignity" makes one of its highest priorities for people with Alzheimer's disease to maintain function at the highest possible level. It is the constant attention to detail—in this case, strong visual contrast—that provides opportunity to maintain independence and dignity.

Specific effects that visual impairments produce on color vision are diverse, ranging from no effect to complete loss of hue discrimination. Most color vision losses that occur with visual impairment can be described in terms of a combination of the following general types of loss: (1) contrast sensitivity, (2) saturation discrimination loss, (3) wavelength discrimination loss, and (4) luminosity loss at one or both extremes of the spectrum.[23]

Careful consideration of color, for function as well as for beauty, is a must for a well-designed environment. The use of color as a cue to enhance visibility of critical environmental features is often

Design professionals should be aware that the deficits that prevent residents from interpreting the environment accurately impede function.

recommended, but these recommendations are usually very general and limited to emphasizing only the need for strong contrasts. Because of the wide range of color vision defects found in low vision, however, color is perceived very differently, and colors that contrast optimally for one person may actually be indiscriminable to another.

To accurately specify color it is important to understand the three most important perceptual attributes of color: hue, lightness (or brightness), and saturation.[24]

- *Hue*
  This term identifies how we name the basic colors, red being at one end of the spectrum with a long wavelength, violet being at the other end with a short wavelength. In most color deficits, the ability to distinguish colors on the basis of hue is diminished.

- *Lightness (or Brightness)*
  These words refer to the degree of apparent light intensity. Lightness is determined by the proportion of light reflected from a surface, rather than the absolute amount of light coming from the surface, which is brightness. In many color deficits, particularly those related to aging and eye disease, the ability to discriminate colors on the basis of lightness is reduced.

- *Saturation (or Chroma)*
  These describe color intensity, or the degree to which a surface color differs from an achromatic (white) surface of the same lightness. Congenital and acquired color deficits usually cause difficulty in discriminating colors on the basis of saturation.

Individuals with normal vision can often perform everyday tasks under conditions in which color contrast is substantially reduced, but the performance of those with low vision is substantially reduced by even small reductions in contrast. Visual impairment also affects chroma (saturation) sensitivity, as well as the ability to distinguish hues from adjacent regions in the color spectrum.

Normal aging generally causes the lens inside the eye gradually to increase in yellowness, concomitantly filtering out certain (short) wavelengths of light and preventing them from reaching the retina. This causes loss of sensitivity to lightness for spectrally extreme colors. As a result, violet, blue, and blue-green surfaces (which reflect light mostly from the short wavelength region) often appear darker to older individuals. Similarly, certain other eye disorders result in loss of sensitivity to long wavelength light. For individuals with these types of disorders, red and brown surfaces appear darker. This type of loss is more typically referred to as a *luminosity loss*.[25]

The Lighthouse, Inc., the world's leading resource on vision impairment, has developed guidelines to provide assistance in designing effective color contrast for people with low vision. For designers, who are often confronted with making difficult color choices affecting people with many visual impairments, these guidelines are not meant to describe what is seen by a visually impaired individual, but instead to outline a framework for the choice of color contrasts that will maximize visibility to visually impaired people.

In designing environments for those who may have either congenital or acquired color deficit, there are three important guidelines to keep in mind.

Design Guidelines for Using Color

1. Exaggerate lightness differences between foreground and background colors, and avoid using colors of similar lightness adjacent to one another, even though they differ in saturation or hue. The lightness that you, the designer, perceive will most likely not be the same as the lightnesses perceived by people with color deficits, but you can generally assume that they will see less contrast between colors than you will. If you lighten the light colors and darken the dark colors, you will increase the visual accessibility of the design.

2. Choose dark colors from hues of blue, violet, purple, and red against light colors from the blue-green, green, yellow, and orange hues. Avoid contrasting lighter shades of the dark colors against dark variations of light colors (blue-green, green, yellow, and orange). Since most people with partial sight and/or color deficiency tend to suffer in visual efficiency for blue, violet, purple, and red, this guideline helps to minimize the ill effects of these losses on effective contrast.

3. Avoid contrasting hues from adjacent parts of the color wheel, especially if the colors do not contrast sharply in lightness. Because color deficiencies make colors of similar hue more difficult to discriminate, try to contrast colors from very different locations on the color wheel.[26]

An overall loss in the ability to distinguish hues of low saturation from white or gray is a common feature in defects arising from visual impairment. To increase visual effectiveness, designers should avoid using pastel colors altogether, and avoid placing white or gray against any color of similar lightness.[27]

Good Color Choices for Contrast	*Poor Color Choices for Contrast*
• Light color against black	• Dark green against bright red
• Dark color against white	• Yellow against white or similar lightness
• Light yellow against dark blue	
• Dark red against light green	• Blue against green or similar lightness
Additional information and accurate color simulations are available from The Lighthouse Inc.	• Lavender against pink

The way we see color is dependent on two factors: the way the surface absorbs or reflects light and the type of light source that lights the object.[28] While light has an effect on color, surface color also affects the quality of the lighting—an effect known as the color's light reflectance value. Light colors reflect light, while dark colors absorb it. White, followed by pastels, has the highest light reflectance; black allows no reflectance.

A color's light reflectance value contributes significantly to task visibility. Objects are discerned only in contrast with their surroundings, and the most effective contrast can be obtained by selecting colors for their light reflectance characteristics.[29] Reflections from painted surfaces—ceiling, walls, and floors—act as secondary light sources. With the skillful use of color and light reflectance values, work surfaces can maximize the use of available light and reduce shadows. A high level of lighting that is mainly reflective has a more positive effect than a high level of direct lighting.

No discussion of color would be complete without a reference to the role lighting plays. The purpose of a light source, besides giving good vision and acuity, is to represent color in as true a manner as possible. Color is visibly modified by different light sources. The perception of any color can vary depending on the type of light source under which the color is seen; the truest color can be seen under daylight. Carpet, wall color, fabrics, furniture, and accessory colors will all look much brighter in direct natural daylight than they will under artificial light.[30] The variety of lighting systems currently in use can alter the appearance of color, as can moving from one light source to another. This makes it particularly important to consider the effects of a facility's lighting system when selecting colors for building interiors.

Because of the difference in lighting, colors change. Since the light source tends to reinforce certain colors, the selection of paints and fabrics, which ultimately affect the success of color in rooms, should

The Effect of Light on Color

The selection of paints and fabrics, which ultimately affect the success of color in rooms, should be chosen under the same type of light source ihat they will be seen under.

be chosen under the same type of light source ihat they will be seen under. Most women have experienced how makeup applied under fluorescent light can change dramatically when seen in natural light, and any designer will tell you that fabrics perfectly matched to another swatch of fabric under showroom lighting may look entirely different when placed in the room where they are to be used.

Incandescent light is very warm and radiates almost all red and yellow; the basic *warm white fluorescent* has an abundance of red, yellow, and green. Under these light sources, the percentage of color is warmer; warm colors will be intensified and cool colors will be neutralized. Natural light also tends to effect changes in colors. Light changes at different times of the day and different times of the year. The afternoon sun is intense white light, which incorporates all colors, and tends to intensify color. Later in the day colors will take on a rosy glow from the sunset, and when there is a lack of light or low light, colors tend to appear darker.

It is a good idea to test possible color selections in the setting where they are to be used, in both day and evening light. The color will appear differently in the same setting at different times of the day. The risk is a quart of paint to insure good choices and eliminate surprises.

Putting Color to Work

Using knowledge and skill to take advantage of the value color offers costs no more than selecting color purely at random; the results, however, can be dramatically different—beautiful colors are no more expensive than the ones that don't work.

Color can submerge objects that intrude into the field of vision, making necessary but visually distracting elements seem to disappear and reducing visual clutter. Columns, beams, and pipes can be camouflaged by painting them the same color as adjacent walls or the ceiling. This can be a particularly important and useful technique in many settings—especially in renovations—when trying to visually clean up and enlarge space with limited dollars.

The size of a space, what it is used for, and the available light all contribute to the effect color has on the people using the space. Color can draw attention to physical details and make a room or a space visually warmer, more interesting, and inviting. The illusion of larger or smaller space can effectively be created by using lighter colors to create the illusion of spaciousness and calmness and can provide a psychological lift. Dark, saturated colors, conversely, often tend to make surroundings appear cramped.

Color preferences are not static and particular colors may affect individuals differently. Many factors play a role in what colors people enjoy

> **Beautiful colors are no more expensive than the ones that don't work.**

—social roles and responses, culture, family, past work experience, climate, and geography. We have much in common in our learned responses. Most people in similar social and economic circumstances share many of the same experiences and learn some of the same color responses. For instance, we associate certain rather subdued colors with lawyers and bankers and more flamboyant colors with entertainers.

Locale is also important in considering appropriate colors for the environment. Some colors are more appropriate for different parts of the country, due to differences in light qualities. In a predominately overcast area, such as Seattle, the color blue, though it provides calming, tranquilizing qualities, could be depressing. Likewise bright, brilliant reds and oranges might not achieve desirable results in the hot Southwest, though softer variations of those hues are often used.

When making selections for special healthcare settings, expectations for these settings are serious. Some of the most controversial issues in settings serving Alzheimer residents are related to color and architectural design. Color can make a powerful impression and it is often discussed as an environmental variable relevant to dementia; however, color, by itself, may have less impact on older people than do other features of the environment such as lighting, acoustics, or seating and seating arrangements.[31]

The quantity of a particular color used in an environment may do wonders in improving the light and life, but too much of a good thing can be exhausting. The question becomes how to apply color appropriately in these specialized settings. It is important to achieve a balance in the number and intensity of colors used, and to choose a range of color combinations and palettes that complement each other. Experience suggests that too many colors used together can be distracting. Elderly residents with cognitive impairment are at particular disadvantage, since they find it difficult to process a large number of stimuli at one time, yet using a single color provides no visual relief and becomes monotonous.

The interaction between color, lighting, and human behavior holds particular significance when designing for residents with dementia and should be integrated in any design to aid residents in their day-to-day living. Clear colors, not necessarily primary or bright colors, but those which do not have grayed or muted properties (mauve, gray blue) are more easily distinguishable.[32] Research suggests bright red, orange, and yellow are the most visible hues, and used effectively these colors can enhance visibility and encourage

Color in Specialized Settings

> *The interaction between color, lighting, and human behavior holds particular significance when designing for residents with dementia.*

motion and activity. Warm colors such as reds and yellows are also more stimulating than cooler colors.

Color selection becomes a balancing act between colors that work behaviorally and those that can be seen visually. Though cool colors such as blues and greens can reduce stress and tension and provide a comfortable, calm, nondistracting environment, they are not seen as easily by the elderly. These are beautiful and pleasing colors to many, however, and this is not a suggestion they be removed from the color palette. With careful attention in selecting how, where, how much, and in what strength and intensity these hues are used, the results can be improved. The extent to which colors are saturated can be even more important than the hues themselves. Studies consistently show that moderate saturation levels, regardless of actual colors, have a calming effect.[33]

Color can influence human behavior; consciously or unconsciously, people respond to the colors around them. The right colors can help to change moods from sad to happy, help to dispel loneliness, encourage conversation, and create a sense of peace and well-being. Speaking at the National Symposium on Healthcare Design, Lorraine Hiatt cautioned, "What I take issue with is the notion that there is one color scheme that is going to return the memories of older people; color that will make them dance again or for the first time."[34] Though the environment and function within the environment can be dramatically improved with knowledgeable use of light and color, we have still not found that it will cure Alzheimer's disease or dementia.

Color for Cueing

Color can help in wayfinding. Lisa Gwyther, Director of the Bryan Center on Aging at Duke University, says that color can provide a latent clue for orientation and wayfinding and suggests that the most successful environments for the cognitively impaired provide visual differentiation. Defining space with color in dining rooms and activity spaces is a strategy that can provide visual differentiation and draw attention to special areas.[35]

Calkins has suggested that for some, a room may be recognized more easily by color than by function and that hallways treated with different colors can provide an added

While color is an important element in the overall design and can make a powerful impression, in specialized care settings it must not be depended on as the most significant or the only cueing device.

reminder to residents. She recommends that if color is to be used as a meaningful orientation cue, staff must use the color by name, referring to the "blue hall" or to the color of the resident's door.

This strategy of color coding of corridors and doorways is a fairly common practice in long-term care settings; however, evidence suggests that for people with Alzheimer's disease it is not particularly useful as a cueing mechanism.[36] Since most will eventually lose the capacity to recognize colors, it is suggested that color be used only in connection with other cues.

In the most recent research on color cueing, in the likely presence of cognitive impairments among residents in long-term care facilities, Cooper, Mohide, and Gilbert[37] employed color cues to attract the attention of cognitively impaired long-term care residents. They used large-scale doors and door frames, and observed Cooper's color contrast guidelines.[38] These were found to attract the attention of the residents; however, residents were unable to determine their significance.[39]

In perspective, while color is an important element in the overall design and can make a powerful impression, in specialized care settings it must not be depended on as the most significant or the only cueing device. Use of contrasting colors in reliable hues for sharper definition and higher visibility is highly effective in providing another cognitive clue. Mentally impaired older people, however, are much more likely to use actual objects, shapes, smells, air currents, and tactile cues, rather than color, to orient themselves.[40]

Selecting Colors

The average person feels insecure about making color selections. Most of us aren't sure where to start. Others are still haunted by past decisions that didn't turn out well, and some are simply overwhelmed with the number of choices. But the biggest fear is making an expensive mistake. Sadly, the frequent result of this color anxiety is that lack of confidence causes many people to give up before they start. Designers and color consultants familiar with the special needs of the elderly and cognitively impaired can help to make appropriate choices.

> *Most of us aren't sure where to start. Others are still haunted by past decisions that didn't turn out well, and some are simply overwhelmed with the number of choices. But the biggest fear is making an expensive mistake.*

Color is an integral component of all physical environments and knowing the basics of color and how to use it as a tool are important steps in creating appropriate residential healthcare settings. Imagination and creativity can make spaces interesting, and though there are no hard and fast rules, guidelines can sometimes be helpful.

- When selecting color, decide on a color scheme of perhaps three to five colors. Dominant colors in one room can become accent colors in another. Variety can be expanded even further by using various shades and tints of the selected colors. Possible schemes include:

  Monochromatic: Variations of a single color

  Analogous: Colors close to each other on the color wheel

  Complementary: Colors opposite each other on the color wheel

- Selection can be done in many ways; one of the most basic is to pick a color, then use the color wheel to make additional selections. The colors that harmonize best for the visually impaired will be the colors opposite on the color wheel.

- Start with color selections for the largest areas of color. Begin with the basic color you chose. Floorcovering, whether carpet, wood flooring, or vinyl is a good example. These are usually the most expensive items and used in the largest amounts.

In designing healthcare settings it can be easier to survey the appropriate floorcovering products and select your color schemes and additional color selections from the colors of the floorcovering product chosen. Improvements in the quality of the products themselves have been substantial and manufacturers are paying more attention to color and to color needs of the elderly.

- Select the wall colors next—wallpaper, paint, wallcovering, or other wall treatments. Paint is the easiest and least expensive wall treatment to change, so make this selection last. Wall color in paint can be customized and matched to fabric and carpet colors.

- Choose the colors for the major furnishings, such as sofas and other large furniture pieces.

- Finally, choose the colors for accent pieces, including occasional chairs, window coverings, and accessories. Accent pieces and accessories give each space its own individuality, and accent pieces, like the accessories we use with clothing, can be mixed and matched.

- When choosing colors, whether for paint, wall covering, flooring, or carpet, use large samples. Professional designers don't attempt color selections from tiny samples and neither should you.

- A well-organized color plan allows for moving furnishings from one area to another with confidence that they will work.

A note of caution: don't be influenced by trends, since popular colors and names of colors are cyclical. You make not like a color called sage green or paprika because you don't like sage or pepper; but you might love the identical colors when they're called desert green and pomegranate.

Warm Colors: Red, Orange, Yellow

Red has an energizing quality appropriate for social spaces, such as dining rooms or visiting areas. Diverse cultures use red in different ways. The Chinese have always favored red, traditionally using it for the bridal gown—a sign of longevity. Deeper tones of rose and terra cotta combine the strength and energy of the earth to offer stability.

Orange is capable of emitting great energy in its purest form and as an earth tone it evokes warmth, comfort, and reassurance. Orange and variations of orange, such as peach and salmon, are cheerful colors and are popular in dining rooms and healthcare environments. As a pale tint, it becomes the most flattering color of all to human skin tones. It leads people to believe that time passes quickly.

Yellow evokes a sense of energy and excitement and its brilliance is most often associated with the sun. The emotional effects of yellow are optimistic and bright, yet sometimes unsettling and seldom restful. Yellow reflects more light than any other color and can be used to increase illumination in poorly lighted areas.

In interior spaces, these qualities may need to be subdued through tinting, dulling or combining these colors with others. When tinted, yellow's brightness may be subdued, but it retains an appealing liveliness. The intensity can be lowered through the addition of violet tones, making it earthy and reassuring.

Cool Colors: Blue, Turquoise, Green

Blue, of the three primary hues, is perhaps most universally equated with beauty. Blue is timeless, linking the present with tradition and lasting values, and it is the most popular color with adults.

Psychologically, blue is associated with tranquility and contentment. It is most commonly associated with the sky and the sea. Deep blue is considered to be the optimum color for meditation, for slowing down the bodily processes to allow relaxation and recuperation. Because of its calming effects, blue has long been a favorite for bedrooms.

Be careful using pale blue, however; by itself, blue can seem a bit too cool and unstimulating and for the elderly is more difficult to see.

Color Characteristics and Suggested Uses for Various Colors

Experienced designers counteract these effects by balancing blue with warmer colors such as yellow or peach for freshness or red for an energizing effect.

Green, the color of plants and nature, represents growth and life and is associated with pleasant odors and tastes. Avoid yellow-greens and purples. Yellow-green colors, if reflected on human flesh, will give it a sickly look. Yellow-green is the after-image of purple. If one stares at purple then looks into a mirror or transfers his gaze to another, that person will look pallid.[41]

Light Colors: Off-Whites and Pastel Tints

Light colors can make objects seem lighter in weight and areas seem more spacious. They reflect more light, help to compensate for low light levels, and maximize the use of available light. They usually give people a psychological lift. Small rooms, corridors, and spaces with few or no windows benefit from using light colors.

Dark Colors: Deep Tones, Gray, Black

Dark colors absorb light and can make a room appear smaller and more cramped. Darker tones can be quite dramatic, but in healthcare settings may be better used in lesser amounts. Prolonged exposure to large amounts of dark colors may contribute to monotony and depression.

Bright Colors: Notable Yellow, Yellow-Green

Bright colors, in their purer shades, compellingly attract the eye, making objects appear larger and creating excitement. Bright colors complement basic wall colors and can be used as accent colors for doors, columns, graphics, clocks, and so on. Large amounts of intense shades of warm colors can contribute to confusion and anxiety.

White

White denotes purity and cleanliness and reflects more light than any other color. White can be used on all ceilings and overhead structures and in rooms where maximum light reflection is needed.

Checklist for Color

☐ Select colors that accommodate ease of visibility for the elderly eye.

☐ Provide good contrast—especially between the walls and the floor.

☐ Provide an attractive color scheme and lighting that enhances it.

☐ Select colors and test samples under proposed lighting conditions to verify how they will appear.

☐ Use objects that are visibly bright and distinct.

☐ Use resident-assisted color selection for their rooms.

☐ Use yellow acetate or cellophane to screen color selections.

☐ Consider staff preferences for staff areas.

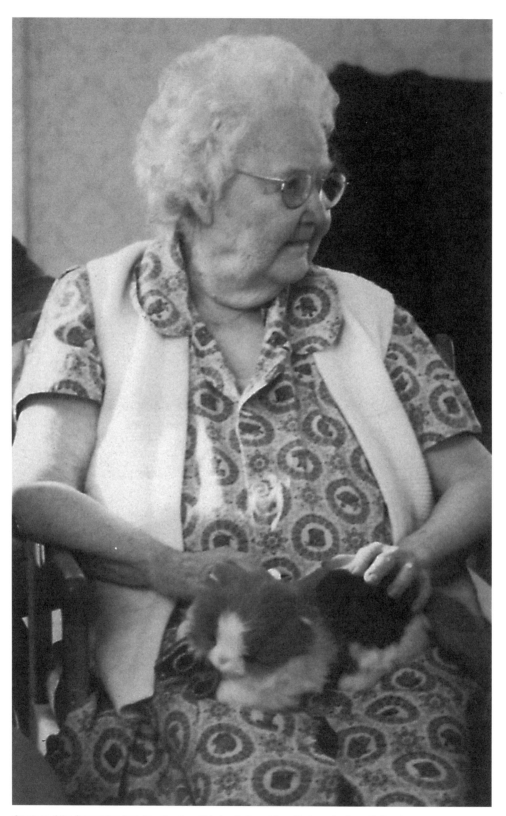

Courtesy of the Greater San Francisco Bay Area Alzheimer's Association. Photography Anna M. Rossi.

CHAPTER 10

Putting Pattern and Texture Back in the Environment

The richness of color and texture, used to full advantage, creates a sense of textural interest that can warm and enliven a room. Color, pattern, and texture are components of every interior environment, but they are used far more successfully in some settings than in others. With imagination there are many opportunities to introduce pattern and texture into the environment; in fact, architects and designers are quite adept at creating interesting patterns using everything from the natural light from clerestories to natural materials used in clever and creative ways to produce texture, pattern, and interest.

Pattern

Today, designers of residential long-term care settings are making selections that will create the greatest level of visual enjoyment for older residents; they are using fewer contemporary colors and patterns. Research has shown that for most elderly residents, the colors and patterns they seem to enjoy and are more comfortable with come from the period when they were in their 40s and 50s, when they were both financially and physically comfortable.[1]

Pattern can be difficult to use effectively, but it can also add a wealth of interest. It should be carefully thought out in residential care settings, since the effects can be unsettling for some. Balance and mobility can be severely impacted. Studies have shown that some people may experience disorientation or vertigo in response to large, bold geometric patterns. Sharp jutting patterns, such as popular flamestitch designs, stripes that can appear as bars, and intertwining patterns can precipitate uneasiness and stress responses.[2] Undulating patterns may contribute to nausea, and some combinations of geometric patterns may actually seem to move, contributing to feelings of unsteadiness and instability.

After noting many apparent reasons to avoid pattern in the environment, let me now say that skilled and conscientious use of of patterns and texture creates a more interesting and stimulating living area, in what otherwise might be a sea of solid colored walls, floors, upholstery fabrics, furniture, and other surfaces. See, for example, Figure 10-1.

> *People with Alzheimer's disease respond on a sensory level, rather than on an intellectual level.*

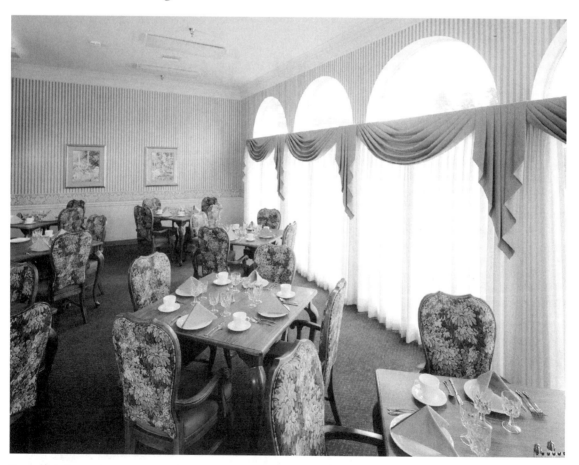

Figure 10-1 Patterns and texture create a more interesting, stimulating, and residential setting in this dining room. Window treatments minimize glare and allow an abundance of natural light. *Courtesy of Spruce Point Assisted Living Community, Florence, OR. Interior design: Cynthia Warner, Warner Design Associates. Photographer: Tom Rider.*

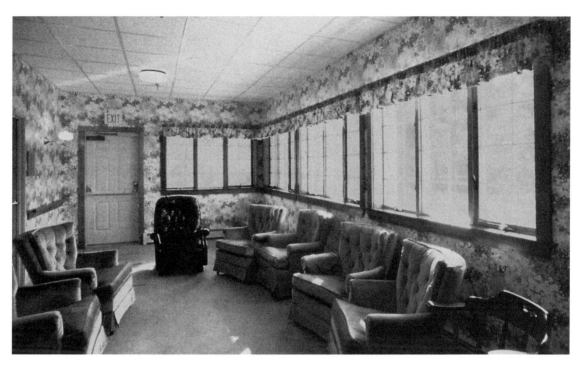

Figure 10-2 Wallpaper adds warmth and contributes to a more homelike atmosphere in this sun room. The distinctive, colorful wallpaper brightens the room and identities this special activity space, which overlooks the garden. *Courtesy of The Alzheimer's Care Center, Gardiner, ME, a program of Kennebec Long Term Care. Architect: SMRT, Portland, ME. Photographer: Robert Perron.*

People with Alzheimer's disease respond on a sensory level, rather than on an intellectual level. There is little information regarding pattern and dementia, a topic that certainly warrants additional research; however, we do know that people with dementia can be overstimulated by too many patterns and designs in one space. While most older people normally experience visual and auditory problems, these effects are compounded when a person suffers from dementia and can profoundly alter the way in which he or she perceives the environment.

Even though all types of patterned wallpapers for Alzheimer's care setting have been used in Europe without problem, there are those who oppose bright, plaid, striped, patterned, or otherwise intricately designed wallpapers.[3] Though simple patterns or solid color fields are safer choices, and may be preferable to complicated or highly unusual designs, healthcare providers at Wesley Hall and at the Alzheimer Care Center in Gardiner, Maine used substantial amounts of wallpaper, because they believed it added warmth and contributed to a homelike atmosphere (see Figure 10-2). Both settings have been studied and neither has reported any serious problems as a result of the patterned wallpaper selections. To the contrary, both were pleased with the "sense of home" that was created.

> *Use pattern, but be aware that too much of a "good thing" can create confusion and agitation. A safer and kinder approach, again, is to be conservative.*

My experience has been that individuals with Alzheimer's disease are less cognizant of selected wallcovering patterns than was previously thought. Poor visual acuity and color contrast may be a a factor, but this generalized experience is supported by findings from a study at Texas Tech University. After analysis of variables, they found no conclusive evidence of an identifiable relationship between wallcovering patterns and the behaviors of residents.[4] Use pattern, but be aware that too much of a "good thing" can create confusion and agitation. A safer and kinder approach, again, is to be conservative. It is helpful to keep in mind that concentration can be improved, however, by limiting the visual distraction of large patterns. Finally, residents with dementia may perceive things that do not exist, which makes it even more important to be alert to patterns—whether in fabrics, wallcoverings, floorcovering, or other materials—that might trigger delusions.

People with Alzheimer's disease have difficulty with spatial relationships, which can impact their sense of balance, leading to greater possibility of falls. The design of the environment must accomodate the special needs and special behaviors of these residents, with strict attention to safety. Impaired depth perception compounded by diminishing cognitive ability makes it more difficult to read and interpret the environment correctly and increases the difficulty of carrying out activities that the rest of us take for granted.

Sharp contrast in color, such as the border design of carpet or the pattern of floor tiles, may be misunderstood and misperceived as a step, a trench, a change in elevation, or a hole in the floor. Large geometric or floral patterns in carpet and other floor covering can be equally confusing, affecting mobility, and producing even more confusion in an already confused individual.[5] The greater kindness might be to exercise conservative restraint with pattern design for floor treatments, so that we don't unintentionally immobilize residents or jeapordize their safety by using pattern as an inadvertent restraint.

Texture and Touch

It often seems we have gone overboard in sterilizing our care settings of both pattern and texture, leaving many residents starved for someone or something to touch. Lorraine Hiatt, one of the pioneers in the study of environment and the elderly, challenges us all, "Our task is to replenish that which has been inadvertently removed, to provide human and inanimate sources of stimulation within each individual's needs, and to consider texture and human contact as resources in our overall program of care and environmental design."[6] With imagination and creative planning, using color, pattern, and texture, the environments we design can stimulate and reassure residents in healthcare settings, and create an atmosphere of warmth and comfort.

Touch comforts us. It reminds us of the time when we were young and safe, when we felt adored and loved. Touch is an ancient healer and critical to health, and it is a continuing mystery why we have failed so miserably in healthcare settings to acknowledge and provide for one of the most basic needs. Sadly, the power of touch is most poignant when it is missing.

Texture takes on added importance in a long-term care environment, where it provides stimulation. There is also some evidence to suggest that it stimulates thinking and responsiveness as well, and can help to recall memories.[7] Quilts, soft surface wall hangings, and velcro compatible, textured wallcovering or wall panels can provide color, visual and textural interest, acoustical value, and opportunities for activity and touching. The door is open for designers to develop meaningful plans to replenish healthcare settings with an abundance of texture and tactile luxury that has been depleted.

Sadly, the power of touch is most poignant when it is missing.

Imagination can stimulate many ways to provide texture in the environment. In turn the creative use of texture can provide many areas of stimulation for residents. Pillows of various shapes and sizes, in multiple colors and textures, can provide something to hold or touch. Commercial or domestic velvets, plain or embossed, satin, wide wale or standard cordoroy, embossed cottons, and many varieties of upholstery fabrics offer interesting surfaces to touch. By using zippers and foam inserts, covers can be easily removed and washed when soiled.

Upholstery fabrics, drapery or other window treatments, bedspreads and coverlets, quilts and other touchable wall hangings, and pillows are items that not only make the setting more interesting, but also improve acoustical conditions and provide clues and cues for orientation.

For those who do not like human contact, the texture of items in the environment may provide their only source of stimulation and touch. Textural variety takes on added significance and it becomes even more important that we assure that these items remain accessible. Soft pillows, for example, or a "well loved" quilt maybe a meaningful connection with life, and the removal of these items, even for cleaning, may trigger a sense of loss, the unintentional by-product of attempting to provide safe and hygienic surroundings.

Even the selection of plants can enhance the texture in a room. The role they play in our well-being is underscored in a well-known hospital study by Texas A & M psychophysiologist Dr. Roger S. Ulrich, who showed that postsurgery patients whose rooms included a view of green, leafy trees—rather than featureless walls—required milder pain-relieving medication and recovered faster.[8] People respond in very positive ways to the wonders of nature. It goes without saying that all plants and trees in residential care settings must be nonpoisonous. A large number of residents in any healthcare setting have dementia, and many people with dementia tend to put things into their mouths.

Pets and Touch

Dogs and other animals can provide alternative means of stimulation and texture. They bridge the necessity for verbal communication, bring warmth, comfort and companionship, and satisfy the human need to touch and be touched (see Figure 10-3). Research confirms that the presence of animals helps reduce depression and increase self esteem in people with Alzheimer's disease. Nonverbal acceptance is especially important to a person who may not be able to communicate verbally. Many care providers and family members have experienced the positive effects of animals on people with dementia.[9]

Aroma and Smell

Smells travel to our brains faster than do sight or sound. Our sense of smell may not be any keener than the other senses, but it often seems to have a stronger hold on our emotions, perhaps because the olfactory system is directly connected to the limbic system, the part of the brain associated with emotion and memory processing.

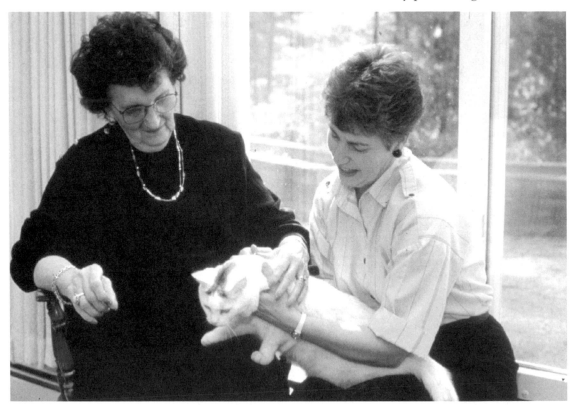

Figure 10-3 Pets bridge the necessity for verbal communication, give warmth and companionship, and satisfy the human need to touch and be touched. *Courtesy of The Alzheimer's Care Center, Gardiner, ME, a program of Kennebec Long Term Care. Architect: SMRT, Portland, ME. Photographer: Robert Perron.*

There is a strong association between smell and emotion. Smell a certain perfume and remember a special person who wore that fragrance or happy events from the past. Alan Hirsch, M.D., neurological director of the Smell & Taste Treatment and Research Foundation in Chicago, conducted a study to analyze memories evoked from certain aromatic simuli. It revealed intriguing generational differences. People born from 1900 to 1930 were much more likely to describe natural smells that made them nostalgic for childhood—trees, hay, horses, pines, meadows, burning leaves. People born from 1930 to 1980 were more likely to describe artifical smells—suntan oil, plastic, even refineries and jet fuel.[10]

The smell of flowers made people from the East nostalgic for their childhood. In the South it was the smell of fresh air, rain, the outdoors; in the Midwest the smell of farm animals; and on the West Coast, the smell of meat barbecuing.[11]

Pleasant aromas are soothing and stress reducing, while unpleasant smells increase breathing and heart rates. Aromatheraphy, a relatively new field that is gaining credence, is used to introduce pleasant scents into a space to increase alertness, decrease agression, and stimulate the body's natural defenses against disease.

The Japanese have been experimenting with scent in public buildings; hotels use a lavender scent to relax guests and a "scent clock" that ejects aroma into the room to awaken a sleeper.[12] Flowers or bowls of potpourri are simple but lovely ways to add fragrance, although the potpourri is not a good idea in settings where residents with dementia might eat it. Flowers, as well as plants, also are effective in cleaning the indoor air by removing toxic pollutants.

Sensory Deprivation

Changes in nature, in color and brightness, as well as variations in temperature and sound, are stimulating. To live in a boring, static, and unchanging environment is unnatural. British psychologist M. D. Vernon, in *The Psychology of Perception,* said, "When there is no change, a state of sensory deprivation occurs; the capacity of adults to concentrate deteriorates, attention fluctuates and lapses, and normal perception fades."[13] Subjects in the study frequently suffered visual and auditory hallucination. Their perceptions of their surroundings were impaired; objects appeared blurred and unstable. Straight edges, for example, such as those of walls and floors, appeared curved; distances were not clear.[14]

A preponderance of white walls is also emotionally sterile and can be visually dangerous; unless stimulated, vision seems to degenerate. If one looks at blank surfaces, such as colorless walls, for too long a time, they tend to fade out and the mind drops into lethargy. Even colors may fade into neutral gray.[15] This makes it very difficult to defend all the white walled environments we find in healthcare settings today, and surely suggests the need for variety in the environment and reasonable exposure to color and other sensations.

Designers of healthcare settings are now beginning to understand that "variety really is the spice of life" and in many respects, necessary to living. Where large numbers of people are being "cooped up" in contrived environments—large housing developments, convalescent homes, and homes for the aged—one thing is certain: color, interest, and variety are needed to counteract sensory deprivation.[16]

Research studies by three Canadian scientists, Woodburn Heron, B. K. Doane, and T. H. Scott, found that a monotonous sensory environment can cause disorganization of brain function similar to that produced by drugs or lesions. Among the effects are impairment of color perception, hallucinations involving color, and distortion of color images.[17] Subjects in studies of isolation and sensory deprivation report difficulty in concentration and periodic anxiety feelings.

According to Herbert Leiderman, another authority, it seems likely that if normal persons can develop psychotic-like states, due to sensory deprivation, then how much more likely it is that sick people, perhaps already perilously near the mental breaking point, could be tipped into psychopathological states by the stress of sensory deprivation. Delirium may be imminent for individuals weakened by fever, toxicity, metabolic disturbance, organic brain disease, drug action or severe emotional strain; sensory deprivation may tip the balance.[18] There seems to be sufficient evidence that sensory deprivation contributes to a sense of dis-ease in otherwise "normal" people, how much more uncomfortable must it be for individuals with dementia?

NOTES

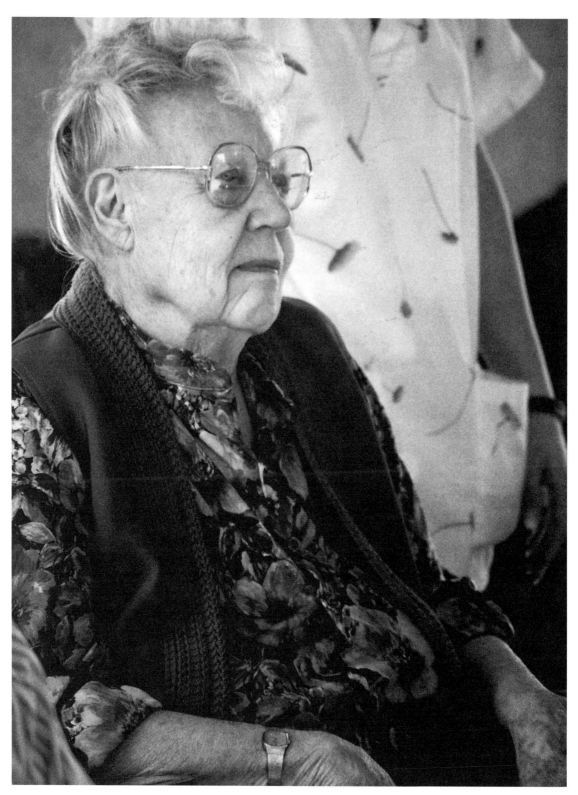

Courtesy of the Greater San Francisco Bay Area Alzheimer's Association. Photography Anna M. Rossi.

CHAPTER 11

Diminished Hearing and the Acoustical Environment

Age-associated hearing loss is the third most prevalent chronic condition among elderly people. It comes on slowly and is handicapping, but it can be less disabling if design professionals use their special skills to incorporate environmental adaptations into building and space design.

Hearing loss is not limited to not hearing clearly. Though all the senses alert us to danger, the ears have been called the sentinel of the senses; they trigger the fight or flight mechanism of survival. With hearing loss it becomes more difficult to separate sounds in the environment and to detect the nature and location of the noise. Anyone with hearing loss may be confused and startled when noise occurs, until they are able to analyze the nature and meaning of the noise and find an appropriate response. Individuals with Alzheimer's disease are unable to make the necessary distinctions or find appropriate responses.

Both the prevalence and the severity of hearing loss increase with increasing age. Between one-third and two-thirds of adults 65 years and older report that they have trouble hearing.

- *33% of adults 65–74 years old have trouble hearing*
- *45% of adults 75–84 years old have trouble hearing*
- *62% of adults older than 85 years of age have trouble hearing*

National Institute of Health Statistics

If present population trends continue, more than 11 million elderly persons will be significantly hearing impaired by the year 2000.

Behavioral Reactions

The onset of adult hearing loss is often insidious, and may not be recognized until someone else calls attention to it. Others are often blamed by the hard-of-hearing person for misunderstandings: "You're mumbling, you're not speaking clearly; speak up, I can't hear you." On the other hand, hearing loss is often misunderstood, accompanied by accusations like, "You can hear when you want to …."

Sound strongly influences the quality of everyone's life, but for the elderly, sound and noise can play an even stronger role. For speech to be understood, volume must be increased, and reflected sound or background noise must be decreased to prevent distortion so speech can be heard clearly. Additionally, disturbing "head noise," known as Tinnitus, often accompanies hearing loss.

Persons experiencing hearing loss frequently loose the easy, intimate communication with persons who are emotionally important, resulting in lowered self-esteem. When noise interferes with understanding speech, hearing music, or taking part in creative activities, many of us become irritable and sometimes disoriented, so it is not unusual to see people who suffer from hearing loss withdraw from activities they formerly enjoyed.[1]

Self-doubt is constantly created as many live with the agonizing fear that they may not be hearing everything, or may be misunderstanding what is being said. Many times the person who is hard of hearing believes others are talking about him. It is easy to understand how missing communication might contribute to the terrifying fear of memory loss. There is no doubt that hearing loss makes coping, and recovering from the stresses of aging more difficult.

> *Sound levels are crucial to the care of people with dementia.*

Most of us have strong emotional responses to sound, and fatigue, anxiety, illness, distraction, some medications, and environmental noise make hearing worse. In addition, excessive noise levels can also cause irritation, frustration, and heightened anger, as well as induce elevated blood pressure levels, heart disease, and ulcers.[2] In today's world noise pollution is of much greater concern.

Sound levels are crucial to the care of people with dementia. Ambient sound is highly stressful and while many older people have some hearing loss, the person with dementia cannot compensate for this. Increased volume in person-to-person conversation is vital. Good sound distribution and acceptable noise levels can produce a more comfortable environment.

Acoustical comfort includes freedom from distracting, intrusive noises, which make concentration difficult for anyone, and especially difficult for the elderly. These noises can seriously interfere with the use and enjoyment of various spaces by residents; however, controlling noise with sound absorption and other techniques can substantially reduce the stress caused by activity noise and routine operations, such as delivery carts.

> *Just as a badly designed room or building can amplify the deleterious effects of hearing loss, thoughtfully designed spaces can facilitate communication, despite hearing loss.*

Design Intervention

Just as a badly designed room or building can amplify the deleterious effects of hearing loss, thoughtfully designed spaces can facilitate communication, despite hearing loss.[3] Good sound control is essential in every residential setting, but it is particularly crucial in healthcare settings, where acoustic treatments seem to be more often the result of habit or formula, rather than thoughtful attention to the unique needs of the hearing impaired older persons who use the space. All too often it seems sound control isn't considered until residents complain.

Noisy rooms effectively "increase" hearing deficit. Long, rectangular rooms, improper sound insulation, especially from adjacent noisy areas, and noisy air flow ducts interfere with hearing and significantly inhibit communication for persons who are hard of hearing.

Lighting also has a strong influence on how well we hear. Because many hard-of-hearing people supplement their comprehension by lipreading, if they cannot see the face of another speaker visual cues are lost. Too little light makes it difficult to *see* well enough to *hear* what others are saying, while too much light or direct exposure to the light source often means too much glare to "hear" well.

The placement of windows and light fixtures should allow the hearing-impaired person to face away from the light while at the same time ensuring that the faces of others are well illuminated. To insure that hard-of-hearing people can see and hear, a speaker or group leader should not be positioned in front of windows; older people should not be looking at the speaker against a background of light.

> *Lighting also has a strong influence on how well we hear.*

A number of challenges, obviously, exist in designing sound solutions, and the best time to address them is in the preliminary stages of concept development.[4] The best sound control plans begin with a process called predesign detailing. While the number and type of design details will depend on solutions suited to the specific needs, with an evaluation and a clear understanding of just how much noise prevention, sound absorption, and sound control are needed, the architect, interior designer, and engineers can design in the appropriate details.

Sound control would be simple if rooms were completely enclosed and uninhabited. Most spaces, however, have windows, doors, recessed ceiling lighting, and air return ducts—all considered to be "basic amenities" and primary sources for sound infiltration.[5]

Some predesign details can be easily incorporated into interior designs and add little or nothing to project costs—space planning, for example, should locate noisy activities away from bedrooms and conversation areas. Door placement is another example. Doors that directly face each other create sound problems, so their placement should be designed to avoid having doors face each other in corridors. Moving doors or other elements that were poorly placed in the design is inexpensive on paper, but becomes an expensive proposition after construction begins. It is also wise to avoid placing any two similar rooms or details back to back or side by side. Elements such as electrical outlets, bathtubs, and medicine chests, if placed back to back, create opportunities for sound to travel from one unit to the next.[6] Anywhere air can pass through, sound can also pass.

Noise is simply unwanted sound. While poor acoustical design will amplify all normal sounds to the level of noise, living in complete silence is, for most of us, uncomfortable. Sounds should be meaningful and give us information. The level and type of noise we are subjected to should be controlled for optimum comfort. Appropriate acoustical design can decrease most noise and diminish the effects of noise problems.

Sound reverberates even more when the floor, walls, and ceiling are all hard surfaces. Low ceilings amplify unwanted and distracting sound. When every surface in the room, except the carpet, is hard, it is a prescription for high levels of noise.

Sound Solutions

Soundproofing is a growing concern. The cost involved, however, is minimal in comparison to the long-range effects of noise on both our physical and psychological well-being. Sound is fatiguing!

Common sounds are not disruptive. In a well-designed space, it is not necessary to speak loudly to be understood, and consequently, the entire atmosphere becomes more comfortable. A room that has both soft (sound absorbing) and hard surfaces placed appropriately within its design makes communication easier by allowing occupants to talk more softly. As a result, residents no longer need to make noise just to prove they exist.

> *Common sounds are not disruptive. In a well-designed space, it is not necessary to speak loudly to be understood, and consequently, the entire atmosphere becomes more comfortable.*

Designers should select interior surfaces and furnishings that do not reflect or amplify sound waves. Creating wall surfaces with niches and ceilings with irregularly re-cessed sections can also be effective in diffusing sound waves. Incorporating an adequate amount of carpet, acoustic tiles, wall panels, and fabric in a space provides a much quieter area. Window glass is a very hard and reflective surface. The effects can be softened substantially by using full pleated sheer draperies and over drapery panels. An added benefit to controlling sound levels is that staff, as well as residents, will be less tired at the end of the day.

When people lose their hearing or cannot hear well, they speak more loudly to compensate. While hearing loss can be improved by using hearing aids, these devices do not work well when the acoustical environment is filled with disturbing and confusing background noises. Most hearing aids in use today are analog units, which amplify all the noises of the room. The recent development of digital hearing aids, which can be designed to each person's particular hearing loss, offers new hope for those who are hearing impaired.

Fortunately, there are a number of practical ways to control the sources of noise. The best results in sound control combine premium-grade ceiling tile for sound absorption with other materials that minimize unwanted sound.

Ceilings

Premium acoustical ceiling tile with high sound transmission class (STC) ratings are specifically developed to reduce sound reflections from the ceiling and to absorb sound in a given space, preventing it from traveling to another space. Panels are made of absorbent materials, often mineral fiber or fiberglass, but may be faced with a variety of materials, such as fabric. With the vast array of ceiling panels available, it is possible to find a high noise reduction co-efficient (NRC) product that complements the design scheme of any space.

Grid systems are available today that make it possible to develop a ceiling design that satisfies both aesthetic and acoustical needs. Panel styles run the gamut from clean unperforated acoustical panels to panel and grid systems that give the look of molded plaster or traditional wood.

Walls

Walls can be constructed in a variety of ways with a variety of sound control capabilities, but it is best to remember: "Not all walls are created equal."[7] Staggered stud construction creates open spaces for insulation; then to the basic "wall recipe" of studs and wallboard any number of sound-controlling elements can be added.[8]

A second layer of wallboard adds mass, and the more wall mass to get through, the greater likelihood that sound will decay before getting to the other side. Using a double thickness of wallboard on one side of the studs and a single thickness on the other will reduce sound reverberation. Soundproofing, or blocking noise from another room or area, can be accomplished in the design of the wall system by adding sound attenuating mineral wool fire blankets (SAFBs), placed in the wall cavity, to help absorb sound. Using irregular shapes also diffuses sound more efficiently than using rectangular configurations.

Generally, walls between living units should be rated a minimum of 45 STC; those separating living units from public spaces and service areas should be rated 50 or higher. Floor-ceiling assemblies separating living units should be rated 45 or higher; a rating of 50 or higher is recommended for floor-ceiling assemblies separating living units from public spaces and service areas, including corridor floors over living units.[9] The floor-ceiling design in multistory structures should be selected both for the appropriate fire rating and also for its high-impact insulation-class rating. Otherwise, even the slightest activity on the floor above will resound through the room below.[10]

Finally, eliminating gaps and other leaks by caulking with acoustical sealant has a dramatic impact on the STC rating. In fact, just one bead of acoustical sealant at the top and bottom edges of the wall board, where the wall meets the ceiling or floor, can improve the STC by 20 points.[11]

Relocatable walls provide maximum flexibility. They aren't permanently fixed to the ceiling or the floor, and ceiling systems and floorcovering can be installed on continuous surfaces, providing cost savings during initial installation. As with fixed walls, SAFBs can be used in the wall cavity of prefinished relocatable partitions to boost sound control performance.

Doors

It is good to keep in mind also that any opening in any wall, movable or not, is a place where sound has the opportunity to move from a place where it should be to one where it shouldn't.[12] Doors and windows are the most obvious openings. Doors are available with gaskets and sound dampening features. An additional source of noise associated with doors is the required panic hardware on exiting doors, for example. It can generate a 90 decibel clang.[13] Less noisy models, available for a slight increase in cost, are well worth the investment.[14]

Windows

Windows and relites (windows between interior spaces) can be glazed with insulated or laminated sound-retardent glass to help control sound leaks from the outdoors. Double or even triple glazing may be required to minimize the impact on the acoustical environment; filling the window mullion with insulation or grout will further boost acoustical performance. This treatment for windows should be employed only if there is disturbing noise from the outdoors; desirable —even delightful—sounds, such as birds singing, may also be blocked by the glazing.

The use of a triple glazing relite in a low-stimulus room will contain the sound of an agitated, noisy resident, preventing the domino effect of alarming other residents. It also allows visual contact with the resident.

Light Fixtures

One of the most often overlooked sources of noise is the light fixtures, which can create unwanted sound reflections. Ceiling fixtures with solid plastic lenses reflect sound and should be replaced with pendant indirect fixtures. Placement of light fixtures in the ceiling grid should be carefully planned, because fixtures placed directly above a partition can reflect sound from one area to another. In addition, space around light fixtures, heating, ventilation, and air-conditioning (HVAC) ducts, and other utilities may allow air and sound to leak through.

Carpet and Draperies

Hearing can be improved and noise levels can be further reduced by using sound absorbent materials on the floors, walls, and window coverings. Both fabric and carpeting absorb ambient noise.

While carpet is useful in absorbing "surface noises" such as dropped items and footfalls, carpeting alone will not provide sufficient sound absorption. Know that while the carpet will absorb sound originating at floor level, it will not impede noise originating at higher levels.

Likewise, drapery fabric does absorb some noise, but it shouldn't be relied on as the only or most effective solution. Padded cornices and thermal drapery lining also absorb sound and help to absorb noise bouncing off glass, but draperies, too, are often overrated as a sound control solution. To prevent sound reflection off of exterior walls, draperies would need to be so heavy they would block light, and would have to be kept closed.

New Sound Technology

Driven by the challenges of new environmental technology, acoustical solutions for controlling "environmental noise" are constantly evolving. Ironically, as interior spaces have become quieter, the outdoors has become noisier. The desire for natural light has resulted in building designs that feature large expanses of glass and windows on exterior walls. As researchers develop new technologies, manufacturers are developing new products to control exterior noise as well as noise from the residents themselves.

Active noise control is a developing concept, certain to see increased use. Rather than absorbing or diffusing sound, active noise cancels it. This is possible because sound moves in waves, just as water does. When the peak of one wave meets the trough of another wave of the same frequency, the two waves cancel each other. Active noise control involves determining the frequency of the noise, then producing another appropriate noise so they cancel each other.[15]

The development of a sound control system that senses existing noises, and manufactures just the right counternoise to keep the space peaceful, should be encouraged for residential healthcare settings. Active noise technology is widely used to remove extraneous noise from large coliseum arenas for musical concerts. It is also being used to quiet HVAC systems.

Though age-related hearing loss cannot be cured, we can technically enhance communication; then it becomes an uncomfortable inconvenience instead of an entrapping handicap.

As computer technology makes the use of active noise feasible, it is likely to find other specialized applications. The use of this technology in healthcare settings would truly be state of the art. As the application becomes more widespread, it could be used to quiet the environment in Alzheimer care settings where calling out and screaming add to noise and confusion.

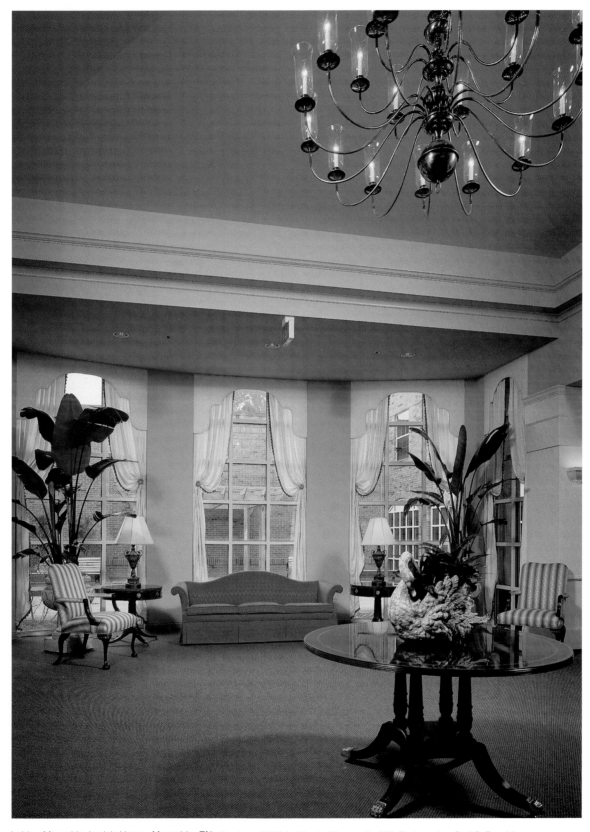

Lobby. Memphis Jewish Home. Memphis, TN. *Courtesy of KKE Architects. Minneapolis, MN. Photographer: Paul G. Beswick.*

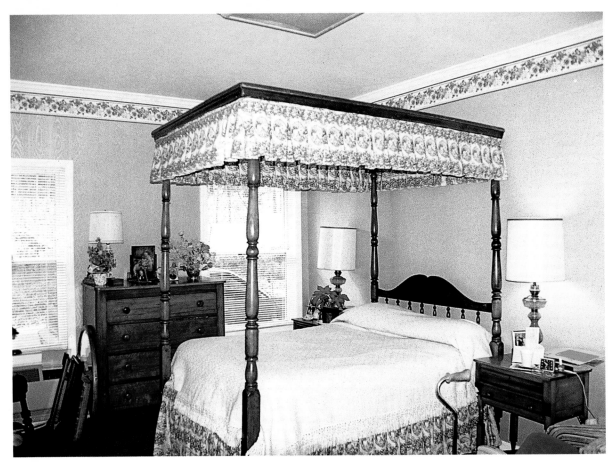

Resident Room. Tulip Garden of Sandy Springs. Atlanta, GA.

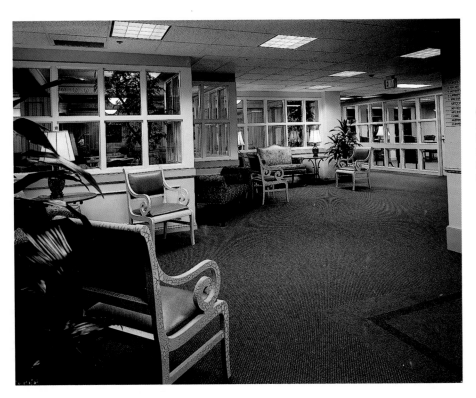

Corridor with seating areas. Memphis Jewish Home. Memphis, TN. *Courtesy of KKE Architects. Minneapolis, MN. Photographer: Paul G. Beswick.*

With thorough, careful planning, desirable acoustical environments can be provided in living facilities for the elderly. Though age-related hearing loss cannot be cured, we can technically enhance communication; then it becomes an uncomfortable inconvenience instead of an entrapping handicap.

Checklist for Hearing and Acoustics

❏ Proper site location insures minimal exterior noise problems such as intrusive freeway noise.

❏ Make a noise survey.

❏ Locate HVAC systems for minimum noise.

❏ Separate operational facilities from sleeping and recreational facilities.

❏ Select building materials that will provide required sound isolation: windows, doors, flooring material, and so on.

❏ Improve effectiveness by using impact-resistant, acoustically absorbing, fabric-wrapped glass fiber wall panel, along with an acoustical ceiling.

❏ Use acoustical materials to avoid background noise that can be disturbing and confusing and to reduce miscellaneous sound.

❏ Lay out interior spaces to separate noise producing activity functions from residential living spaces.

❏ Provide an enclosed area for television to significantly reduce noise and improve the ability to hear.

❏ Design door placement to avoid having them face each other directly in corridors.

❏ Replace public address systems for paging with an electronic paging system.

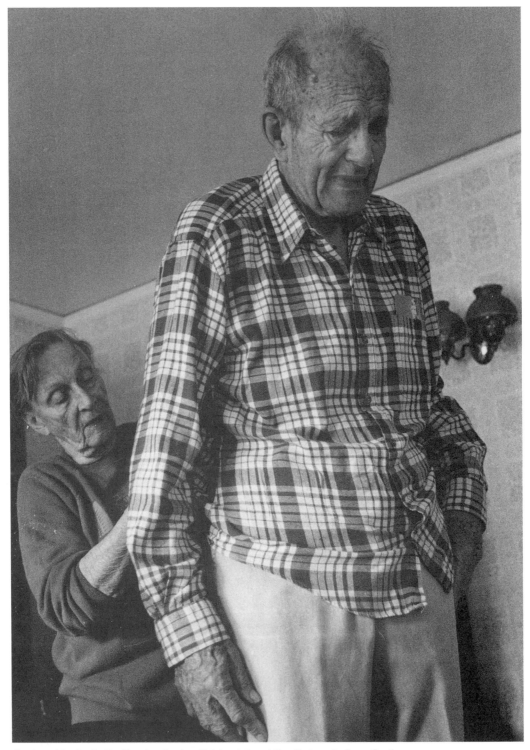

Courtesy of the Greater San Francisco Bay Area Alzheimer's Association. Photography Susan Bradley.

It is within our ability to untangle the web of wayfinding problems presented to the elderly and confused.

CHAPTER 12

Wayfinding Guidelines

Disoriented and unfamiliar with their present surrounding, some residents become agitated and disruptive. Thankfully, greater understanding and research have led to changes that enable residents with significant cognitive impairments to live more peacefully, with dignity, in a variety of care settings that promote independence.

The ability to negotiate through the environment—to know where you are in relationship to where you want to be, and how to get from here to there—is an important part of a person's independence, and self-sufficiency. Age-related changes in sensory abilities, as well as cognitive changes and the loss of short-term memory, contribute to the difficulty some older people have with knowing where they are, where they want to go, and how to get there.

One of the objectives in wayfinding design for aging is to enable elderly people to read their surroundings, allowing them to know where they are, and to make the appropriate decisions about how to reach their destination.[1] "Clues and cues" provide focus and a sense of structure in the environment. People with dementia, in particular, have an easier time in an environment where there are clues to tell them where they are and what they are supposed to do.

Special attention must be given to the orientation information or cues that the environment provides. People with dementia are cognizant of and attuned to different elements and characteristics of the environment at different stages of the disease.

Wayfinding refers to what people see, what they think about, and what they do to find their way from one place to another. It involves knowing where you are; knowing your destination; knowing and following the best route to your destination; being able to recognize your destination; and finding your way back.[2] The cognitively impaired person's ability to remember pathways based on past experience, especially recent experience, is severely limited. The physical environment can either provide a variety of cues to help in the wayfinding process or it can increase disorientation.

Special attention must be given to the orientation information or cues that the environment provides. People with dementia are cognizant of and attuned to different elements and characteristics of the environment at different stages of the disease.

Stress detracts from individuals' abilities to make their way around. Residents who are having trouble finding their way may experience emotional stress from being lost, and those who are weak may suffer physically from going the wrong way and walking further than needed. Research indicates that 90 percent of catastrophic behavior is caused directly or indirectly by caregiver actions or the environment. This is an area where design professionals can have a profound impact on improving the quality of life for confused individuals and their caregivers.

Among the worst examples of interior design for orientation are long sequences of undifferentiated, repetitive elements, such as doors in a long double-loaded corridor. The space is disorienting and uninviting; the distances are daunting; and every door looks the same. For those with cognitive impairment, trying to find the dining room or one's bedroom may be as hard after months or years of living in a particular setting as it was the very first day. They can't remember! With careful planning and attention, architects and designers can provide the support that can allow all but the most severely impaired residents more control over their environment, and consequently, more functional independence.[3]

With deteriorating memory, residents often have difficulty and fail to identify their rooms. Nameplates and room numbers are meaningless guides. Color may be helpful for some, but color alone is not enough for sufficient identification. Art work, a painting, a hanging quilt or tapestry provide stronger cues. Beautiful, colorful quilts add color and pattern, as well as charm, to the environment and provide good sound absorbent material. See the example in Figure 12-1. A problem arises, however, when quilts or any other singular item are used as cueing devices to distinguish different neigh-

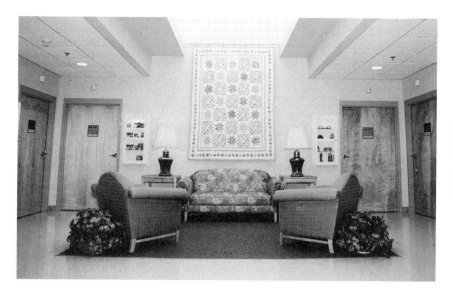

Figure 12-1 A colorful hanging quilt provides a strong cue. *Courtesy of the Fountainview Center for Alzheimer's Disease, Atlanta, GA.*

borhoods or different areas. Because color is not a particularly significant way to create distinction for the elderly and the confused, simply varying the colors and patterns is much too subtle for easy identification. Varying the cue or landmark itself is much more successful. A large, beautiful quilt in one area, for example, a grandfather clock as a focal point in another, a window or distinguishing painting in a third, these cues provide clear distinction and make wayfinding an easier task. See Figure 12-2. Subtle cues for people with Alzheimer's disease are not successful. Cues need to be varied, distinctive, and bold.

Figure 12-2 As a landmark, the grandfather clock makes wayfinding an easier task. Copperidge, Sykesville, MD. *Courtesy of Perkins Eastman Architects PC. Photographer: Curtis Martin.*

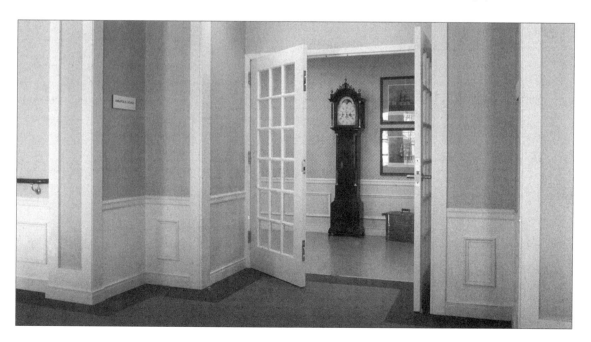

The inability to locate public bathrooms may contribute to the problem of incontinence. Among residents with Alzheimer's disease, there is a need to clearly identify bathrooms. Rather than referring only to signs, wayfinding needs to be thought of a system.[4] It is a myth to believe that signs are all that's needed to help people find their way. The keys to a successful wayfinding system are that wayfinding elements are designed well, that they are mutually supportive, and that they provide accurate and consistent information.[5] Unfamiliar with the environment, people are able to find their way as a result of numerous factors that work together—multiple cueing, or providing the same information in several different ways.

Redundant cueing, landmarks, "neighborhood" decorating schemes, sculpture, paintings, or architectural features such as personalized porches and doorways, changes in illumination levels, and changes in floor surfaces can all be effective cues. Music or sounds from an activity room or fragrances of baking from the kitchen offer additional signals. A cue as simple as the smell of brewing coffee or baking bread from an open kitchen announces breakfast is being served.

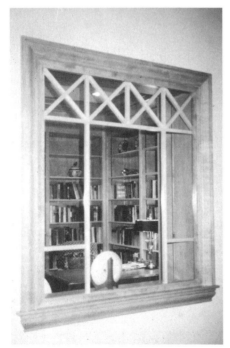

Figure 12-3 An interior window from a hallway into other interior spaces allows residents to see into the room and choose whether to go in. The Hallmark, Chicago, IL. *Used with permission of The Prime Group, Inc.*

Landmarks are physical features of the environment that stand out and are memorable. They aid in wayfinding by helping residents to know where they are and to decide how to reach their destination. Windows with outdoor views give a clue to location. Interior windows from a hallway into other spaces (see Figure 12-3), such as the dining room or various activity rooms, allow residents to identify the space without disturbing its occupants. Creating variety in lobbies and hallways also helps to identify the spaces.

Cues become very important and distinguishing features help: distinctive furniture, clear signage, personalization with photographs or pictures, and even color coding. Familiar cultural cues using color, shape, texture, and lighting are helpful in creating a residential, noninstitutional, nonthreatening, comfortable environment, both pleasing and functional to the user. Residential furniture and window treatments, a small kitchen available to residents, or a piano are all noninstitutional cues as to purpose of the space.

The use of a name plaque, personal photographs, and/or other door decorations are reported by many to help the disoriented resident locate his or her room. One such "bio-board" is shown in Figure 12-4. However, with the progression of the disease, the ability to comprehend written words, even a name, usually diminishes. Since

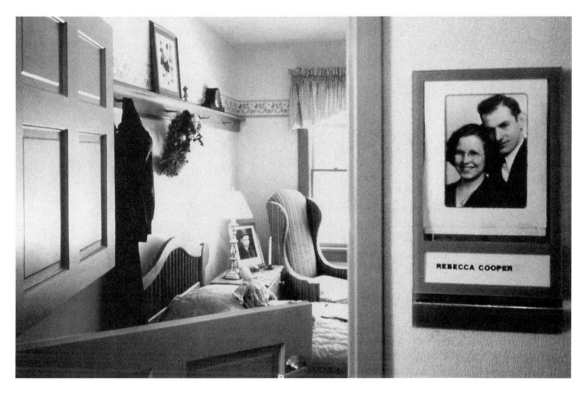

Figure 12-4 The use of personalized photographs, plaques, or other room identification adjacent to the door helps many residents identify their rooms more easily. *Courtesy of Perkins Eastman Architects PC. Photographer: Robert Ruschak.*

there are often relatively few clues outside the bedroom for assisting a confused resident, use this method in addition to others to help with room identification. Results indicate that residents in the early stages of Alzheimer's disease did not encounter any difficulties in locating their bedrooms. Residents in the intermediate stages of disease were less successful.

Cues that require the ability to read and comprehend, such as signs on bathroom doors, are effective only in the relatively early stages of the disease. Signs with simple graphics — for example, a picture of a toilet on the bathroom door — give visual clues for those who can use them.[6] Such aids reduce the amount of direction some residents need.

There are residents who may walk through the hallways and never look into the rooms, so signage or pictures on an open bedroom door will not be seen. Others may be focused only on the handrail, and others on the floor. Margaret Calkins offers good advice when she says, "Do what is necessary to create visually distinctive entries and rooms, even if it means putting the cue at the bottom of the door."[7] Perhaps the best clue to locating one's own room is the individualization or the personalization of the space with the resident's personal

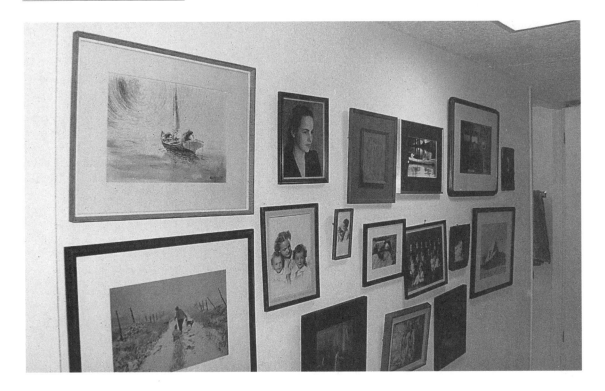

Figure 12-5 Resident's memory wall. One of the best clues to locating one's own room are the resident's personal photographs and possessions. *Courtesy of Vista de Santa Fe, Santa Fe, NM.*

possessions. In all settings, people benefit from having some personal furniture, photos, decorations, and other possessions. Relying only on a few photographs, no matter how meaningful, doesn't personalize a room. Lovely rooms that all look the same, no matter how well intended, don't provide the same nurturing and security as having one's own personal possessions (see Figure 12-5). A favorite bedspread or chest may be the most significant cue when an individual is lost and confused.

Adequate lighting must be provided to insure that signage and cues can be seen and used to ease the journey. Supplemental lighting may sometimes be needed. Signs covered with glass create glare and reflect multiple images on the glass cover plate. They tend to function more as mirrors than for direction. Many elderly people simply will not be able to read them and even more will be blinded by the glare. Matte finishes that absorb reflected light and glare help with this problem.

Views to the outside provide one of the principal architectural methods of orientation for wayfinding.[8] There are cues to location, as well as to time of day and weather conditions and the season of the year. In a presentation at the Third Symposium on Healthcare Design, Jeffrey Rich, M.D. of Stanford Medical Center remarked that from a medical standpoint, patients tend to get very depressed if they lose their orientation to day and night, resulting in depression and profound disorientation.[9]

Figure 12-6 Personal memorabilia displayed in a lighted showcase, adjacent to the bedroom entrance, increases the ability of mildly and moderately impaired residents to locate their rooms independently. *Courtesy of the Corinne Dolan Center at Heather Hill Hospital, Health & Care Center, Chardon, OH.*

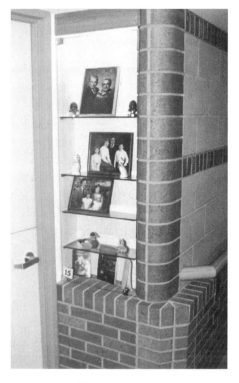

Windows and views to the outside, relative to interior circulation paths, should be to the side of the path and not at the ends of corridors, where they can create glare and confusion. Whether on the inside perimeter, with exposure to a secured or protected garden or courtyard, or on the outside perimeter with views to the outside, this design eliminates the orientation hazards of double loaded corridors, opens the space, and provides window views to the outside world. Creating small seating areas in alcoves with windows to the outside can enhance the experience and the use of interior corridors.

Architectural cues such as personal memorabilia displayed in a lighted showcase, adjacent to the bedroom entrances, increased the speed and/or ability of mildly and moderately impaired residents to locate their rooms independently at the Corinne Dolan Alzheimer's Center.[10] Display cases may be designed in various ways, but if personal mementos are to be meaningful for cueing purposes they must be visible; consequently they need to be lighted. In addition, the single most important requirement is that they be recessed into the wall. This is a safety issue. Residents with low vision may not see, and cognitively impaired residents may be unaware and bump into cases that projects from the wall. If the unit extends more than 4 inches out from the wall, it is in violation of Americans with Disabilities Act (ADA) codes.

Objects holding special memories for the resident prior to the onset of disease, selected by family members, are placed in the display cases, as shown in Figure 12-6. The most reliable cues appear to be items with long-term memory associations that have some personal meaning. Research suggests that personalized cues are up to 50 percent more effective at helping residents locate their bedrooms independently than nonpersonal cues. Symbolic associations such a pictures of vacations or favorite animals are less effective for cueing than more concrete objects. For example, cognitively impaired residents are more likely to understand cues like an old favorite chair.[11]

Attempting to find the most effective cueing devices, research at the Corinne Dolan Alzheimer Center indicates that a single word, such as "Toilet," was more effective than a compound word such as "restroom," or a picture of a homelike toilet. In designing effective signage for wayfinding, residents with Alzheimer's disease respond to signs with dark lettering, contrasted with a lighter background. Signs on the floor that combined the word "Toilet" with short directional arrows were the most effective method of encouraging residents to enter and use toilet facilities in the living areas. At places where the resident must turn a corner, the cue word, "Toilet," should be repeated.[12]

Though pictures may be more valuable than words for cueing and directions, silhouetted figures of a man or woman are not particularly successful cueing devices for residents in the middle to late stages of Alzheimer's disease. One of the more successful techniques is using a bright color for the door, coupled with a canopy to make the doorway to the toilet significantly visable and attention getting. Creativity is invaluable. Combining several cues is more effective for some residents.

Placement of Cues

All cues should be placed so that all residents can see them. Wall decorations or signs mounted at eye level increase visibility and are more likely to elicit response. Signs that identify the location of toilets or other cues and clues should not be placed on the upper portion of a wall or above the door. They will never be seen. Most elderly residents don't have the range of head motion characteristic of younger people. Short wayfinding arrows on the floor appear to be the best indicators in directing residents to the correct location.[13] Directional signs should be in large print, and repeated frequently for reassurance.

All cues should be placed so that all residents can see them.

Not all signage is to cue residents. Identification signs for the staff room, janitorial supplies, medication room, and so on, should not be "attention seeking." The distinction is designed for resident safety.

Wayfinding is often an afterthought in the design process and is not addressed until the end of the building project. The wayfinding needs of the elderly and particularly the confused need to be assessed and integrated into the design plan as one of the most critical issues. Treating the ability of residents to live in and use their environment as if it were an insignificant afterthought is inhumane and insures problems in delivering quality care. It is within our ability to untangle the web of wayfinding problems presented to elderly residents.

Guidelines for Signage

The ADA now mandates that signs designating permanent rooms, as well as signs that provide information about functional spaces, for example, dining rooms, resident bedrooms, laundry, toilets, and so on, must meet guidelines. These guidelines are presented here in layman's language to familiarize you with the signage requirements of the ADA.

ADA Signage Requirements

1. **Raised Letters and Numbers Accompanied with Grade 2 Braille**
   Temporary inserts, as for resident names, do not have to comply.

2. **Contrast**
   Characters and symbols must contrast with their background. This refers to lettering and numbers. Further the background must provide strong contrast with the wall or door color. An eggshell finish is recommended. In addition, research indicates that signs are more legible for people with low vision when characters contrast with their background by at least 70 percent. The greatest readability is usually achieved through the use of dark letters or symbols on a light background.[14]

3. **Height**
   Signs should be mounted 60 inches above the finished floor to the centerline of the sign.

4. **Location**
   Signs (including bio-boards) must be installed on the wall adjacent to the latch side of the door and 2 to 3 inches from the door jamb, as shown in Figure 12-7.

5. **Width-to-Height Ratio**
   Letters and numbers should have a width-to-height ratio between 3:5 and 1:1. The minimum character height is 3 inches and should be determined by the appropriate viewing distance from which the sign is to be read.

More information affecting new construction and alterations as of January 26, 1992 is available from the Federal Register (U.S. Government Printing Office) and from Intersign Corporation.

Installation Tips

1. The Americans with Disabilities Act (ADA) requires all signage to be mounted on a 5 ft. center (see below).

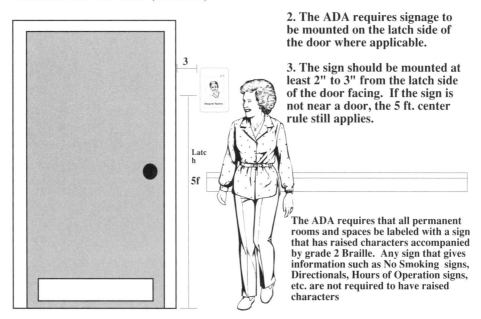

2. The ADA requires signage to be mounted on the latch side of the door where applicable.

3. The sign should be mounted at least 2" to 3" from the latch side of the door facing. If the sign is not near a door, the 5 ft. center rule still applies.

The ADA requires that all permanent rooms and spaces be labeled with a sign that has raised characters accompanied by grade 2 Braille. Any sign that gives information such as No Smoking signs, Directionals, Hours of Operation signs, etc. are not required to have raised characters

4. Always use a level to insure proper installation

5. To insure a secure installation , clean the surface that the sign is to be mounted on & press firmly on the sign surface. This will help the adhesive to bond securely.

Figure 12-7 Signs, including bio-boards, must be installed on the wall adjacent to the latch side of the door, 2 to 3 inches from the door jamb. *Courtesy of Intersign, Inc.*

SECTION III

Special Care Settings

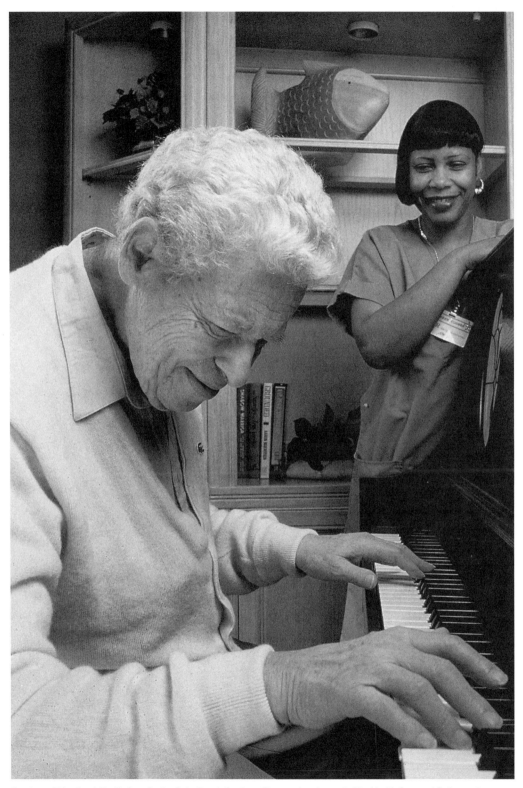

Courtesy of Heartland Health Care Center, Palm Beach Gardens, FL, owned and operated by Health Care and Retirement Corporation, Inc.

CHAPTER 13

Creating a Feeling of Home

One of the most welcome changes in healthcare is the recent trend toward deinstitutionalization of care environments. Care settings are adopting a more residential flavor, beginning with the exterior and moving through the front door into distinctly more inviting "homelike" and humane settings—settings designed to comfort, to support, and to heal both body and spirit in a physically and emotionally safe space.

People of all ages cherish their independence. Yet the changes in our bodies as we age—in vision, hearing, strength, dexterity, and even mental competence—mean that we need to make little adjustments in our environment from time to time. Unless we do, our quality of life may suffer and living comfortably may become harder and harder—perhaps even unsafe.

To accommodate long-term care needs, more architects are utilizing cluster design to redesign large building into small-scale elements or units. The cluster concept reduces the scale to a more familiar size, similar to a home, making life more manageable, particularly for people with Alzheimer's disease. Woodside Place, in Oakmont, PA, and Sedgewood Commons, in Falmouth, ME, both deliver more than

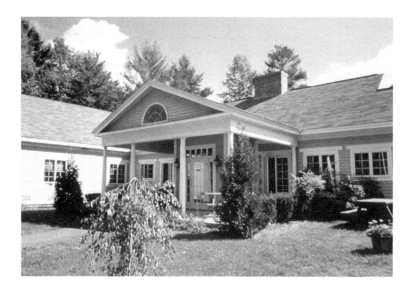

Figure 13-1 The residential nature of the building is emphasized through exterior finishes, window treatments, and landscaping. *Courtesy of Alzheimer's Care Center, Gardiner, ME, a program of Kennebec Long Term Care. Architect: SMRT, Portland, ME. Photographer: Robert Perron.*

superficial illusion of residential scale. To reduce the scale, each of these settings used three connected houses or "homes," with each cluster composed of living room, dining room, kitchen, and bedrooms for 10 to 12 residents. The residential nature is also emphasized through exterior finishes, window treatments, and landscaped gardens and planting areas, as shown in Figure 13-1.

The average resident in assisted living today is a frail woman in her mideighties, who may find the distance to the dining room, in more traditional healthcare settings, an impossible task. Designing smaller scale clusters eliminates the need for long, institutional, double-loaded corridors of resident bedrooms and long travel distances. Well-designed cluster homes respond with understanding to the residents' intimate needs.

The Language of Home

There are many ways to create a homelike environment; they range from changing the way we speak about the environment, to using the language of home, using residential style furniture for a less institutionalized look, and genuinely encouraging residents to bring furniture and other personal items for their bedrooms to keep them in touch with that which is familiar to them.

The language of home is quite different from the language of healthcare or the language of facilities and institutions. We can never hope to achieve homelike environments as long as we continue to refer to corridors, rather than halls or hallways, as long as we build activity rooms, rather than a music room, library, laundry room, or bedrooms. Multipurpose rooms or day rooms, used for dining, craft activities, television viewing, and every other activity with no designated space, are

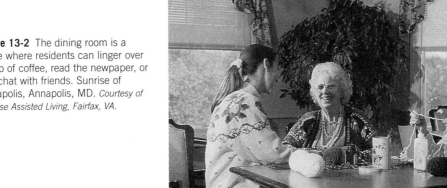

Figure 13-2 The dining room is a place where residents can linger over a cup of coffee, read the newpaper, or just chat with friends. Sunrise of Annapolis, Annapolis, MD. *Courtesy of Sunrise Assisted Living, Fairfax, VA.*

not homelike and are becoming less acceptable for residential settings. Different parts of the country and different cultures may designate household rooms differently, but almost no one grew up with a day room or a nurses' station as part of their traditional home environment.

Ideally, each household has a dining room that looks like a dining room, dedicated solely to meal-related purposes—including lingering over a cup of coffee, reading the newspaper, or just chatting with friends, which is much more in keeping with home and much less confusing for confused residents. Consider, for example, the dining room shown in Figure 13-2.

What is Homelike?

While research does not indicate that a homelike environment will delay the deterioration process caused by Alzheimer's, when the environment at home makes us feel cozy and comfortable, safe and secure, the very quality of life improves.

People with dementia are confronted with an ongoing series of changes in themselves and their world. It is important, to the extent possible, to maintain their ties to that which is familiar and comfortable. Every effort should be made to pattern the environment after the familiar—the home and the past. This will help to provide a "soft transition" into the new setting.[1]

Because people with Alzheimer's disease do not adjust easily to change, the homelike qualities of a setting take on added importance. If the environment seems familiar, residents are more likely to be able to under-

> *While research does not indicate that a homelike environment will delay the deterioration process caused by Alzheimer's, when the environment at home makes us feel cozy and comfortable, safe and secure, the very quality of life improves.*

stand and cope with the change of relocating to a new place to continue their lives.[2] A homelike environment adds continuity and familiarity to the lives of those in Alzheimer's special care settings.

My memories of helping my mom move, first into an intermediate care setting and later into a skilled care environment, are still extremely upsetting. The truth is that I didn't help her move. I not only moved her out of her lifetime home, I moved her from one state to another and into a nursing home. It was clearly not what she wanted. She didn't want to move at all, and certainly not to a nursing home!

It was, at the time, better than most, particularly in terms of care and some understanding of their increasing population of residents with dementia. It was, however, not home. In fact, with the single exception of the furniture my sister and I insisted on putting in her room to make her comfortable, there was nothing homelike about it. In retrospect, insisting on the furniture was probably the only thing I did right.

My first impulse was to improve the aesthetics, to make things prettier. This was not a new experience for me. Gloomy, colorless, uninteresting places push my brain into overdrive—redesigning, rearranging, recoloring and accessorizing everything in sight—and it goes without saying that most long-term care settings are in great need of creative intervention and improvement.

My memories are still all too vivid of the day my brother-in-law and I moved some of Mom's furniture and personal belongings into the room she would share with a roommate named Jewel. In spite of our best efforts, the ambience was still dismal and institutional. As we were leaving, Ed promised Jewel, "I'll be back on Sunday and I'll bring you some flowers." She just continued to stare out the window and finally replied, "Why bother? They'll only die." And then more softly, "I only wish I could."

Leaving Mom was awful, and worse still, I hated going to visit. I always found it difficult and painful. Fortunately, times have changed. Today healthcare settings are much more aware of the impact the environment has on both residents and families. Families desperately want to feel they are making good decisions and doing the best and most appropriate thing for their loved ones.

Creating settings that are more like home helps families feel more positive about their decisions. The environment delivers an important message when the front door of any healthcare setting is opened, and that message should be: "Here is a safe, accepting, nurturing place to live." A homelike setting encourages continued family involvement and strengthens family ties.

The word "home" recalls feelings of warmth and memories of family and friendships. But home is not just a place; it's a concept of comfort and familiarity that nourishes body and soul and etches indelible memories in the mind.

How can people with Alzheimer's remember home? Home is in our minds. It's an emotional memory, and such a comforting idea that it doesn't require a lot of thinking and reasoning. People with Alzheimer's disease often dwell on home. Sitting in their own homes, they may turn to their own family members and say "I want to go home." They are constantly looking for mother. Mother and home seem to mean the same thing—being secure, being loved and nurtured, feeling positive, feeling safe. If we can build our caregiving and our care environments around those needs, then we can support the quality of life.[3]

> *The word "home" recalls feelings of warmth and memories of family and friendships. But home is not just a place; it's a concept of comfort and familiarity that nourishes body and soul and etches indelible memories in the mind.*

Home can be reassuringly familiar—a living room, dining room, kitchen, bedrooms, and bath, with all the familiar traditional elements—a comfortable and convenient environment that provides options for social interaction and the routine of daily living. Residents need to maintain a sense of the dignity of their own homes. Attention to details, such as tasteful wall coverings, fabric, furniture, carpeting, moldings, and plants, all humanize the environment, making the inside warm and cozy and making the house a home.

Selecting colors, fabrics, furnishings, and finishes is the fun part of the job, but the choice of interior finishing materials may seem confusing, with thousands of options available in flooring, wallcovering, window treatments, fixtures, and furniture, and it can be difficult to know what the best choices are. The most homelike environments are not always perfectly coordinated looks. Lest we forget the overriding importance of those selections, many residents are depending on you to make good selections so they may function better. Don't forget for a moment how necessary and important your choices are. Eighty-year-old residents in healthcare settings will appreciate your efforts to provide good lighting and good seating.

In a traditional home setting the entry or reception hall is an invitation to the living space and an introduction to the family within; in a residential healthcare setting it should be the same. The entrance is the first impression. It should be warm, friendly, and inviting to all, and for residents with dementia, it should serve as a transition space to decrease confusion and disorientation.

Entry

A covered entrance can help to equalize illumination levels, providing a transition area between outside daylight and interior light levels at entryways and exits. Careful planning of the light control systems will make the interior lighting design flexible enough to provide a deliberate transition to lighting levels specified for interior spaces. A small seating area in the entry area allows residents time to adjust to changes in light and to hang coats.

A coat room in the entry prevents residents from rummaging through their own belongings or those of others. Once they are beyond this space, it allows residents to be spared the distractions and constant reminders of the comings and goings of the outside world. A disguised entry will also decrease attempts to wander away.

Personal observation and new technology allow more sensitive surveillance than disturbing alarm systems or humiliating "beeper" devices.[4] For example, if an administrative office is situated adjacent to the entrance, an employee can unobtrusively monitor the door. Noisy alarm systems may alert staff, but the noise contributes to disruption, confusion, and agitation among residents. New technology for security, including automatic door locking mechanisms that effectively prevent unsupervised exiting, are available.

Living Room

Cluster design is effective in scaling down the overall size of a setting into manageable parts, and interior design can do the same thing for larger rooms. Living rooms or lobby areas also can be visually broken down into smaller spaces. Breaking up the space and creating additional conversation areas makes the living room more inviting and more likely to be used and enjoyed, like the one shown in Figure 13-3.

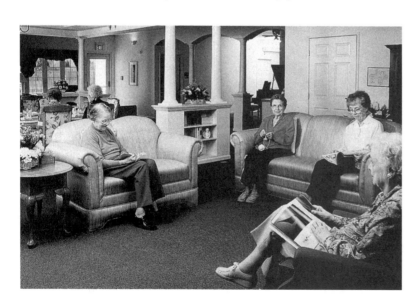

Figure 13-3 A smaller living room setting, designed for intimate conversation, promotes socialization and interaction between resident and visitors. Garden Square of Greeley. *Courtesy of Living Centers of America, Greeley, CO.*

Large spaces can be overwhelming and intimidating; they do little to encourage socialization. A living room–type setting that is designed for entertaining family and friends, that includes intimate conversation spaces promotes interaction between residents. Thoughtful color and fabric selections, construction detailing—including fireplaces, and furniture and furnishing scaled down in size—speak of home and extend a homelike feeling to residents and their families and visitors. Warm nurturing color palettes, especially colors from the autumn harvest and fall flower colors, add warmth. Include a range of lights and darks, but avoid muddy colors.

Unlike grand-scale lobbies that rarely seem to be used, the smaller living rooms found in cluster design are less intimidating in size, which encourages their use. Using a library, a room for watching television, and other special spaces ensures that the group remains smaller and that the spaces are used. Families find these more intimate areas more enjoyable for visits, as well.

Sunrooms

Sunrooms and, in the south, Florida rooms, are enclosed porches filled with windows and an abundance of natural light. For examples, see Figures 13-4 and 13-5. They are places to have a cup of tea or coffee, read, visit with friends, or just sit and enjoy and be nurtured. These spaces are designed to capture sunlight and to be used as living spaces and a place for plants. A well-designed sun space does not trap heat and the temperature doesn't rise above the outdoor air temperature during the summer. Operable windows can provide natural ventilation in warmer weather.

Sunrooms and indoor atriums can take advantage of a new window glass from PPG called "Starphire," which transmits 90

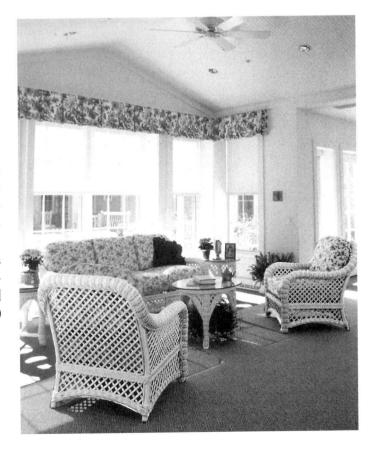

Figure 13-4 The windows fill the sunroom or sunporch at Copperidge with an abundance of natural light. Copperidge, Sykesville, MD. *Courtesy of Perkins Eastman Architects PC. Photographer: Curtis Martin.*

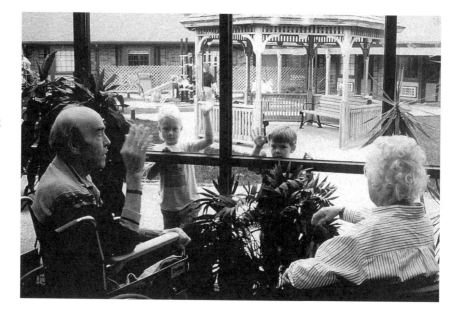

Figure 13-5 This is a living space designed to capture sunlight and provide a closer connection with the world outside. Foxwood Springs Living Center, Raymore, MO. *Courtesy of Foxwood Springs Institute.*

percent of the ultraviolet light, as opposed to typical glass that absorbs ultraviolet.[5] Sunrooms and interior atriums can be lovely additions and would be welcomed anywhere.

Dining Rooms

Mealtime is an especially important time, often the most anticipated highlight of the day for the elderly. It's an opportunity to socialize, to visit with other residents, to gossip, and enjoy good food, but if the ambience is not conducive to socialization, mealtime will not be a pleasant experience.[6]

For residents, dining is the most frequent activity and offers opportunities for socialization as well as nourishment. The dining room energizes a facility—yet it is often found in a central location, away from the residents rooms. This may showcase a lovely dining room, and be convenient for dining staff, but it can be inconvenient and even hazardous for residents, particularly those who have mobility problems.

A large dining room can be overwhelming. Multiple small dining rooms, serving smaller numbers of people in quiet settings, are more conducive to a pleasant dining experience. The smaller room size allows more flexibility in designing rooms of different shapes and sizes, and this change makes dining spaces feel more familiar and homelike, and far easier to infuse with warmth. The reduced room size also helps to reduce noise, presenting less of a challenge to older adults. It becomes much easier to minimize distraction and concentrate on the task at hand—eating.

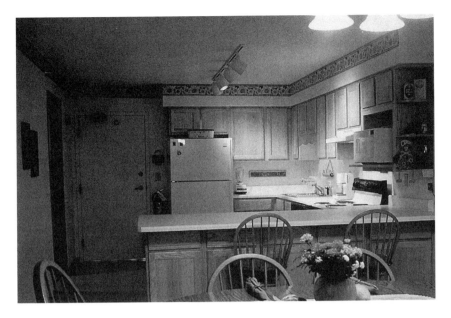

Figure 13-6 A kitchen eating area is a less formal mealtime setting and allows family visitors to cook a special dinner for Grandma on her birthday. Kensington Cottages of Mankato, Mankato, MN. *With permission of Kensington Cottages Corporation, Golden Valley, MN.*

Family dining rooms in a smaller scale setting provide congenial spaces for any meal and are more flexible for small groups of people. A kitchen eating area, like the one shown in Figure 13-6, is a less formal mealtime setting and allows family visitors to cook a special dinner for Grandma on her birthday. Smaller dining areas are preferable. Though it may not always be possible, dining areas should be distinct from activity spaces to help minimize confusion. More intimate dining areas allow residents to:

- Converse as well as enjoy the sensory stimuli provided
- Experience a quieter environment with less excess auditory stimulation (noise)
- Enjoy a more homelike atmosphere, more family-like in scale
- Experience less distraction, making it easier to concentrate on the task at hand

The meal is the most basic reason that people are attracted to assisted living. Nourishment is vital to maintain health and wellness, and dining should be a relaxing experience. If there is too much noise, however, the social dining experience becomes a very stressful experience.

Speech communication in the dining room is important—meaning there must be no echo and the reverberation time should be within limits. Fine restaurants consider good acoustics a prerequisite to fine dining. Loud noises have no place in dining settings, and that includes intercoms and television noise, which distract and frighten residents, contributing to unacceptable behavior.

Residents, especially those with Alzheimer's disease, may have trouble eating if they are distracted by noise or poor lighting conditions. Even a heavily patterned tablecloth can interfere with a resident's ability to concentrate on eating. Smaller dining areas, however, do help to prevent the confusion that many Alzheimer residents experience in large groups.

Dining areas must be well lit. The criteria for lighting dining space can be developed based on the visual tasks to be performed and the needs of aging eyes. These visual tasks range from circulation within the space, to seeing the faces of table companions, and safely using sharp utensils.

Millions of dollars are spent in market research in the restaurant industry to discover what is appealing to customers, what colors, what type of lighting, what ambience makes them comfortable, what makes them eat more, spend more, and keep coming back. By paying attention to what successful restaurants are doing, we may get some valuable clues in how to better encourage residents to eat.

An ambient lighting system used in combination with decorative lighting is often the best solution. The ambient light allows for an even distribution of light on room surfaces, while chandeliers and wall sconces can be added for their decorative effect and to add a little "sparkle" to the space. They should be located above eye level and frosted, filament-wrapped, or shaded bulbs should be used to control glare, as shown in Figure 13-7.

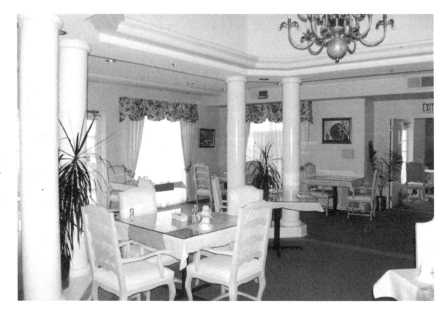

Figure 13-7 Chandeliers with shielded lamps are used as a design feature in residential dining, while needed light levels are provided by indirect cove lighting. *Courtesy of The Hallmark at Palm Springs, Palm Springs, CA.*

The minimum light level for the dining room is 50 fc. A high ceiling makes it more difficult to provide high levels of evenly distributed light. If adjustable controls are used, illumination levels can be raised for maintenance tasks and lowered for a change in ambience. Light-deprived meal settings can also be enhanced by orienting breakfast areas and other morning activity areas toward the east. Then the beginning activities of the day are designed to take full advantage of the morning light.

Warmer, stronger colors in social dining rooms encourage conversation and interaction. Restaurants, especially fast food restaurants, use red-orange and yellow to increase appetites and encourage eating. An appetite color scale, in which the effects of color were measured, placed red-orange at the top of the appetite scale. Bright warm colors like red, yellow, and orange tend to stimulate digestive juices, while soft cool colors tend to retard them.

Studies show there are peaks and valleys when appetite levels are connected to color. The low point is in the yellow-green area. Appetite appeal is restored in cool-green and blue-green, and shows a definite drop in the purple area. This means that purple-red, violet, yellow-green, green-yellow, gray, olive, or mustard are poor color choices for promoting appetite and encouraging eating.[7] If the goal of the setting is to encourage eating, then color selections should be made in the warm color range, but with more residential hues such as coral, peach, or soft yellow.

In a cafeteria that had light blue walls and was air-conditioned, people complained of the cold though the temperature was 72°. Later when the temperature was raised to 75°, they still shivered and complained. Finally a color consultant advised repainting the walls orange. Diners then complained that the 75° temperature was too warm. Finally it was reduced to the original 72°, and everyone was happy again.[8]

In dining spaces for dementia residents, focus may be an added challenge. Selections of warm hues, but less intense shades — soft peach, for example — would be less distracting. The wall color should contrast with the floor, and color selections for tables and chairs should provide strong contrast. Matte surface finishes reduce glare and reflections from shiny surfaces and large windows.

For the benefit of residents with reduced vision, when choosing table settings and preparing food presentation, consideration should be given to optimizing contrast.

- Highly visible borders around the edge of the table enhances visibility.
- Place mats provide contrast with the table top or plates and utensils and provide a more homelike ambience.

- Highly visible borders around the rims or edges of cups and plates enhance visibility.
- Plates, utensils, and containers should have good contrast in color or brightness from the usual background.
- If residents are pouring their own beverages, it is preferable to have light-colored containers for dark liquids and dark containers for light-colored liquids (e.g., milk).
- Skillful use of color on a white plate for contrast makes the food easier for residents to see and encourages them to eat.
- If menus or place cards are used, they must be clear, high contrast print of appropriate size. Menus placed on bulletin boards use larger print.[9] (See the discussion of signage in Chapter 12.)

Social interaction is fostered by seating residents at small tables of four in the dining room for all three meals of the day. Both the furniture arrangement and the tables themselves must accommodate wheelchair access. Tables that allow wheelchairs and conventional seating are now available, as shown in Figure 13-8. Stable chairs that glide easily can be pulled back from the table to sit down, and then moved up to the table while the person is seated. Make sure that the chair arms fit under the table. Residents have difficulty eating when they can't get close enough to the table.

Chairs with arms are essential for support. When rising to a standing position, stability is important! Casters on dining chairs should be avoided, for all too often chair backs become supportive devices for the frail elderly.

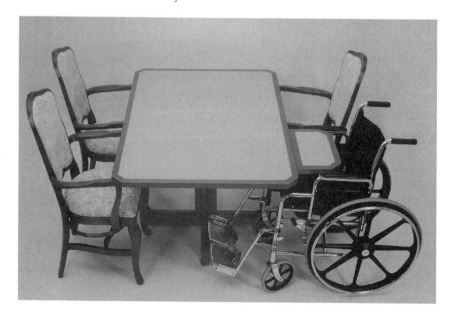

Figure 13-8 Tables with flip-up trays allow wheelchairs and conventional seating. The contrasting border provides definition to the table edge. *Illustration courtesy of L&B Contract Industries, Inc.*

Last but not least, an often overlooked necessity when designing dining rooms is an accessible bathroom. Resident rooms are often located some distance from the dining location—too far to reach in time. Fear of needing the bathroom facilities, which may not be available, can be a disincentive for residents participating in activities outside of their rooms, and that includes dining. An accessible toilet increases the potential for controlling incontinence and preserves self-esteem.

Kitchens

In the home, the kitchen is where food preparation takes place and meals are prepared. Though not intended for regular meal preparation, small-scale kitchens in residential settings are designed to provide meaningful therapeutic activities and experiences for people with dementia. Familiar household tasks such as washing dishes, setting tables, sweeping, and folding towels are activities that are associated with the kitchen and small family households. Accessible and safe kitchen areas facilitate this kind of activity, as well as group activities such as baking and decorating cookies, making ice cream, or washing vegetables.

Good design planning can allow access to the kitchen, even in the absence of a caregiver. Dangerous equipment can be stored in a locked cabinet, leaving the kitchen accessible to residents to get a cup of coffee, a soft drink, or a glass of water. Responding to changing abilities, simple adjustments in shelf height and depth should be made. To provide accessibility for older residents with limited range of motion and for wheelchair users, wall mounted upper cabinets should be lowered several inches; shallow shelf depth minimizes accidents resulting from attempts to exceed one's safe reach. Under counter cabinets, which require bending, should be minimized.[10] Smart stoves that turn themselves off, or a hidden switch or control lockout feature prevent unwanted operation and allow the kitchen to remain accessible.

Induction cooktops, manufactured by General Electric, have no exposed coil, open flame, or heated surface. They have a high frequency induction coil below the cooktop's smooth surface that heats the cooking utensil by magnetic friction, without directly heating the cooktop surface. The only heat on the cooktop is that which it absorbs from the pan. Even if the element is turned on accidentally, no heat is generated unless a utensil of 5 inches or greater in diameter, is placed on the heating element. When you remove a pan from the heating element, the heating coil is de-energized and will automatically turn itself off.

In addition to the familiar tasks associated with the kitchen, this is also an area that provides opportunities for socialization.

Residential kitchen workspace should be designed to include small kitchen tables with plenty of seating. The ambience of the setting encourages comfortable, informal socialization and the kind of reminiscence that often takes place at the kitchen table.[11]

Resident Bedrooms

The transition from one's own home to a group living situation can be very stressful. Being removed from the familiarity of physical and social settings that have been part of one's life for years, and being forced to relinquish the right to privacy that most of us take for granted, is not easy.[12] The bedrooms in these care settings assume added significance because they may be home to residents for many years. The additional time necessary to insure that they are comfortable, satisfying rooms, designed to meet the functional needs of their residents in the best way possible, personalized and highly reflective of their residents, is certainly worth the effort.

Rather than design rooms for the absolute minimum amount of space possible, we must expand our thinking and design rooms that are sufficiently spacious to encourage a normalized lifestyle. Enlarge spaces to a room size that accommodates a sofa or a small sitting area.

> The bedrooms in these care settings assume added significance because they may be home to residents for many years. The additional time necessary to insure that they are comfortable, satisfying rooms, designed to meet the functional needs of their residents in the best way possible, personalized and highly reflective of their residents, is certainly worth the effort.

It is interesting that budget motels and even maximum security prisons provide far more square footage for their "guests" than do most healthcare settings. Space within the resident's room should respond to the needs of higher functioning residents, as well as the more frail.[13]

Assisted living settings are taking the lead in increasing room size and will likely see increased benefits in happier residents with fewer behavioral problems. Residential healthcare environments are quite different from acute care settings, where most people have a short stay. As design professionals and providers we need to remain sensitive to both the need for privacy and the need for adequate space. In addition to sleeping and dressing in the bedroom, many older people also spend time there, reading, watching television, resting, or pursuing hobbies. There is an added measure of comfort and security in being surrounded by one's own personal possessions.

While it is generally thought that private rooms and private baths are a better idea, some feel that private rooms increase isolation and hasten decline. Others feel that all individuals have a need for privacy and that social stimulation is better provided in areas other than the bedroom.[14] Many providers feel private rooms positively impact

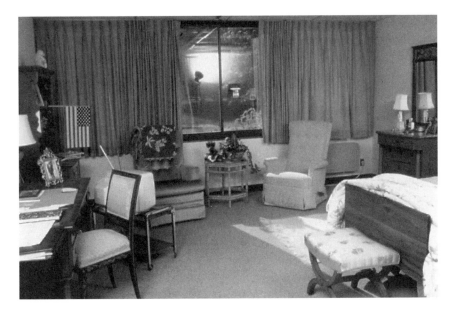

Figure 13-9 Resident bedroom filled with personal things that look as though they were just removed from home and magically recreated in this setting. *Courtesy of Alois Alzheimer Center, Cincinnati, OH.*

the quality of care. Some feel there are fewer sleep disturbances in private rooms, and that staff assistance with toileting functions can be provided more easily. The privacy of a resident's own room is more inviting to visiting family members, and noise is more easily controlled. Some residents, however, derive comfort and security from sharing, and a number of shared rooms should be provided for couples and for those who prefer to share a room.

Personalization

Residents should be able to bring some of their own belongings and furniture into their new home to create a more familiar environment. In shared rooms, a partial privacy wall to divide bed areas can provide opportunities for individualizing space with items from home. The ideal, particularly in a long-term care setting, is to have fresh, interesting bedrooms, filled with personal things that look as though they were just removed from the resident's house and magically recreated in this setting.

Using the resident's personal furniture and bedspread, wall color or wallpaper, and accessories to recreate their bedroom from home, as shown in Figure 13-9, would ease the transition for some. Duplicating the furniture layout of the bedroom from home as closely as possible could make the environment feel more familiar and help confused residents feel comfort in new surroundings. Families who are actively involved in the replication effort also experience the relocation in a more positive way and

> *The ideal, particularly in a long-term care setting, is to have fresh, interesting bedrooms, filled with personal things that look as though they were just removed from the resident's house and magically recreated in this setting.*

feel a part of the resident's life in the new setting. Personalizing the bedroom not only makes it a comfortable and homelike place to spend time, but also reinforces the concept that the resident is an individual deserving of personal space that reflects his or her own individuality.

Life safety codes (fire regulations), which vary from state to state, must be honored. Bedspreads and drapery fabrics should be flame-retarded, but a better idea may be to select one of the many FR fabrics now available in a large variety of patterns, colors, and textures. These fabrics are inherently flame-retardent and most are washable. Other fabrics can be flame-retarded; however, this is a custom finish, which must be executed and certified by a fabric finisher. It is not available from a spray can. A variety of patterns and solid colors are available in FR fabrics—everything from plaids to florals, even lace patterns similar to old-fashioned lace curtains are available with an FR rating.

When I think of room personalization, I'm reminded of one of the scenes in a nursing home in the movie "Fried Green Tomatoes," a scene that I found personally touching. Mrs. Threadgood had her own ideas about personalizing her space. She completely covered the two walls adjacent to her bed with pictures of flowers cut from magazines, books, and greeting cards and lovingly pasted them over every visible surface as a reminder of her gardens at home and the flowers she loved. A poignant reminder—the wonders of nature heal the soul. Give each resident a garden by putting a flower box outside every window.

Greater sensitivity and careful design planning will keep us from continuing to unintentionally "sterilize" the environments of the elderly, deleting important reminders of their lives and severing meaningful ties to the past. Depression and disorientation seem obvious and predictable responses to such trauma, but sensitivity and good design can reap visible positive benefits for the same individuals.

Color

A balance of color is essential to keep a room interesting and, when residents spend large quantities of time in one room over a long period, to prevent sensory deprivation. Color can help to lift spirits and make rooms cheerful, and residents can be involved in the decision making for colors used in their environment, particularly in choosing their own room color. This process offers an important opportunity for each resident to feel included, to participate in the personalization of that most important living space—his or her own room.

Rooms should be painted periodically and apricot, peach, sunny yellow, or any of a variety of warm earth-colored paint colors are no more expensive than white. This is a departure from the various hues and tints of white that many long-term care facilities have featured, but it is a distinctly more humanistic approach and could be easily implemented with careful planning. Again, these are the details that help to make institutional setting more like home.

Develop a palate of three to five colors from which residents can make their choices. Provide large sheets of color for selection—a minimum 9×12 inch standard paper size. Even skilled designers, used to working with color, can sometimes be fooled by small color chips from a paint deck. Remember that in long-term care settings, failing eyesight and the availability of natural and artificial light significantly impact which colors are selected and how they will appear.

The preselected palette of harmonizing colors offers variety, insures that the rooms are coordinated, and also provides a distinct appearance to help each resident identify his or her own room. By not placing rooms of the same color side by side, the uniqueness of each individual bedroom is emphasized. A mix of contrasting tones can relieve monotony, create a high level of visual enjoyment for elderly residents, and provide clearly defined visual cues. Yellow-based pinks, such as salmon, coral, or a soft yellow-orange, as well as many other colors, can provide warm pleasant surroundings.

A few people with dementia retain the ability to recognize and attach importance to colors long into the progression of the disease.[15] These cognitively impaired residents can still be included and assisted in the color-selection process. For a population that does not understand a direct question about color preferences, this can be accomplished by giving them a variety of colors (crayons, markers, paint chips, colored paper) and then observing which ones they use most often.[16]

Using pattern and color in a resident's room does require special care. This is their personal space, and in most cases, their *only* personal space. It is important that the color and pattern selections not conflict with the resident's personal tastes.

Lighting

Typical of the increased sensitivity to how lighting affects residents, designers are attempting to find a new balance between a noninstitutional appearance and effective lighting. For a good example, see the before and after photos in Figures 13-10 and 13-11.

To prevent lights from shining directly down into a resident's eyes, many healthcare settings are now using indirect pendent lighting and lighting concealed behind valances and coves for increased levels of even ambient illumination. This is supplemented with table lamps, or in some cases, wall-mounted swing lamps for task lighting. Wall sconces can be used for decorative purposes, but are not sufficient as primary light sources.

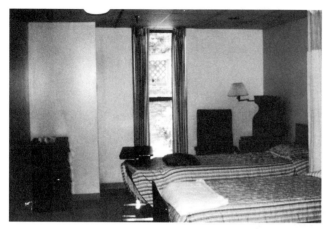

Figure 13-10 Resident room (before). One of the goals of the resident room renovation was to improve the lighting. *Courtesy of Lenbrook Square Skilled Nursing Facility, Atlanta, GA.*

Figure 13-11 Resident room (after). The best face-lift you've ever seen! Light level was increased from 8 fc to 40 fc and the space visually enlarged. *Courtesy of Lenbrook Square Skilled Nursing Facility, Atlanta, GA. Interior design: Linda Watson, ASID, Watson Limited Planning and Design.*

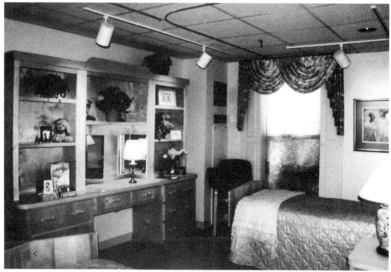

Wall-mounted fluorescent over bed fixtures are not appropriate for the elderly. They are bright, often unshielded, sources of light that produce glare and shadows and contribute little to even illumination. With the lighting technology available today, wall-mounted over-bed lights are stark reminders of medical settings.

A Light in the Night

Night-lights are necessary. Many elderly residents will need to use the bathroom one or more times during the night. Night-lights and a clear pathway facilitate safe trips to the toilet and help to avoid falls and unnecessary incontinence.

Locating the bed to accommodate direct visual access to the toilet, as shown in Figure 13-12, helps to prompt those with cognitive

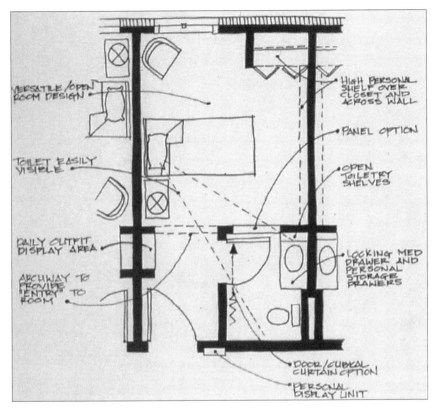

Figure 13-12 Locating the bed to give direct visual access to the toilet helps to prompt those with cognitive impairment. *Courtesy of Folgers Architects & Facility Design.*

impairment. A bedside table or night stand can have a light installed under the apron of the table to provide a nightlight. The light can be wired with a motion sensor, or as a shielded, indirect light source, remain on all night without disturbing the resident.

Older residents are highly vulnerable both to drafts and to changes in temperature. Thermostats that are operable by the residents allow self-regulation for thermal comfort. If this is a problem with cognitively impaired residents, an inexpensive clear plastic cover can be placed over the controls.

Temperature Control

Both closets and drawers should be available for clothing and other personal possessions. Chests, armoires, or more conventional closets that can be adapted for specific uses all provide efficient storage. Built-in furniture is not as recognizable for residents with dementia. If open vinyl-coated wire baskets are used as drawer/storage within a closet, be sure they are sturdy and secure. Furniture used in healthcare settings must be constructed to withstand more than normal residential abuse.

Storage and Independent Dressing

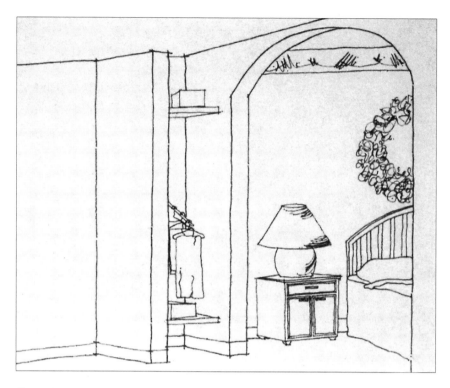

Figure 13-13 Closet modification placing clothing in sequence assist residents to dress independently. Nebraska Masonic Home, Plattsmouth, NE. *Courtesy of Folgers Architects & Facility Design.*

Many residents with Alzheimer's disease have difficulty getting dressed by themselves. Confusion and a short attention span, as well as cognitive dysfunction and physical disability, conspire to turn the routine of dressing, including clothing selection, into a complicated series of actions.

A special closet modification developed at the Corinne Dolan Alzheimer Center increased the level of independence by 19 percent. The closet modification restricted access to only the selected set of clothing, which was displayed in the order in which it was to be put on (see Figure 13-13). In this way, the resident's attention is directed to a specific article of clothing, which he or she must correctly put on. The clothing is in sequence, so they see which article of clothing to put on next. For example, the resident sees underclothing first and pants or a skirt last. Socks placed on top of shoes cue that they should be put on before the shoes.

The need for direct physical assistance was reduced by one-third to one-half, and the number of verbal prompts were increased. Residents were better able to dress independently with simple verbal directions or reminders when attention was centered on dressing; they were less dependent on their caregivers for physical assistance.[17]

Each bedroom should provide a window with views of the outside. If you believe that health and environment are closely connected, it is important to bring a feeling of sunshine, fresh air, and light—much like a garden—into the bedroom. Gardens, lawns, and woods are a source of sunshine and a connection with nature. Low windows increase visual access to the outdoors and provide natural light and brightness in the room. Window seats can provide cozy seating, as well as extra storage, if they are the correct seating height and not too deep.

Shared balconies and gardens add to the residential appeal and offer opportunities to enjoy privacy as well as to socialize in shared spaces. Architects should be encouraged to provide access to outdoor spaces near resident rooms, allowing them access to fresh air and natural daylight for vitamin D. For individuals with Alzheimer's disease, a shared balcony or porch on ground level, opening into a secure courtyard, provides freedom to choose—to view from inside or go to outside; balconies on upper levels for this population, however, are dangerous and inappropriate.

Access to the Outside

Design considerations for private bathrooms for older users should include accessibility, adaptability, proper lighting, flooring, and contrast. Since toileting activities are often carried out with the assistance of nursing home staff, enough space to accommodate a wheelchair as well as an assistant must be provided.

Bathrooms

Doors should have minimum clear width of 2 feet 8 inches to accommodate wheelchair access and should swing outward to permit access from the outside in case of a fall or other emergency. An adaptable bathroom provides flexibility and support for continued usage by older people as they experience age-related disabilities, yet it does not intrude with support when it is not needed.[18] Door locks are not recommended for bathroom doors. If assistance is needed a locked door could waste valuable time, and residents with Alzheimer's are likely to be trapped inside the bathroom.

Residents with Alzheimer's disease are often aware and frustrated by their failing memories, realizing too late, for example, that an embarrassing episode of incontinence happened simply because the need to urinate was forgotten. It is important to use every available design opportunity in the environment to reinforce skills the resident still possesses.

The toilet itself can present many design dilemmas—too high or too low. For easier wheelchair transfer choose a seat adjustable to wheelchair height (15 to 19 inches). A standard toilet with seat height of 15 inches to the top of the seat, with appropriately placed grab bars, is recommended for general use by the elderly. The seat height can be raised by attaching an elevated seat if necessary. Toilet seat covers offer flexibility for using the toilet as a seat. Whether to leave the cover up as a visual reminder for the resident with Alzheimer's disease or to put it down to keep that individual from attempting to flush wash cloths and other items is still an unanswered question. Toilet seats are available in a multitude of colors other than white. Good contrast between the floor and the fixture, the wall and the fixture, and the toilet seat and the toilet all help to cue use and insure accuracy.

Grab Bars

Grab bars should be included in bathrooms to provide solid handholds for getting on and off the toilet, and for entering or getting out of the tub or shower if they are included. Grab bars must be secure, have no have sharp or abrasive edges, and must not rotate in their fittings. An oval design requires less strength to grasp than a circular bar.[19] Grab bars are available in color, and should contrast with the wall for maximum visibility. Chrome and metallic bars may produce reflected glare or blend in with the walls. Lightly textured powder-coated finishes not only refract light and add color, but allow for a better gripping surface. There are beautiful bright colors available, but high gloss finishes produce glare and keep them from being good selections for the elderly or visually impaired persons.

People with strength differences prefer grab bars on both sides of the toilet, and people in wheelchairs need one side clear for the approach. A swing-up assistance bar can meet both of these needs.

Inclusion of a tub or shower in individual resident bathrooms is a subject of much debate. At minimum a toilet and lavatory with vanity must be provided. Raising the bathroom vanity to a height of 36 inches, rather than the standard 32 inches, saves bending and back pain for many. The vanity surface offers an opportunity to introduce color and provide contrast with the lavatory bowl to increase visibility. An edge detail with a slight lip helps to contain spilled water; the edge itself should be bullnosed to avoid sharp corners and edges. Grab bars can also be mounted on the front face of the vanity top.

Sufficient, even light distribution in the bathroom is essential; the Illuminating Engineering Society (IES) recommendation is 30 fc. Be particularly alert to all the possible glare-producing finishes in this small space and design to produce sufficient light levels and minimize glare. Glare is a hazard for the elderly, especially in the bathroom, where it can contribute to balance problems and falls (see Figure 13-14).

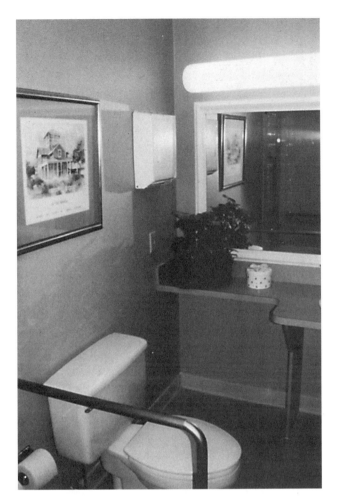

Figure 13-14 Achieving even light distribution that minimizes glare requires controlling surface finishes in this small space. *Courtesy of Lenbrook Square Skilled Nursing Facility, Atlanta, GA. Interior design: Linda Watson, ASID, Watson Limited Planning and Design.*

The use of sheet rubber or a cushioned no-wax sheet vinyl floor surface minimizes the number of seams and the opportunity for fluid to find its way into the underlayment, making offensive odors less likely. Floorcovering should have a nonslip, nonglare surface. No-wax sheet vinyl with a textured surface reduces glare by refracting light and has an easily cleanable surface. The floor color should provide contrast with the toilet. Carefully selected floor covering and vinyl wall covering add interest and give the feeling of a more residential space.

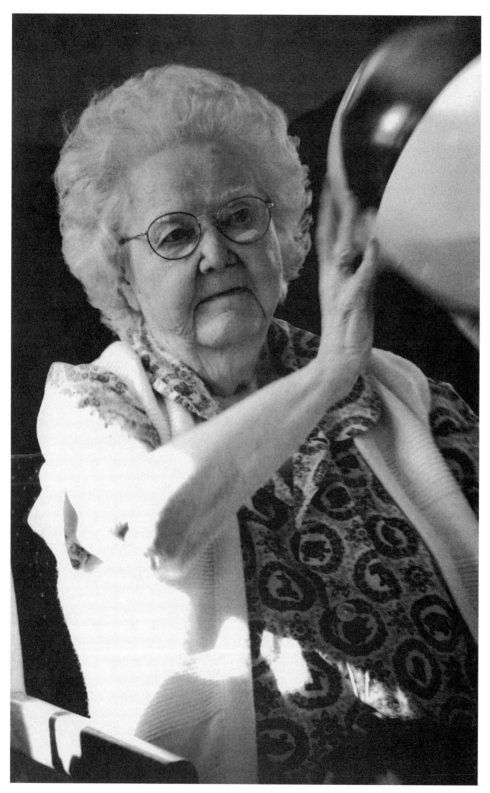

Courtesy of the Greater San Francisco Bay Area Alzheimer's Association. Photographer: Anna M. Rossi.

14

Designing Spaces for Special Activities

Persons with Alzheimer's disease have special needs. Most remain physically healthy well into the course of the disease. But as Alzhemer's steals their memory, judgment, and ability to reason, these people need more and more care to perform the most basic activities of daily life and to prevent harm. In addition, appropriate therapeutic programs can help support their remaining functional abilities and prevent excess disabilities that unnecessarily occur with the disease.

Activities

"Life" exists in the activities of being and doing. Working, playing, sleeping, eating, exercising, and other aspects of everyday living require an inclusive, refined frame of reference—a frame of activity that encompasses all of life. Residents with dementia are often more capable than either they or their caregivers realize or expect. When daily living is simplified, broken down into small steps, or adapted to meet specific needs, residents can be more involved and better able to respond. If these special residents live in an environment that does not encourage participation or one that assumes that they cannot do for themselves, they easily fall prey to feelings of inadequacy and a role of passive involvement.[1]

The "activity" of life is a search for meaning and purpose. Dignity and the inner sense of worth arise from work and other occupational skills, daily living relationships and endeavors, recreation, and other meaningful productive activities. Well-designed environments support these residents to function at "their best," to participate, and to find value in living and in themselves.

Activities make up their lives, including the basic activities of daily living (ADLs), arising for a new day, bathing, dressing, grooming, eating, and sharing experiences with friends. Activities and activity spaces frequently play a major role in establishing the noninstitutional atmosphere of a setting,[2] bringing more community and normalcy to a home setting. Including a small-scale kitchen, living room, dining room, family room, and a small laundry room reinforces the sense of "home" for those living in residential healthcare settings. This environment supports involving residents in meaningful activities, in a home setting that encourages success and a sense of self-worth.

Innovative Changes

Perhaps one of the most remarkable and positive recent changes in healthcare design has been in the area of activity programming. The creative and therapeutic use of activity areas has expanded from one large communal space to a variety of smaller activity spaces. In some cases, activity areas are clustered in the core of each unit, maintaining a separate identity, with clear boundaries existing between each activity space; in others, they are scattered throughout. The dining room, kitchen, and living room are the source of many domestic activities and integral parts of each residential cluster.

There are clear advantages to dispersed activity areas, among them greater variety and location choices for the activities provided. With smaller spaces, it is much easier to maintain a residential scale, both in room sizes and furnishings. Many of the spaces accommodate varied use and flexible scheduling of activities; for instance, a small library can also serve for music therapy and family visits. Stimulation and noise are easier to control, and there is greater ease in separating an agitated resident from the rest of the group.[3] A "quiet room" where an agitated individual can be calmed and comforted by staff in privacy can be considered another activity space. A small room or alcove is often sufficient.

Most activities are now directly accessible to all residents and are no longer limited to a few conventional offerings of arts and crafts, music, and bingo. In addition to the normal activities of the day, residents now have opportunities to take part in a variety of activities ranging from taffy pulls and ice cream making, to snowman construction and trips to local points of interest. Music, walks, gardening, and other meaningful, failure-free activities should be emphasized.

Activities in Alzheimer's special care programs must support remaining abilities and minimize failures, support dignity, and enable pleasure (see Figure 14-1). This type of activity program provides meaningful opportunities for residents to give to others and to have a role within "their community."[4] For persons with Alzheimer's disease or other cognitive impairment, the inability to continue initiating activity causes many to feel less productive and less useful, and opportunities for each person to be productive through meaningful activities must be provided.

The majority of people in long-term care settings are women, and most are of an age that they were typically wives, mothers, and housekeepers. For these residents, familiar productive activities might ideally involve participation in some food preparation activities. Many residents feel at home helping with such domestic activities as housekeeping tasks, as shown in Figure 14-2, meal preparation, helping to set the table, or clear the dishes, sweep the floor or dust. If it

Opportunities to Be Productive

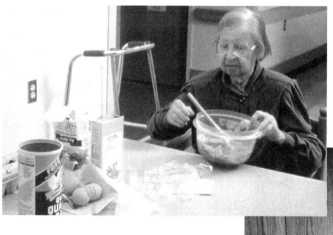

Figure 14-1 Many residents enjoy making cookies and participating in domestic activities. *Courtesy of The Norma and Joseph Saul Alzheimer's Disease Special Care Unit at the Jewish Home and Hospital for Aged, Bronx, NY.*

Figure 14-2 Household tasks and meal preparation help residents feel useful and reinforce self-esteem. *Courtesy of Frances McCandless Center for Alzheimer's and Related Disorders, Wesley Manor Retirement Community, Louisville, KY.*

makes them happy, it's therapeutic activity. This activity does suggest the need to have a kitchen in an area where residents spend the majority of their day. Remember to plan space to store equipment and to include necessary safety devices, such as hidden shut-off switches for the stove and dishwasher, when appropriate.

Folding towels and other laundry is another common activity, as shown in Figure 14-3. It makes more sense, however, to fold towels in the laundry room, where there is a washer and dryer.[5] These are basic activities that engender contribution. They allow individuals to contribute to meeting the needs of "their family" in ways that are respected and that they are able. Life is about relationships and giving, and in these activities residents are able to give and to feel included—emotional needs being met with dignity. Many residents derive great satisfaction and self-esteem from contributing to housekeeping activities within a homelike setting, and these activities help to maintain a sense of normalcy and routine.

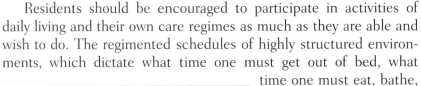

> *Life is about relationships and giving, and in these activities residents are able to give and to feel included—emotional needs being met with dignity. Many residents derive great satisfaction and self-esteem from contributing to housekeeping activities within a homelike setting, and these activities help to maintain a sense of normalcy and routine.*

Figure 14-3 Folding towels and personal laundry in the laundry room. *Courtesy of The Norma and Joseph Saul Alzheimer's Disease Special Care Unit at the Jewish home and Hospital for Aged, Bronx, NY.*

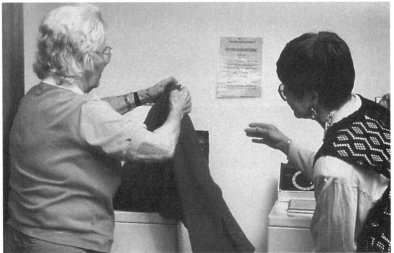

Residents should be encouraged to participate in activities of daily living and their own care regimes as much as they are able and wish to do. The regimented schedules of highly structured environments, which dictate what time one must get out of bed, what time one must eat, bathe, and retire, minimize freedom of choice and the opportunity to express individual control. Meals, bathing and grooming, and other activities can be organized in such a way as to be integral to the activity program and to allow residents the freedom to make choices about when they get up in the morning and what they have for breakfast.

The goal of Alzheimer's special care is to achieve and to maintain maximal levels of functioning for the longest period of time. Studies done by Barry Rovner, M.D., at Johns Hopkins show that there appears to be a positive impact, in relation to the activities program of special care units, on the level of care of residents. Many challenging behaviors can be decreased and/or controlled by the structure provided through the activity program and by the carefully designed environment of a special care setting.[6]

The most successful programs emphasize activities with structure and flexibility. The ability to contribute is important. Structured activities should provide sensory, cognitive, and physical challenges that are appropriate to each resident. Music therapy is a lifeline for people with dementia. Through music, residents can take part in activity that provides sensory input, cognitive activity, and can be physically active. It is important, however, to remember that residents are not only robbed of their memories of people and events, but also are robbed of their memory of how to move their bodies.

Picture books and magazines are of great interest to and used frequently by residents. It is common for residents with dementia to thumb through them, responding primarily to the pictures rather than the text. Caregivers often report that individuals with Alzheimer's disease receive pleasure from engaging in old familiar activities, such as a former avid reader looking through books even though he can no longer comprehend the words.[7] Old magazines from the 1940s — the *Saturday Evening Post, Colliers* and *Life* — are particular favorites. Flea markets and attics are great resources.

Programming Value of Activities

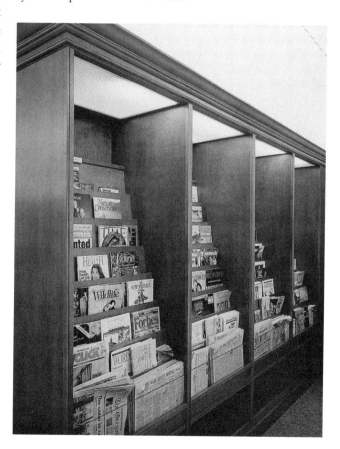

Figure 14-4 Well-designed lighting enables residents with low vision to make selections more easily in this library. The room is also suitable for other small group activities. *Courtesy of Holladay Park Plaza, Portland, OR. Architect: WEGroup Architects. Interior design: Center of Design for An Aging Society. Lighting design: Center of Design for An Aging Society and Interface Engineering. Photographer: Charlie Borland.*

Entertaining Activities

All residents, especially those with dementia, need both privacy and interaction and socialization. Special settings should provide for specific types of small group or individual activities, such as a music room or alcove. These small activity alcoves can be multifunctional spaces. A library like the one shown in Figure 14-4 can also be a place for family visits, a setting for afternoon tea, or a place to chat with friends or read the newspaper in privacy—all small group activities that provide opportunities for intimacy, while encouraging at least passive participation from residents with dementia.

Special care settings need not mean that all people are of one level of mental functioning, nor that all groups or socializing is with people of the same degree of alertness. Providing multiple, simultaneous activities enhances residents' control by increasing options.

Creative therapy—art, music, dance—offers many residents with Alzheimer's and other dementias nonverbal methods of expression, as shown in Figure 14-5. Joyce Simard, national director of Alzheimer's and Special Programs for Marriott Senior Living Services, said, "With this type of programming, we can help residents express feelings they cannot express verbally."[8] In the crucible of dementia, there are many painful daily agonies. As days and weeks and years go by, expressive verbal language and the ability to think coherently are compromised.

Figure 14-5 "Memories in the Making" is an art program used to enhance the lives of individuals with Alzheimer's disease. *Courtesy of the Alzheimer's Association of Orange County. Photographer: Robert Bell.*

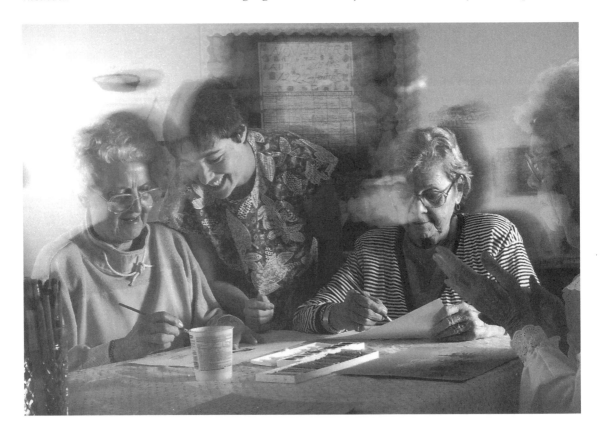

So we carry a greater burden to listen more carefully, to attend to the person more fully, to try to appreciate the greater importance of nonverbal and symbolic forms of communication.[9]

Art is being used to enhance the lives of individuals with Alzheimer's disease in ways that could not have been imagined even 10 years ago. It can help to link residents with family and professional caregivers when words may no longer carry meaning. The process of painting allows stories and emotions trapped inside to surface. The following experiences from the "Memories in the Making" program are shared with the permission of the Alzheimer's Association of Orange County:

> *A woman, who suffered from Alzheimer's disease, cried much of the time at the care facility where she lived. No one seemed to be able to console her for long. On the days when the Memories in the Making art teacher came, the woman painted pictures of her family and her past. When the art teacher talked to her about the colors and splashes of paint in her paintings, the teacher learned of the tremendous guilt the woman was feeling about difficulties and problems she had encountered while raising her children. She felt she had not been a good mother. She revealed this guilt through her painting.*

> *"When her daughters learned about these feelings, they were able to respond. They told their mother that they forgave her and that they understood. They hugged her and demonstrated their forgiveness. Afterwards, her periods of weeping stopped. The impression of all those involved was that the woman was able to communicate intense feelings which were still impacting her life, through the language of art. Her paintings opened a door of communication when words no longer could suffice.*

> *"Alex is one of the more dramatic examples of the effects of the "Memories" art program and how effectively therapeutic programs can affect residents behavior and their lives. His paintings all were dark and troubled. His behavior was often agitated and troubled as well. During one of his art sessions he was asked what bothered him, he broached a subject in class about which he had never before said a word to his family or friends. He painted a dark, expressive painting and said:*

> *"We landed on a beach. There were bullets and bombs everywhere. There was so much smoke everywhere we got scared because we couldn't see what we were shooting. There were green soldiers' bodies everywhere and there was so much blood. It was terrible, just terrible, you can't imagine. That's enough —that's the story.*

> *"After Alex shared his nightmare memories, his paintings changed to a surprising degree. He has become more vocal now and his troubled mood has gone. He now uses bright colors in the art he makes. His paintings allowed him to use the language of art to release trapped emotions. The "Memories method" can open channels of communication for Alzheimer artists. This is truly therapeutic activity at its best."* [10]

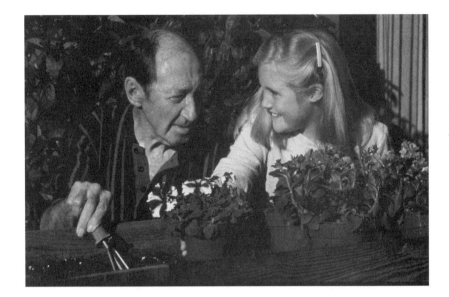

Figure 14-6 Many residents are grandparents and derive great joy from children. *Courtesy of Heartland Health Care Center, Palm Beach Gardens, FL, owned and operated by Health Care and Retirement Corporation, Inc.*

Using a resident's life history is essential to providing proper care. Take advantage of interests, past work, and the leisure experience of the residents. Joyce Simard remembers one resident who rummaged through other's clothing on a regular basis. Once staff found out that she had been a sales clerk, they set up a rack of clothes for her. For other residents who had enjoyed shopping, the same rack of clothing, sporting price tags, provided a safe, familiar activity.[11]

Many residents are parents or grandparents and derive great joy from children, as is evident in Figure 14-6. Small children give hugs, climb on laps, sing to the residents, and do not seem to mind if the answer provided to a question is inappropriate or irrelevant. Some residents who show little responsiveness to any other activity will enter a ball game with enthusiasm when enticed by a child.

Pets are also good residents. They give endless affection and are good company for many elderly people. Residents are often involved in feeding and caring for animals, whether birds, colorful fish in an aquarium, Maggie the cat, or Pal the retired Seeing Eye Dog. Bird watching is another interesting activity.

Group Socialization

Encouraging social activity in small groups helps residents feel they are members of a community that cares. Typically, most groups are fewer than 12 people and provide yet another opportunity for socialization. In some settings, groups are designated as a special "club," for example, the breakfast club, the morning out club, or the men's club.[12] Activities generate friendships, pride, and membership. For example, activities for men might include woodworking, fixing appliances or cars, or gardening for vegetables or flowers in a greenhouse. These clubs nurture friendships for the lonely, encourage members to feel useful, and above all stimulate purposeful engagement as a means to combat social lethargy.

Involving community garden clubs to help with creating and maintaining gardens, or setting up activities such as mixing potpourri and making dried flower arrangements can, with sensitive planning, be a source of physical and social stimulation for residents, and an opportunity to foster community understanding and involvement.

Exercise is a good small group activity. The cumulative effects of even light exercise performed a few minutes at a time throughout the day are beneficial, and regular exercise is vital to maintaining maximum range of motion and use of the joints. Walking can be one of the best all-around exercises, and a moderately paced walk of just five minutes can help maintain or even increase flexibility in the joints of the lower body.[13]

> *"Creative activities within a community contribute to a sense of vitality and to a sense of belonging, and their nurture should be the goal of healthcare designers and administrators."[14]*

"Creative activities within a community contribute to a sense of vitality and to a sense of belonging, and their nurture should be the goal of healthcare designers and administrators."[14] It is extremely important that those who design and develop living facilities for the elderly incorporate life-enhancing activity programs in their designs, for these programs are crucial to the elder person's quality of life.

Stimulating creativity and inclusion requires a special attitude—one of receptiveness to new ideas. Variety and flexibility are key and encouraging new initiative is essential. Activity development and

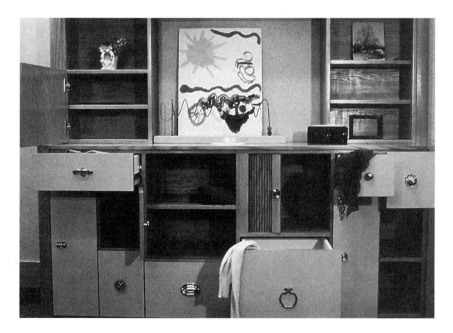

Figure 14-7 Residents with Alzheimer's disease may satisfy their compulsion to rummage or manipulate objects at a special cabinet with locks, drawers, levers, and other gadgets. *Courtesy of The Norma and Joseph Saul Alzheimer's Disease Special Care Unit at the Jewish Home and Hospital for Aged, Bronx, NY.*

planning are vital to quality of life for the elderly, especially for those who are cognitively impaired. It is an area that today is receiving greater and much needed attention. Design professionals must work closely with activity program specialists to ensure that environmental design for the elderly is driven by their ability and activity needs, and that residents are not forced to adapt their activities to a less than supportive environment. We would all do well to remember that creative activities flourish best where the residents themselves are encouraged and physically supported to participate.

Hallways

Corridors in residential facilities are at least five feet wide and usually eight feet wide in nursing homes, with handrails on either side. The width is prescribed but it is the length that is problematic. Many residents in long-term care settings are frail and come to live in a residential care setting as a result of poor ambulation. Long corridors are completely inconsistent with providing physical and emotional safety, increased mobility and function, or a homelike setting.

Using cluster design, architects have begun to more closely replicate the home environment. They are using creative design skills to shorten the distances and transform corridors into more residentially scaled hallways. Corridors are institutional; hallways are reminiscent of home. This should help to increase familiarity with the environment and increase the confidence levels and the mobility of residents.

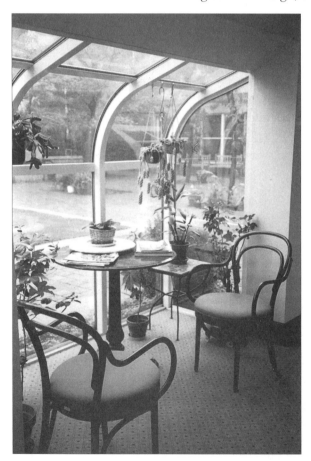

Hallways are also meeting places. Where we are not able to physically shorten the distance, more skillful design must be applied to varying the size, shape, corners, heights, and views to provide better circulation space. Opinions on recommended rest spaces are diverse, ranging from every 15 feet to every 60 feet in corridors or walkways. To accommodate the physical limitations of frail elderly residents, seating niches (like the one shown in Figure 14-8) should be

Figure 14-8 Small alcoves or nooks provide places to rest in a long hallway and pleasant spaces to visit with family and friends. *Courtesy of Duncaster, a Life Care Retirement Community, Bloomfield, CT. Photographer: Dianne Davis.*

available every 20 to 30 feet along lengthy corridors. Without seating, elderly residents may be reluctant to travel any distance.

Nooks

Whenever possible, break space visually into small areas and use even the smallest bit of unused space. A closet or an indentation in a wall can be used to create a stopping point as a resting place. I once used space where an unused water fountain had been removed to place a chair and a small table. These points of respite can mean the difference between older residents getting out to walk and socialize or sitting in one spot all day. Even very small areas should accommodate a chair or wheelchair, and with an attractive wall lamp, a picture, and wallcoverings, you have a place to pause in a long corridor.

Point of Interest

Features of the environment often contribute to unsatisfactory behaviors in mentally impaired people. This population needs variation in design, such as texture, touchable surfaces, and points of interest (perhaps a display like the dolls in Figure 14-9) to help reinforce cognitive skills like wayfinding. Because many corridors are long and lack any residential landmarks, they provide little stimulation for conversation. Without anything meaningful on which to focus, many cognitively impaired persons explore inappropriate places—like a neighbor's room or the utility closets.

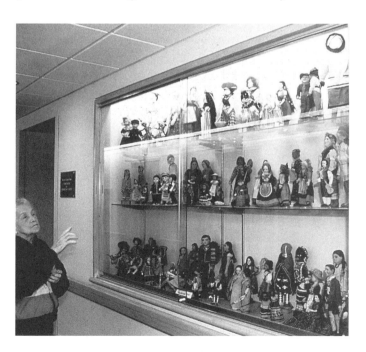

Figure 14-9 Landmarks and points of interest in hallways and long corridors, such as the display of dolls, help to reinforce cognitive skills in wayfinding and make walking more interesting. *Courtesy of The Norma and Joseph Saul Alzheimer's Disease Special Care Unit at the Jewish Home and Hospital for Aged, Bronx, NY.*

Lighting

Many settings now use cove lighting in hallways to give the illusion of a wider space. It produces a soft, evenly distributed light if the ceiling is a matte finish with a high reflectance value. Continuous fluorescent downlighting where the ceiling and wall meet will also produce an even illumination at eye level and along the walls.[15]

Using fluorescent lamps concealed in architectural molding to provide indirect light is a successful method for corridors. Lighting, wall mounted 12 to 18 inches below the ceiling, provides a continuous light valance that allows light to wash down the wall as well as providing up-light to reflect off the ceiling.[16] Since reflective light takes on the color of the surface it bounces off, a white ceiling finish with a matte surface provides the best reflective value.

Higher light levels in narrow corridors produce a more secure feeling.

When recessed ceiling luminaires are used to light corridors, the fixture brightness and the brightness of the ceiling surrounding the fixture should remain close. Bright patches of light, produced by lamps that are placed low in the fixtures or close to the lens, produce spots of glare, since the visual distance is extended in corridors. Lighting should be arranged so that luminaires provide broad diffuse illumination with no pronounced illumination differences and do not become bothersome sources of glare. Illumination levels of about 30 fc are recommended by the IES.

If wall sconces are added to corridor lighting for a more residential feeling, the Americans with Disabilities Act (ADA) requires that they be placed at or above 80 inches from the floor, and they may not project more than 4 inches into the room cavity. Fixture selection becomes very important when projecting diffused light into the pathway, rather than directing the light upwards toward the ceiling. Since alternative levels of high and low illumination require constant eye adaptation, spacing is even more important. Higher light levels in narrow corridors produce a more secure feeling.

Where window walls are used, controls can also be used to balance lighting within the space, accommodating for changes in daylight levels. The lamp color should be specified to blend with daylight, in addition to balancing levels of illumination. Blinds, or some other means of shading, should be available to avoid or reduce glare (see the example in Figure 14-10). Avoid windows at the ends of corridors. The glare from a large window combined with a shiny floor can create serious difficulties.

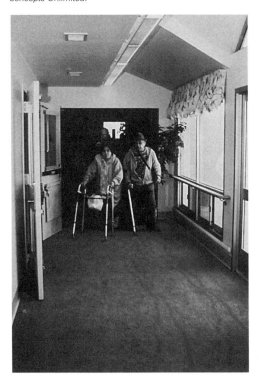

Figure 14-10 Pleated shades on these windows in a corridor help to prevent glare and balance the lighting within the interior space. *Courtesy of On Lok Senior Services, San Francisco, CA. Architect: Barker Associates. Interior design: Elizabeth Brawley, IIDA, Design Concepts Unlimited.*

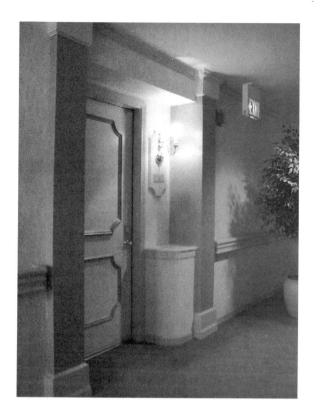

Figure 14-11 This entrance to a resident room is well defined architecturally, well lighted, and includes a place to put a purse or other belongings while opening the door. *Courtesy of Oakbrook Common, Southfield, MI. Interior design: Bridget Bohacz. Photographer: Jeanne Halloin, Michigan State University.*

Adequate lighting should be provided for seeing keyholes, room numbers, and name plates on doors, as shown in Figure 14-11. Supplemental lighting will sometimes be needed. Glossy and highly reflective floor surfaces, especially near large window areas, can create problems with glare and should be avoided. Carpet is the solution of choice but stay away from strong or highly visible patterns that could be interpreted as changes in height, as shadows, or as objects on the floor.

By carpeting hallways and corridors, considering window location, and using diffused light, glare can be reduced dramatically. Better lighting, reduction of glare, and the selection of nonslip surfaces will minimize the likelihood of falls and create a safer environment for aging residents.

Carefully select the placement of chairs, tables, or indoor pots and plants in corridors for visibility. Wheelchairs, waste bins, and other hallway clutter should be banished to built-in storage units.

Handrails

All long-term care settings designed for older people should have handrails designed to enhance balance, encourage movement, and allay fear of falling. Most handrails, however, are hard to use with the limited range of movement, low energy levels, and loss of handgrip

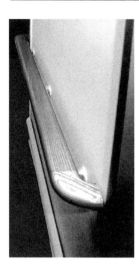

Figure 14-12 A broader, oval handrail, flat on top and bullnosed on each side, offers better support for mobility and balance. *Courtesy of On Lok Senior Services, San Francisco, CA. Architect: Barker Associates. Interior design: Elizabeth Brawley, IIDA, Design Concepts Unlimited.*

strength that characterize many elderly residents. A small round hand "pole" can be particularly difficult for residents with arthritic hands to grip. A well-designed handrail, a broad oval, flat on top and bullnosed on each side, is easier to use as support (see, e.g., Figure 14-12). It allows residents to grasp the rail and permits them to glide along the rail, leaning on their forearms. Perhaps its most important feature is that it enhances mobility.

Well-designed handrails do not detract from the homelike image; to the contrary, they send a message of support and alleviate the fear of losing one's balance and falling. Powder-coated finishes provide color, texture, and a hard finish. Wooden handrails offer a warm finish and residential look.

Handrails should be provided on both sides of corridors so that older people with impairments in one hand or arm can still utilize a handrail to negotiate the corridor. Although a mounting height of 33 to 36 inches from the floor to the top of the handrail is standard, the height may vary according to need. I have mounted handrails at 41 inches to make them easier to use.

Finishes

Professional designers use color and imagination to bring vitality to spaces that are really "pass throughs." Imaginative color planning in a hallway helps to convey friendliness and an invitation to further exploration. Using colors with high reflectance values will maximize the available light to offset low lighting levels. Intense shades of warm colors should be used sparingly in hallway locations to avoid contributing to residents' confusion or anxiety.

Wall and ceiling finishes should address acoustics and aesthetics; wall finishes must be designed to withstand high levels of traffic, including contact with wheelchairs and walkers. Surface finishes must be smooth enough to avoid abrading or cutting fragile elderly skin as residents brush against walls. Fabric walls, wallpaper, and acoustical wall fabric with a Velcro-compatible finish add interest and texture. Acoustical wall fabric used in panels above a chair rail can create interesting activity areas. Crocheted doilies or fabric shapes cut to form a quilt design can be adhered to the wall with Velcro and can be moved or redesigned by residents. Someone with a more creative mind could develop a myriad of fun patterns, shapes, textures, scenes, and designs. Acoustic wall fabric is available in a wide variety of colors and textures from several manufacturers, such as J M Lynne Co., who carry specialty wallcoverings.

Checklist for Corridors

❏ Provide clear contrast and definition where the wall meets the floor.

❏ Use materials that reflect the light in a diffused manner.

❏ Establish lighting levels that are even and consistent throughout the distance to be traveled.

❏ Provide appropriately placed seating opportunities along the way.

❏ Provide points of interest to engage residents.

❏ Use handrails designed to support and assist mobility and balance.

Rough textured paint should not be used, nor should slick surface finishes that reflect glaring light. Brick, concrete block, and tile resist abuse, but hardly engender the ambiance of home.

Since the corridors also serve as the principal means of egress in case of fire, walls, doors, hardware, ceilings, finishes, and openings must be selected to protect against fire and smoke as required by applicable codes.[17]

Television Lounge

Televisions and radios are played very loudly quite often. The treble level rises when the volume increases. With new technology this situation can be resolved by rerouting the TV or radio through a stereo monitor and appropriately increasing the bass—allowing the hearing impaired the opportunity to listen.[18] Lightweight headphones may also be appropriate for some residents; their use avoids disturbing others sensitive to loud noise.

Televisions, VCRs, and audio equipment can be stored in an entertainment unit, which can be closed when not in use, as shown in Figure 14-13. Housing audiovisual equipment in an entertainment unit not only improves the aesthetics of the room, but it keep cords and outlets out of sight and out of reach, and also removes the possibility of tripping over loose cords.

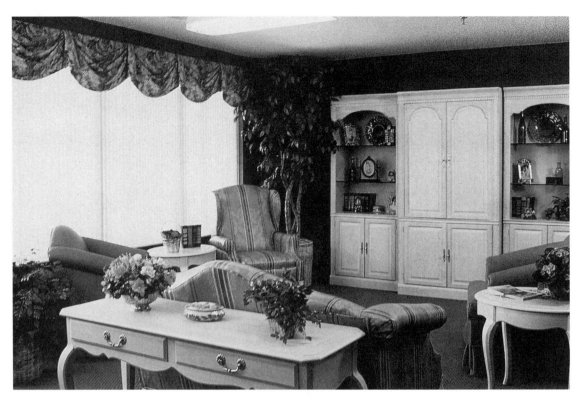

Figure 14-13 Televisions, VCRs, and audio equipment can be stored in an entertainment unit, which can be closed when not in use. *Courtesy of Life Care Center of Charleston, Charleston, SC.*

Bathing Rooms

Bathing—one of the most common activities in our lives and one that gives most of us great pleasure—is virtually guaranteed to provoke agitation among many residents with dementia. Typically, residents with Alzheimer's disease become agitated due to a combination of environmental overstimulation, caregivers impinging on their personal space, and physically painful experiences.[19] Bathing rooms can be dangerous; it is not uncommon to find residents on the bathing room floor.[20] While all of the problems may not be attributable to the physical environment, there are interventions that would foster great improvement. Until recently, little attention has been given to the role of the physical environment, environmental adaptation, or design in influencing residents' behavior.

In some of the first studies of issues related to bathing in Alzheimer's SCUs, Dr. Philip Sloane, professor of family medicine at the University of North Carolina, Chapel Hill, found that 43 percent of residents with dementia were considered disruptive during bathing. Problematic behaviors took the form of physical and verbal resistance, hitting, slapping, grabbing, swearing and cursing, as well as yelling and screaming.[21]

As assistant professor of nursing, Joanne Rader, also involved in research of bathing issues and dementia, took an active role in a research study. She was the subject of a nursing home bathing experience—with very interesting results. Her description of the experience identifies many sources of problematic behavior. As the assistant began to bathe her, Rader grew cold. The unexpected spray on her face distressed her; soon after she began sinking through the hole in the shower chair, her dangling legs and feet turning blue. As she was wheeled back to an empty resident's room, she felt a cool breeze fan her bottom, and although a towel covered her, she felt publicly naked.[22]

Convinced that the bathing environment has a critical impact on residents' behavior, Ann Marie Monahan, a clinical nurse specialist, who studied under Rader at Oregon Health Sciences University, renovated a tub room. She made the space smaller by enclosing each tub to ensure privacy and hung artificial plants and pictures, such as Renoir's bathers, to cue residents to bathing. Color added to the walls was a welcomed addition, as were privacy curtains, cane furniture, and towel bars. Though this renovation was not part of an organized study, it's not hard to believe that the residents responded positively. More interested in the environment, they were distracted from their anxiety as they talked about the pictures.

As approaches are explored for improving the environment in bathing rooms, many of the design strategies already discussed can be applied. While there is little agreement on whether a more spacious room or a smaller, cozier environment is preferable, everyone agrees the bathing room needs help. Breaking up the space creates privacy and more intimate areas.

Acoustics

Designing noise abatement throughout the bathing area is important. Agitation, confusion, and fear cause the highest level of screaming in bathing areas, making it possibly the noisiest place in an Alzheimer's special care setting. Ceramic tile walls and floors reflect the noise generated by running water and exhaust fans, creating a cacophony that produces hypertension and stress, and triggers ancient survival strategies of fight and flight. The noise of the shower, in addition, is a further irritant to persons with hearing deficits. Eurostone, a moisture-resistant, sound-absorbant acoustical ceiling tile mitigates much of the noise, making it an excellent product for use in environments with high humidity and moisture levels.

Pretty fabric shower curtains of several layers and many folds, lined with a clear plastic shower liner, absorb sound, as well as creating a softness in the room that is both residential and familiar. Double rows of colorful towels on towel bars mounted on the wall also help combat the reflected sound.

Other Factors

In addition to the problems already mentioned, a steam-filled room compounds the problems of low vision. Is it any wonder that bathing is such an unpleasant experience for residents and staff alike?

Though changing floor surfaces it is not usually recommended, this is one area that might benefit from combining unglazed ceramic tile or sheet rubber in the shower area with nonflow-through moisture barrier carpet throughout the balance of the space. Careful design detailing can ease the transition, and using the same color and color value for tile and carpet—for example, deep rose or raspberry unglazed tile in the shower area, combined with carpet of the same color and value—will ease the visual transition. Remember to provide sharp visual contrast between the floor and wall to assist with balance.

Wallcovering or attractive wallpaper borders used above a wainscoting gives the bathing room a warmer, "more inviting" appeal.

Temperature Control

Independent temperature controls for this room, along with heat lamps and radiant floor heating systems, would help residents stay warm, especially those with cold feet. Having a towel warmer or a warm terrycloth robe on a hook close by would be welcomed. When the residents come out of the bath or shower and put on thick terrycloth robes, they can pat themselves dry or dry in the robe while their hair or makeup is being done. It is much better for fragile skin to be patted dry than to be rubbed, and it's warmer, softer, and much more like home. Using warmer color choices in combination with effective lighting can affect the perception of warmth in the room.

Light and Lighting

Most bathrooms at home have a window. Why not have a window in the bathing room? If the space is an interior space, there are wonderful lighted artificial windows with views that are hard to distinguish from the real thing. They are a point of interest and a means to distract agitated residents. When possible the warmth of the sun from a skylight is also pleasant. Glare can be easily controlled.

Indirect cove lighting, a softer lighting source, removes some of the harshness from the space; decorative sconces also enhance a more residential look. Imagine a pretty armoire for storage instead of the standard utilitarian storage cabinet. Adding two chairs to form a conversation area in the corner of the room provides a place to sit and talk or calm a resident while removing clothing or robes. An old fashioned washstand could hold a pretty tray of talcum powder, body lotion, fragrances, and other nice smelling amenities that belong in this room. Make the bathing room inviting, make it feel like a treasured space from home. Redesigning, or more accurately designing this space, should be viewed as an investment, rather than an expense. As in any other space, if residents feels at ease, safe, and cared for, behavior is substantially different from behavior inspired by fear and loss of control. Currently, behavior in bathing environments could hardly be more difficult. Change takes imagination and a willingness to do things in a different way, but it is possible. While the environment can't change the behavior problems caused by the ravages of Alzheimer's disease, it can minimize fear engendered by threatening surroundings.

Grooming Area

A space for grooming, with an attractive vanity, including a mirror, and comfortable seating should be the focal point of the bathing room, as shown in Figure 14-14. A wall-mounted mirror in a pretty

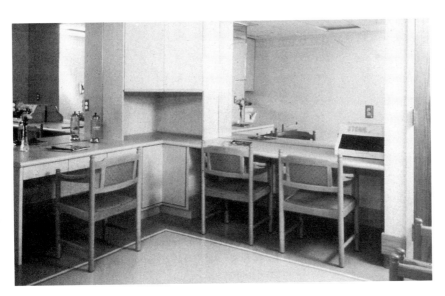

Figure 14-14 The grooming area is an area for pampering and taking care of one's self. *Courtesy of The Norma and Joseph Saul Alzheimer's Disease Special Care Unit at the Jewish Home and Hospital for Aged, Bronx, NY. Architect: Perkins Eastman PC.*

frame is familiar. Most of us respond very favorably to personal attention, especially having our hair arranged and makeup applied. Many women had a special area for makeup and fixing their hair in their homes, and even those who didn't may have dreamed of it.

For many women bathing and grooming was a ritual; it represented taking care of oneself, pampering. Perhaps if we are more sensitive to the "way things were" in this area, pleasant memories might be recalled, opening the possibility for pleasant experiences and less difficulty. Bubble bath, herbal bath fragrance, and scented soaps increase the pleasure for anyone. Bath oils, however, create slippery surfaces and should not be used.

Transforming this area offers a positive way to refocus attention in a more sensitive way. It sends an entirely different message. The bathing space is no longer a cold, functional, highly impersonal space for clinical hygiene, but a warm, welcoming, highly personalized space, where the expectation is for nurturing, increased personal attention, pampering, and sensitivity in attending to personal care needs. The picture is very different. The attitude that creates this visually and emotionally supportive space acknowledges the need for good hygiene, and the equally important emotional needs of the resident to feel safe and cared for.

Bath and Shower Areas

Since towel bars are often used as grab bars, use pretty colored grab bars for towel bars, complete with pretty colored towels. Temperature control mixers prevent scalding hot water from reaching the faucets; showerheads can also be fitted with devices that automatically shut off the water if the temperature exceeds a safe level. Dual shower heads at different heights for tall men and short little ladies are a thoughtful addition, but not a costly one. For residents with more progressed dementia, handheld showers are easier to control and less anxiety producing. Showers must be equipped with grab bars that contrast with the wall for visual identification and should be equipped with a seat or a shower chair. Shower chairs should have soft seats, and their color should contrast as well, either a color to contrast with light shower wall, or white to contrast with a color on the walls and floor.

Which Tub Is Best?

Residents in early and midstage dementia are usually able to transfer in and out of the tub with limited assistance, and are also usually capable of significant participation in washing. Tubs for these individuals should allow them to enter independently and to sit upright while bathing. Residents with advanced dementia, by contrast, often have problems remaining upright and need partial or full assistance getting in and out of the tub. They will also require substantial assistance with washing. To accommodate all residents with dementia, tubs should allow sitting up or reclining positions and provide ready access for the caregiver to all body areas.[23]

Height adjustable tubs allow the tub to be a comfortable working height for staff. Lifts can be frightening for anyone, especially someone with dementia; consequently it is better to minimize elevation changes during transfer for nonambulatory residents. The more unfamiliar the tub, relative to a resident's memory, the more likely it is to cause agitation.

These tubs should have a slip-resistant floor. Temperature control systems prevent scalding, and knobs and controls should not only be out of reach for residents, they should be out of sight. The tubs themselves are oversized and frightening for many residents, as are the controls. Though necessary, and recognizable to staff, they present yet one more threat to a confused resident. The controls should be designed for safety—to minimize the risk of injury to residents or staff. Controls can be disguised or preferably relocated to a wall and hidden from view.

All tubs must be disinfected between each bath; many tubs have automatic disinfecting systems.

Certain features most likely to cause agitation with residents were identified including: loud noises, excessively noisy faucets or whirlpools, lifts (especially high ones), and lengthy filling or emptying times (residents often become cold). Transfer devices or seats that do not feel secure and water levels that rise close to the resident's head during whirlpool use were also issues.[24] Creditable studies, such as Sloan et al.'s, which identify problems, provide substantial information to designers and manufactures, so that products and environments can be substantially improved for residents.

Features included on some tubs that were found to be helpful were: hydrosound, a method of agitating water without using whirlpool jets; foot, head, and back supports or pillows; built-in soap dispensers; and warm air jets when the tub is empty. In some settings a tub of adequate size to accommodate large residents may be needed.[25]

Finally, of the tubs surveyed, the ones found to be most suitable for persons with early and midstage dementia were: Ferno Recline-A-Bath Two, GTT Freedom Bath, Parker Bath, and Silcraft Access. For persons with advanced dementia the following tubs rated highest:

ARJO Serenade, Amada Smart Tub, Ferno Recline-A-Bath Two, and Parker Bath.

In creating environments for residents with Alzheimer's disease, facility policy and design criteria often make the difference between a limiting environment and a healing environment. The bathing room is one of the biggest challenges for designers in special care settings. Knowing that people with dementia may be especially responsive to even modest changes in their environment leaves no doubt that more than a humanitarian gesture is needed to improve and humanize this environment, and in doing so, contribute substantially to improving quality of care and quality of life.

Staff Retreat

Environments for people with dementia should include a space or spaces for staff retreat, like the lounge shown in Figure 14-15. Caring for people with dementia is an extremely demanding and draining job, and staff members, no matter how dedicated, need an occasional break. The staff retreat should be designed to provide a quiet, comfortable, and uplifting space, and a convenient work area where tasks

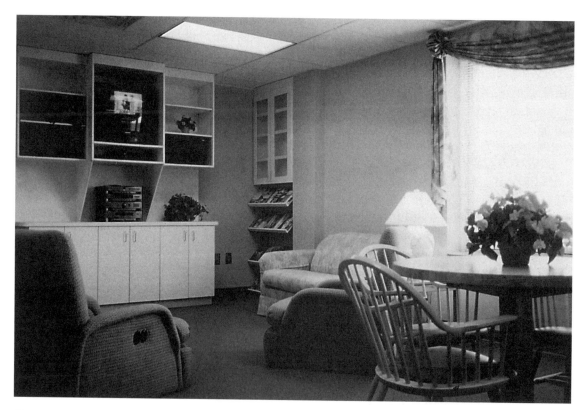

Figure 14-15 The staff retreat offers comfortable seating and a quiet place for uninterrupted conversation and decompression, as well as a pleasant spot to work. *Courtesy of Promina Cobb Hospital, Austell, GA. Interior design: Linda Watson, ASID, Watson Limited Planning and Design.*

such as charting can take place. Comfortable seating, a view to the outside, a place where private conversations can take place without interruption, all encourage decompression as well as socialization.

Sufficient storage space is essential and should include storage for coats, purses, and other personal items, as well as any equipment needs, medications, or supplies. A bulletin board, for policy changes and upcoming events, staff mailboxes, and journals are other items that might be located here.[26]

Providing for staff needs delivers the message that staff is valued, and reinforces staff members' perception of themselves as valuable people. Staff access to a private place for temporary retreat can increase the quality of life and of caregiving.

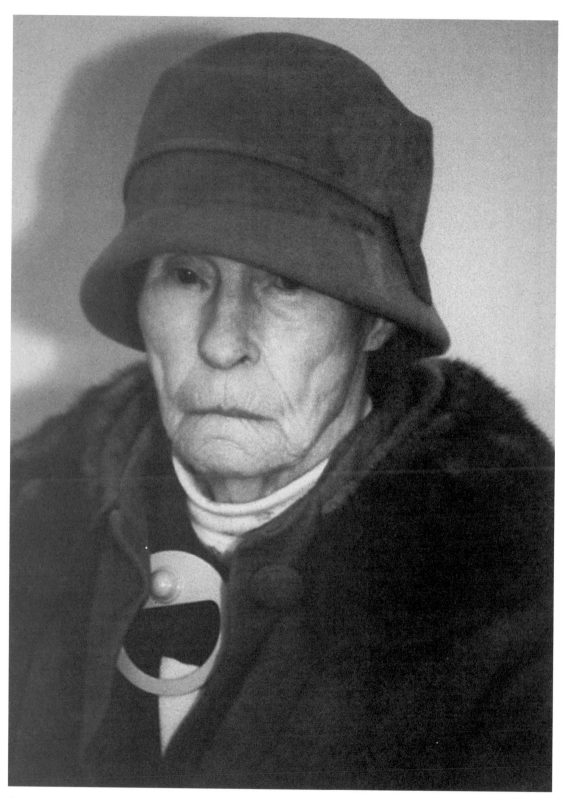

Courtesy of the Greater San Francisco Bay Area Alzheimer's Association. Photographer: Anna M. Rossi.

15

Therapeutic Gardens and Outdoor Space Design

Confined, enclosed spaces are often upsetting for people with dementia.[1] Low levels of stimulation, long corridors lined with identical doors, and the lack of windows, conditions that might prove disorienting to less impaired people,[2] often result in aggressive or hostile behavior from disorientation. Access to safe and secure areas provides an opportunity for fresh air, walking, privacy, and a literally a different view of the world—it is certainly less confining.

Carefully planned outdoor environments are particularly valuable for the cognitively impaired. These outdoor spaces can help to maintain a connection with the natural environment, and provide added opportunities for socialization and a wide range of activities that allow participation at different levels of skill and ability (see the lovely example in Figure 15-1). Many activities can be designed to stimulate residents' long-term memory of their previous home life—mowing the lawn with a push mower, raking leaves, gardening, and hanging clothes on a clothesline. Outdoor areas can also offer places of solitude, which are hard to find inside.

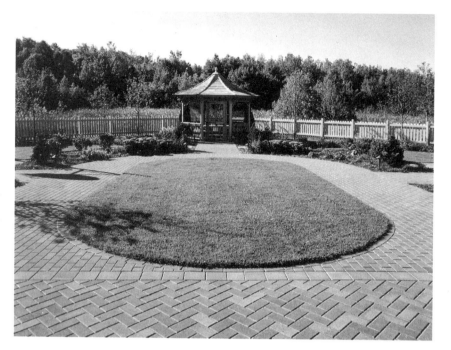

Figure 15-1 The gazebo in the Hawthorne garden at Sedgewood Commons provides space for outdoor activities and shelter from the sun. *Courtesy of Sedgewood Commons, Falmouth, ME. Landscape architect: Robert Hoover, Studio L.A., Portland, ME. Architect: SMRT Architects. Photographer: Jim Daniels, Portland, ME.*

Being outside is necessary for well-being and for life itself.

Too often, lovely gardens and outside spaces are not included as part of the overall space design of the care program, but instead are often added as decoration, without serious thought as to how they might be planned and used to add to the residents' quality of life. Even when they are part of the design, as construction or renovation budgets are overrun, the landscaping and design features that make these therapeutic outdoor spaces accessible for older adults are often eliminated. Being outside is necessary for well-being and for life itself.

One of the most common requests from residents and their families is for more outdoor spaces with partial shade or filtered light. Adjustable umbrellas, shade-producing arbors, and other structures and plantings help to control sunlight and extend the use of the garden into several seasons.

Designs for outdoor space will vary according to location, microclimate, availability of space, and existing features. There is also a growing interest in creating outdoor spaces to complement the interior spaces. Hallways and corridors are carefully planned, including the floor and ground surface colors, leading into gardens. Recognition of the part the wonders of nature play in healing environments is responsible for increased window surfaces and more inspired placement. Bringing the outside into the interior spaces by providing sunlight and abundant views of gardens, flowers, groves of trees, mountains, birds and animals, and other interesting sights, is healing to the soul. For cultural familiarity, we might look to the garden styles of the 1930s and 1940s for inspiration, since that is when current residents with Alzheimer's disease were perhaps gardening in their own backyards or walking the public parks.[3]

To better adapt the outdoor environment to compensate for the physical and sensory changes related to aging, designers must be familiar both with the needs generated by the aging process and with the special needs of residents with Alzheimer's disease.

Safety and Security

In addition to being physically safe and secure, it is extremely important that an outdoor space be perceived by staff, family, and residents as safe and secure. The single biggest barrier to free use of accessible outdoor space is staff concern that a resident may wander away or be injured.[4] Increased visibility often helps staff comfort levels. If residents are to have free choice about going outside, it is the challenge and the responsibility of design professionals to be sure the outside spaces are as safe and secure as they can possibly be.

In order to adequately address safety concerns, design must accommodate the diminished visual acuity and the physical capacity of the elderly residents. With the high incidence of osteoporosis in the aged, safety in relation to physical mobility is a crucial aspect of design. Falling, the most common safety issue with the elderly, can result in serious fractures in elderly individuals. It cannot be completely avoided in any setting, however, if a resident is to be allowed freedom and autonomy. Decreased visual acuity, strength, endurance, balance, and coordination also contribute to the safety and accessibility problems of most outdoor environments.[5]

Falls can be minimized by ensuring that paving surfaces are glare-free, nonslip, and of uniform texture and color. As Alzheimer's disease progresses, lack of coordination and balance can be a problem. Some individuals tend to shuffle rather than walk, which reinforces the conclusion that a garden for these residents must be level, with just enough slope to avoid puddles.[6] Surfaces should remain "nonslip" in wet or dry conditions, and be free of irregularities such as cracks, potholes, or uneven spots. The walkways should have clearly distinguishable borders and good contrast between the pavement and its immediate surroundings.

The greatest concern after falling is exiting. While we want to use outdoor areas, those areas must be secured with plantings and fencing. For some residents the urge to leave is strong, and physically able residents can be very agile and quite clever in climbing, vaulting over, or crawling under. Parking lots and staff and family comings and goings are powerful cues, and these views should be screened away from residents.

As designers we are faced with creating what Hall, Kirschling, and Todd referred to as "sheltered freedom,"[7] which allows residents a greater degree of freedom and dignity within the bounds of a safe and protective environment. This setting actually enlarges the scope of daily experience. A study of exit behavior conducted at the Corinne Dolan Alzheimer's Center indicated that agitated behavior decreased when residents had free access to the garden.[8]

While fenced or walled gardens may be necessary, the challenge is to create an enclosure without the feeling of confinement. Fencing requires special thought and can be an attractive design element, as shown in Figure 15-2. It can be partially obscured with plantings, or a black vinyl clad chain-link fence can be nearly invisible in the right location. A six-foot high fence that can not be easily climbed is usually required.[9] Trees and garden structures should be located far enough away from the building to discourage their use as climbing aids. Gates and locks also require camouflage to minimize attention by the residents.[10] In Japan a stream with water only 5 inches deep was used as a landscape barrier.

Older people have expressed strong preferences for physical features that compensate for physical impairments and support safe passage—nonslip walkways, handrails, and wide walkways that accommodate two-way traffic without physical contact. Handrails provide additional safety and security for frail residents. They serve as supports, as well as a guide to return the confused resident to where he started, and should have clear visible contrast against the background.

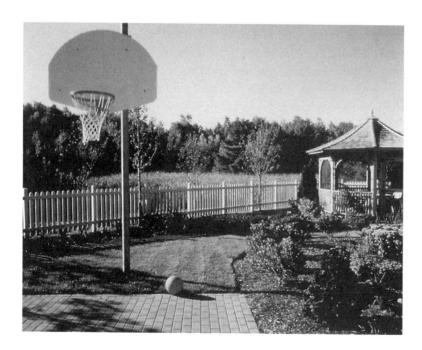

Figure 15-2 The basketball hoop in this garden provides activity for residents and visiting grandchildren. The garden fence can also be an attractive design element. *Courtesy of Sedgewood Commons, Falmouth, ME. Landscape architect: Robert Hoover, Studio L.A., Portland, ME. Architect: SMRT Architects. Photographer: Robert Hoover.*

With diminished visual and auditory acuity, physical mobility, strength, and endurance, there is risk of injury from hazards not seen or heard. In designing outdoor space it is essential to maintain an adequate level of light while minimizing glare. Most older adults have extreme sensitivity to glare and reflection from shiny surfaces. Glare from bright white paving reflecting up into the eyes creates particular problems. Using a material of a medium to dark value to reduce the glare is a better solution. Residential lawn furniture that meets the needs of the elderly can be attractive and relatively inexpensive, and by using furniture of nonreflective materials, glare can also be minimized effectively.

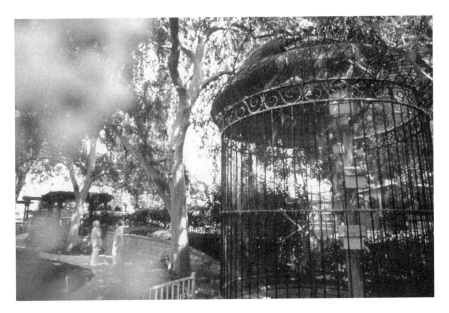

Figure 15-3 The aviary in the Wanderer's Garden in "Harry's Haven" stimulates the interest of those who walk through the beautiful gardens. *Courtesy of the Motion Picture Television Fund, Woodland Hills, CA. Photographer: Douglas Kirkland.*

Just as in planning the interior, the outdoor environment should be designed to provide variety and flexibility of use (see Figure 15-3). Private spaces are needed, as well as accommodations for group activities. Small courtyards or garden spaces that relate to a house or family groups are frequently used design solutions. It is a rare outdoor space that can provide for everyone's needs. A variety of gardens and outdoor spaces is more likely to meet the needs of early stage and more active residents, while other spaces are more specifically designed for the needs of the midstage and late-stage residents. Limiting outside experiences to only one space becomes less stimulating. Orienting outside spaces to the south will provide warmth from the sun and shelter from the winds. Shade trees or structures such as porches, pergolas, awnings, and umbrellas provide shaded areas and protection from the sun. These structures can also provide shelter from showers.

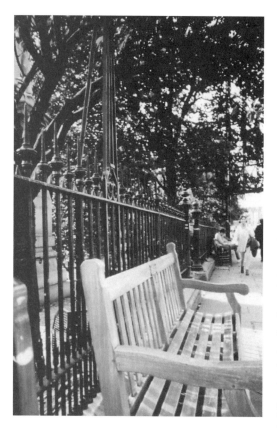

Figure 15-4 Benches and chairs provide an opportunity to rest. In Edinburgh, Scotland, benches are not restricted to parks, but located at convenient intervals along the main streets. *Photographer: Elizabeth Brawley.*

Wandering paths often provide the design device to link smaller spaces with larger spaces and to link various selected elements in the environment.[11] Clearly defined pathways that circle back to the starting point will assist residents in finding their way. The physical and emotional well-being of the individual and the need to feel safe and secure must be addressed,[12] as well as the potential problems arising from the cognitive deficits associated with Alzheimer's disease. For example, well-designed areas that allow for wandering while ensuring that an individual is safe and can be supervised easily, and pathways that flow in loops, bringing residents back to where they started, allow a safe outdoor journey. Trees and plants that drop fruit could create a walking hazard and should be placed away from walking areas.

Benches or chairs located along the way offer an opportunity to rest or to just sit enjoy the garden. Seating areas located under trees or trellises can filter the sunlight and give the illusion of privacy, as shown in Figure 15-4. Interestingly, accommodating the need for privacy may actually encourage socialization.[13]

Wayfinding and Orientation

It is vital to maximize awareness and orientation and reinforce the residents' ability to exercise freedom of choice through movement. Distinctive landmarks, familiar items from the past, and self-contained looping paths are a few examples. A porch like the one in Figure 15-5 can serve as a large visual landmark for a safe return. It not only provides a transition area from inside to out, expanding interior space, but it also allows for sitting and walking in the outdoors in a wider range of climate changes than would a space that is unsheltered.[14]

Nontoxic Planting

Individuals with Alzheimer's disease often put things in their mouths and eat flowers and plant material. Funkenstein points out that ingesting plants is not typical of early to midstage dementia, but it is

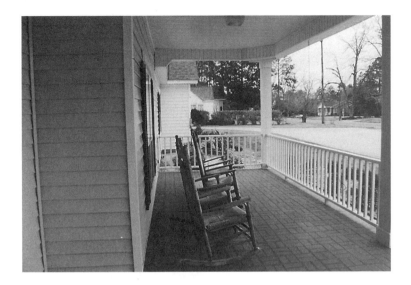

Figure 15-5 The front porch is a familiar place to relax, rock, and watch the activities of the neighborhood. The porch also serves as a large visual landmark for a safe return. *Courtesy of Willowood, Edison, GA.*

more common in the later stages of the disease. All plantings for mid-stage and late-stage residents must be nontoxic; plantings for early stage allow for discretion.[15] There are many beautiful, fragrant, and delicious varieties from which to choose. The bright colors and velvety texture of pansies made them very inviting; they are my personal favorites from my mother's garden.

The Corinne Dolan Alzheimer's Center provides easy access to a fenced two-acre park and garden featuring wandering paths and landscaped with 90 species of nontoxic plants to protect residents who may pick and eat the garden contents.

Sensory Stimulation

While persons in the middle to late stages of dementia respond to a peaceful, calm, quiet environment,[16] many early stage residents delight in a more active and stimulating environment. Dull, monotonous surroundings encourage adverse reactions such as anxiety, fear, and distress; however, with beautiful gardens and a variety of outdoor spaces available, residents, able to move about during the day, can be treated to a desirable and pleasing change of pace and space. Gardens (like the one shown in Figure 15-6) are a lovely and interesting way to provide a wonderful source of sensory stimulation and to avoid monotony — a virtual symphony of sight, sound, light, color, fragrance, birds, and small animals.

Creating interesting focal points within the outdoor space, such as fragrant gardens, bird feeders, garden ornaments, weather vanes, and flower gardens will provide diversion, destination goals, and a relief from the interior environment, motivating residents to go outdoors.[17]

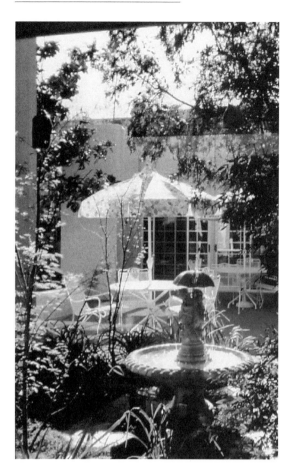

Figure 15-6 Gardens provide a wonderful source of sensory stimulation, with sight, sound, light, color, and fragrance. *Courtesy of Heatherwood Alzheimer's Assisted Living, Walnut Creek, CA. Photographer: Elizabeth Brawley.*

Outdoor spaces offer unique opportunities for a wide range of stimulating, potentially life-enriching activities, such as assisting a resident who has been a lifelong gardener to maintain some form of small outside gardening spot; raised planting beds that are wheelchair accessible can provide residents another opportunity to garden, as shown in Figure 15-7.

Accessible gardens can also be created on an enclosed terrace or a porch by using several large pots of plants with chairs grouped in the center for conversation. Roof gardens are not one of the more desirable solutions for providing outdoor space for dementia residents. Because they are not areas where residents can safely wander unaccompanied, their use is staff intensive, and they are, consequently, not available for spontaneous use.

Figure 15-7 Raised planting beds that are wheelchair accessible can provide residents with an opportunity to garden. *Courtesy of Heatherwood Alzheimer's Assisted Living, Walnut Creek, CA. Photographer: Elizabeth Brawley.*

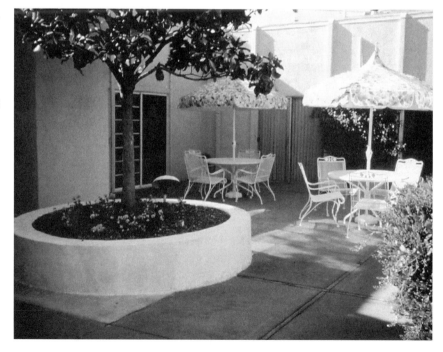

Using the Outside Environment

The most important factor in determining whether outdoor spaces are actually used is staff motivation. Well-designed outdoor environments provide the potential for numerous casual and organized events that can complement ongoing indoor activities. They offer opportunities for residents to both observe and participate in activity, and to observe changes in seasonal landscapes.[18] The use of well-designed and accessible outdoor spaces has been shown to significantly reduce problems of exiting, agitation, and violent behavior.[19]

Therapeutic gardens and well-designed outdoor spaces (see the examples in Figures 15-8 and 15-9) are being adopted and used in more and more residential care settings. We need to ensure that they don't go unused. Residents in healthcare settings are generally frail and at risk for a variety of problems; in most cases that's why they are there. What families are looking for is not a guarantee that "no harm" will come to their relative, but a guarantee that staff will access the problem in an individualized way and evaluate the risks and benefits with the resident and the family. Staff, family members, and administration will need to have open discussions and mutually develop a care plan and an agreement of shared risk for the residents' safety and well-being. Even with the most careful planning and the most vigilant staff, falls may occur. Although the changes that take place as a consequence of aging make one more prone to falling, quality of life may be as important, or even more important, than safety to the frail or impaired individual. Risks must be weighed, family members must be included in the process, and we can work together to encourage an atmosphere of living and enjoying life to the greatest extent possible.

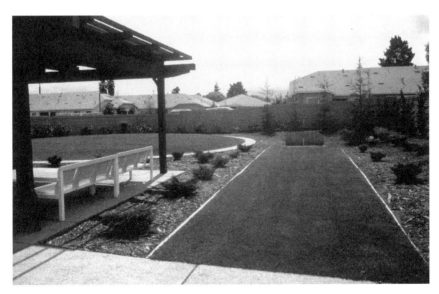

Figure 15-8 Good planning provides safe, secured outdoor spaces with places to walk, to garden, and to sit in the shade and enjoy the view. *Courtesy of Alzheimer's Activity Center/Respite, Research for Alzheimer's Disease, San Jose, CA.*

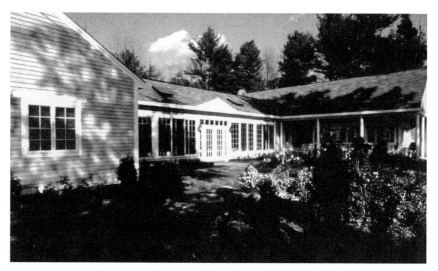

Figure 15-9 The patio overlooks a large flower and vegetable garden. The open layout encourages walking on a pathway that leads each resident safely back home again. *Courtesy of Alzheimer's Care Center, Gardiner, ME, a program of Kennebec Long Term Care. Architect: SMRT, Portland, ME. Photographer: Robert Perron.*

Checklist for Outdoor Spaces[20]

❑ Include flowering trees, shrubs, and perennials to provide a sense of seasonal change that reinforces one's awareness of life's rhythms and cycles.

❑ Incorporate features to attract birds—a fountain or birdbath, a bird feeder, trees appropriate for roosting or nesting, and bird houses. Stimulating the senses helps to lift people's spirits.

❑ Use plant species that attract butterflies as a gentle reminder of how precious life is.

❑ Select paving surfaces that are smooth enough to accommodate wheelchairs.

❑ Arrange entrances to the garden and the width of pathways so that individuals can be accompanied, side by side, with ease.

❑ Arrange seating near the entrance into the garden for social interaction.

❑ Use seating with backs for sitting in comfort. This is especially important for someone who is weak.

❑ Provide tables and chairs for a picnic or a cup of coffee.

❑ Consider adjustable umbrellas to allow to people to control the amount of sun or shade.

❑ Provide one or more eye-catching and unique features for wayfinding.

Implementing Effective Interior Design

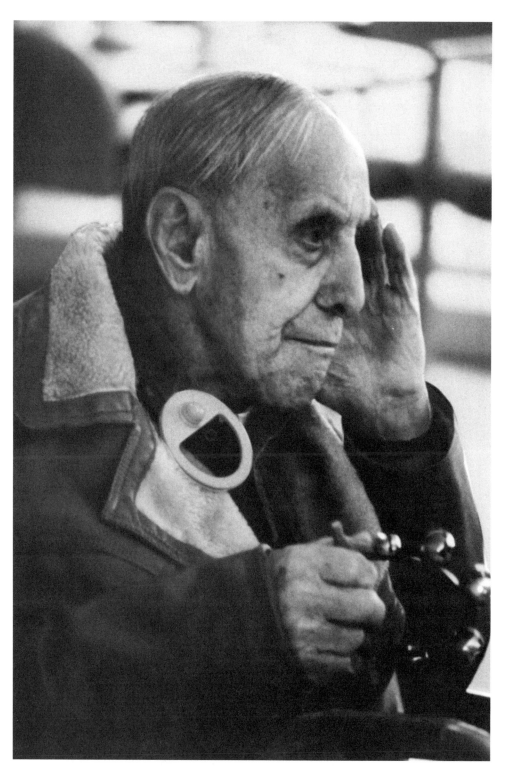

Courtesy of the Greater San Francisco Bay Area Alzheimer's Association. Photographer: Anna M. Rossi.

CHAPTER 16

Furniture and Fabrics

Why do some rooms seem so comfortable for people to gather in while others seem to cast a pall on social interaction? We may never have all of the answers to that question, but for residential healthcare settings where social interaction contributes to residents' quality of life, we must make every effort to promote easy interactions.

For easy conversation, group chairs at right angles when possible, as demonstrated in Figure 16-1. Being seated at right angles to another person has been shown to be psychologically more comfortable than being face-to-face. The face-to-face position may be too confrontational for some, and sitting side-by-side makes it awkward to make eye contact. For elderly residents seating configurations are especially important, because many have hearing impairments that should be accommodated and mobility limitations that must be considered.

Seating arrangements should be flexible enough to accommodate social gatherings of varying degrees of intimacy. Sofas, found in everyone's living room, are the worst seating for comfortable socializing. They are designed to make occupants face forward, not toward each other, and regardless of providing seating space for three people, you will rarely find more than two sitting on the sofa at one time. The frail elderly often find it difficult to rise from a sofa, particularly if there is

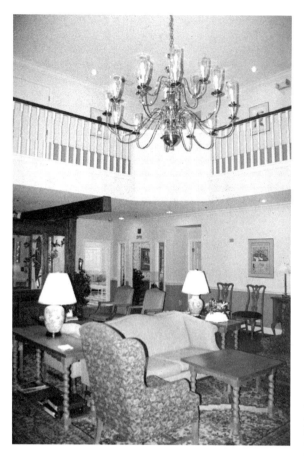

Figure 16-1 Being seated at right angles makes conversation easier. *Courtesy of Tulip Garden, Decatur, GA.*

no arm for support. The same can be true of chairs; they are often too low, too soft, and too deep—a deadly combination for mobility. A loveseat or a settee for two provides the same ambience and is much easier to use.

Don't make seating too far apart, or residents will not feel a part of the social circle. If the room is too large, smaller seating groups are friendlier than a single large one. When arranging furniture for socialization, be thoughtful and plan well. Seating near windows and natural light is always used if the light is diffused to eliminate glare.

Unless residents move furniture on their own initiative, it is important not to constantly rearrange furniture after it has been placed. Individuals with Alzheimer's rely on a familiar environment. If it is constantly changing, the familiar is removed and they are left with more uncertainty and confusion. If residents rearrange seating, pay attention and discover why it works better for them. We are still learning; we don't have all the answers, particularly in working with people with dementia.

Social interaction is important and appropriate color, texture, and arrangement can increase meaningful social activity. Most families want to remain actively involved with residents. Significant importance should be placed on their role and accommodations provided so that family and other guests feel welcome and included.

Mobility and Seating

The processes of aging, with arthritis, loss of balance, fatigue, and rheumatic inflammation, makes movement more difficult and more uncomfortable, often producing its own disincentives to maintaining mobility. Loss of mobility is a gradual process, except, of course, in instances of catastrophic loss such as stroke or a broken hip. As abilities decline and people become less able to get up on their feet, their sense of balance decreases, steps become less sure, and a process of deterioration begins to accelerate. Occasional falls take place, and a terror develops regarding the eventual incapacitating fall that will result in a broken hip.

Lack of mobility causes further deterioration as unused muscle groups atrophy and a downward spiral accelerates. Each day that muscles are not used approximately one-thirtieth of a person's strength disappears, resulting in "orthostatic hypertension" or low blood pressure.[1] Upon standing upright, residents are at risk of getting dizzy and falling. Nowhere is the old adage "Use it or lose it" more true than with the elderly.

Incentive to move is a complex issue that depends on adequate mental stimulus as well as on the proper equipment. Creating the incentive for people to want to move about, however, requires imagination and insight. Opportunities for socialization, and the visual interest as one moves from one point to another, are obvious stimuli to travel movements. Sensitive design—the smells of coffee brewing, the new bloom of a courtyard fruit tree, the opportunity to feed a communal pet—all can encourage people to move about for more than the customary feeding rituals.[2] In an environment where people's ability to move lessens, there is a very real need to create new incentives to keep residents active and mobile.

In order to help residents feel secure in moving about, we must provide places to sit. Mobility for many frail elderly residents is dependent on knowing there are reliable resting places available. Hallways, for example, frequently lack properly spaced resting places. This often compels "marginal walkers" to stop walking, and some resort prematurely to wheelchairs, which provide them a seat.

Wheelchairs, however, are really designed to transport individuals and were never intended as resident seating, especially for long-term sitting. The construction of a wheelchair's seat rotates the hips inward, causing the person to slump forward, compressing the lungs.[3] This is a problem that can be corrected with proper back support, but it makes infinitely more sense to keep residents mobile by providing adequate seating opportunities, rather than forcing them into wheelchairs. There is abundant evidence that even seemingly inconsequential levels of exercise are useful to older people, and any movement provides some level of exercise and benefit in maintaining muscle mass and preventing atrophy.

Seating

It is important to specify chairs with the right seat height, pitch of the back, and arms that make them comfortable and easy to get in and out of. What we need are chairs that fit and support. Chairs should be sized to the person; a resident's feet should be flat on the floor when seated. A chair that is comfortable for a six-foot-tall man will most likely not be comfortable for a five-foot-tall woman. Just as you might find in the home, a variety of chair styles and sizes should be available.

The importance of selecting seating for older people cannot be overemphasized, and Figure 16-2 provides some badly needed guidelines. Typically the elderly tend to sit for extended periods and to have poor blood circulation and difficulty getting into and out of seating. If

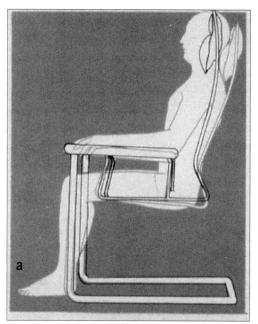

(a) Rocking chairs should redistribute and cycle the pressure between the resident's seat and back, as shown, while alternately reducing the pressure on the seat, allowing capillaries in the skin to open up and facilitating better circulation.

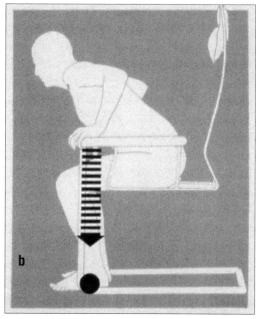

(b) Extended arm rests enable the sitter to first pull himself or herself forward in the chair with hands and feet aligned. The resident thus engages the stronger lower-body muscles in the task of rising to a standing position.

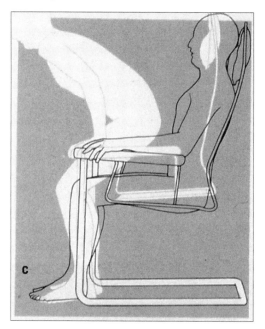

(c) Chairs can provide a support surface in the front of users, such as the extended armfront shown. This serves as an axial prop for pushing against by keeping the front of the armrests motionless. Once standing, an individual can safely support himself or herself until ready to walk.

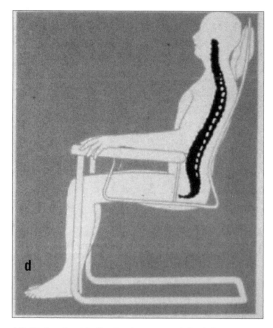

(d) Chairs should offer lumbar support, lordotic curvature, as well as support to the neck or "cervical" area so that the resident's weight is evenly supported.

Figure 16-2 *Illustration designed by and courtesy of Roger Leib for ADD Specialized Seating Technology, Los Angeles, CA.*

Figure 16-3 Good chairs can be hard to find. When products don't satisfy needs, creativity finds a way. "Tennis ball shoes" make it easy to move. *Courtesy of Nevins Family of Services, Methuen, MA.*

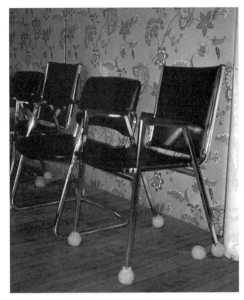

appropriately designed chairs were available, with arms extending beyond the seat so that residents could just stand, instead of being forced off balance as they propelled themselves forward to get up from their chairs, we might find more residents getting out of their chairs and walking.

People breath more easily when they are sitting erect or standing, and when chairs provide much needed lower back support, breathing is easier. Senior chairs must outperform all others in comfort and quality.[4] Good chairs can be hard to find and not all chairs are appropriate for all uses (see Figure 16-3). Rocking chairs, dining chairs, lounge chairs, game table chairs, wingback chairs and others, all have different functions.

Rocking Chairs

Rocking chairs, like the one in Figure 16-4, can redistribute and cycle the pressure between resident's seat and back, stimulating circulation. The rocking motion also stimulates the vestibular canal in the ear, which not only gives us our sense of balance, but also creates a calming effect. For residents with Alzheimer's disease, who can be aggressive rockers, a rocking chair with a stable base can be calming and therapeutic.

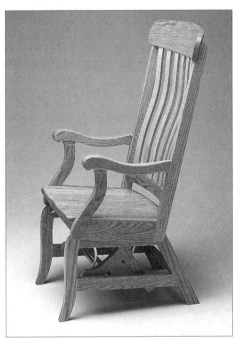

Lounge Seating

Hip fractures caused by inappropriate lounge seating were identified by former U.S. Surgeon General, Dr. C. Everett Koop, as a major safety issue. It's

Figure 16-4 Olive's chair. Rocking chairs are always a favorite. *Courtesy of Adden Furniture, Inc., Lowell, MA.*

amazing how many people get stuck in chairs. Unfortunately, hip joints can be shattered or broken when frail elderly individuals attempt to rise from an inappropriate chair. Most upholstered club type chairs are too low, too soft, and too deep.

The elderly experience great difficulty trying to push themselves up and out, a problem further exacerbated by arms that are too low

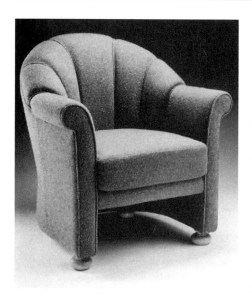

Figure 16-5 Manhattan Lounge Seating provides comfort and easy support for rising from a seated to a standing position, and is available with removable, washable slip covers. *Courtesy of Senior Style, Ltd., Portland, OR. Designer: Eunice Noell. Photographer: Paul Gentry.*

and do not extend out to the front of the seat. Chairs with arms placed well forward for safety and ease of exit enable residents to engage their stronger lower-body muscles in the task of rising to a standing position and also safely support themselves while standing until ready to walk. Take a look at the example in Fgure 16-5.

Without an opening under the front of the seat, a less stable person experiences difficulty standing. The opening allows one foot to be placed underneath so the individual is able to push up to a standing position. Stability is greatly improved when there are four points of support, one foot under the seat, one foot forward, and both hands on the arms of the chair.[5] Chairs of different sizes and varying seating heights should be offered to accommodate "the long and the short of it." To assist older residents in rising from their chairs, seating heights should be slightly higher than standard, between 18 and 19 ½ inches.

Lounge chairs and club chairs, when properly constructed with an 18-inch seat height, firm seat, and arms for support, can be comfortable and supportive. It can be difficult to rise from an upholstered chair if the seat is too deep. Moisture barriers prevent penetration of fluids that are a source of odor and cause mildew and rot. Well-designed and properly engineered seating can provide comfort and independence for older residents and contribute to an enhanced quality of life.

Dining Chairs

Stability is important in a dining chair. Chair backs become a means of support for many frail elderly residents. Arms are essential for support while rising, and those arms should easily fit under the table (see Figure 16-6). Though dining chairs must pull away easily from the table, casters are too unstable. Chairs on wheels or seating that is unstable is dangerous and should be removed, particularly when residents use it for support.

Special Features

Specially designed chairs can provide unique advantages. Providing dry seating surfaces with no heat buildup can be a particular chal-

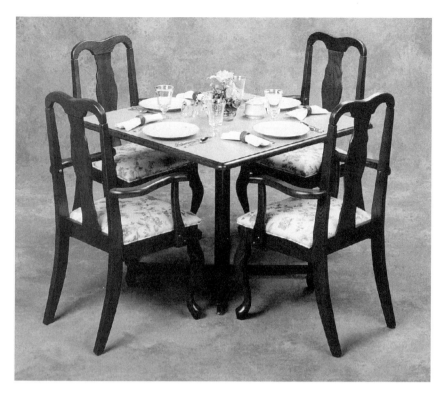

Figure 16-6 Arms are essential for support while rising and should fit easily under the table. *Courtesy of Akin Industries, Inc.*

lenge. Special features such as mesh seats and backs for chairs bring greater air circulation that also helps prevent decubitis ulcers. Because they are easy to clean, sanitation is improved and there is no odor buildup from fluid trapped in fabric or upholstery materials.

Chairs that offer highly refined lordotic curvature and correct lumbar support provide comfort and support for residents. When a variety of chairs are offered, these are usually the first ones to be filled. A flexible chair back offers staff personal back protection as they assist residents in rising.

The Warren chair, from ADD Specialized Seating Technology, is available in three sizes (small, medium, and large), with extra width (two inches wider) for heavy residents. It is shown in Figure 16-7. The Rose chair, from the same manufacturer, in a high or low back, nonrocking version, is approved for a 550-pound weight limit.

Wicker furniture is now available with a special finish to withstand exposure to moisture and sunlight. The protective acrylic finish, formulated from outdoor resins, requires little maintenance, though how much varies with exposure. All materials for the furniture and frames are mold and mildew resistant and clean with soap and water. The acrylic finish provides a much smoother finish to the touch and provides another option for furnishing sunrooms and living rooms, as shown in Figure 16-8.

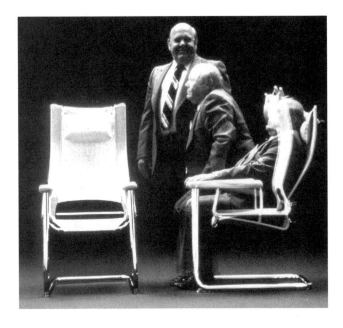

Figure 16-7 The Warren chair was specifically designed to meet the special needs of elderly users. It is available in three sizes. *Designed by and courtesy of Roger Lieb for ADD Specialized Seating Technology.*

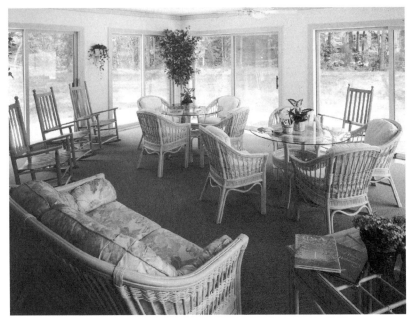

Figure 16-8 Wicker furniture gives a feeling of lightness to a pretty sunroom. *Courtesy of The Oakes, Thomasville, NC and Thomasville Furniture Industries.*

California Technical Bulletin 133 (TB 133)

In order to protect the public, upholstered furniture is subject to fire regulations in every state; the laws protecting residents in healthcare environments are even more stringent. California Technical Bulletin 133 is not "just one more fire retardancy test." It is a full-scale fire test for furniture manufactured for use in certain public buildings. It shows what happens when the components are used together. The specific types of public buildings vary from state to state, depending upon local regulations; however, in

California, TB 133 applies to prisons, jails, hospitals, healthcare facilities, board and care homes, old age convalescent homes, licensed child care facilities, stadiums, auditoriums, and public assembly areas of hotels and motels. It was first introduced in 1984 and upgraded in 1991, and is now considered state-of-the-art in upholstered furniture flammability standards.

TB 133 standards require that seating be tested as a complete unit, rather than as individual components, to ensure that, when exposed to open flame ignition, the product self-extinguishes and contributes little fuel or heat. The amount of smoke and toxic gases generated is also measured. Only the manufacturer can certify that the upholstered product meets California TB 133.[6]

Though TB 133 has not been adopted in every state, the standards it sets are law in some states and pending in others. It is endorsed by the furniture industry, as well as by governmental and fire fighting organizations, as state-of-the-art. Using TB 133 standards assures that you are specifying the safest available products. For professional designers specifying COM (customer's own material) there are many materials and COM fabrics available now to create TB 133-compliant products, helping to ensure the safety of residents in healthcare settings.

Furniture and seating for healthcare use should be specified to the more stringent commercial or contract quality standards. Contract quality has higher specification demands and sturdier construction than residential products. Residential seating, for example, is not made to withstand the same weight tolerances or abuse standards to which contract seating must to comply. There may be no recognizable difference in the residential look of a chair, but a great difference in construction.

Whether you're looking at dining chairs or upholstered seating, always sit in chairs to check for stability, height, fit, and comfort. Buyers should be cautious of manufacturer's designations such as "healthcare chair" or "for use by the elderly." These catchy phrases can be just that—far from reliable and certainly no guarantee. Most reputable manufacturers will provide seating products for onsite performance testing. Being familiar with selection criteria will also save many costly mistakes.

Tables

Chairs and tables should work comfortably together. The arms of chairs should fit under the table, to allow residents to get as close as possible for dining or for working on a task or project. Standard table height is 29 inches and, to accommodate for wheelchairs, 34 inches high. Though it is not necessary that all tables be adjustable, tables are available with adjustable height bases to increase flexibility.

Checklist for Seating

❑ Specify chairs of contract, versus residential, quality. Proper construction, stability, and good pitch are assets to residents' mobility.

❑ Use chairs with arms in all areas—dining room, activity rooms, living rooms, and bedrooms.

❑ Use chairs whose arms extend beyond the seat.

❑ Provide a variety of chair styles and sizes.

❑ Size the chair to the person—people come in different sizes.

❑ Make sure that chairs fit and support. Good back support holds an individual upright and helps to prevent incontinence and fatigue.

❑ Select chairs that are not too low, too soft, or too deep to exit easily.

❑ Make sure that a person can sit comfortably, with feet flat on the floor.

❑ Make sure that seat heights are appropriate for the elderly, 18 to 19 ½ inches.

❑ Choose seating with smooth edges, rounded corners, and a generous feeling.

❑ Look for a crumb space around the inside, back, and arms to assist in cleaning.

❑ Look for specially treated fabrics, which afford extra protection and durability without sacrificing beauty, quality, and choice of design.

For socializing and dining, tables seating two or four residents are preferable. Square or rectangular table configurations allow combining to expand surface size when needed. The straight sides of a table also allow residents to have their own territory. Placemats help to define the space even more.

Elderly residents often use furniture for balance and support, and tables with four legs are more stable than those with a pedestal (see Figure 16-9). A 42-inch square table should provide adequate room for wheelchair accessibility, as well. Table tops are available in wood, laminate, and a variety of other materials. Wood is warm and residential. Laminate tops can provide color and the opportunity for a contrasting border, which is helpful to many residents in identifying the boundary of the table. All edges should be bullnosed or rounded to prevent injury from sharp edges.

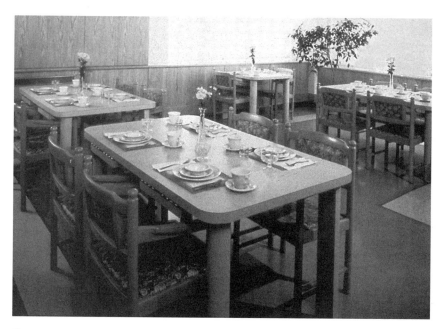

Figure 16-9 Elderly residents often use furniture for balance and support; tables with four legs offer support. The Cafe in the Norma and Joseph Saul Alzheimer's Disease Special Care Unit. *Courtesy of The Norma and Joseph Saul Alzheimer's Disease Special Care Unit at the Jewish Home and Hospital for Aged, Bronx, NY.*

Tables with "spill-free" edges help to restrain spills and keep food and liquid spills on the table rather than in the lap. The raised rim with a rounded, soft edge is soft and warm to the touch of delicate skin.

Many accidents in the bedroom occur as the resident is getting out of bed. The one table that often seems to be missing is a bedside table with a light underneath to be used as a night-light. This light could be turned on when needed or left on through the night for the same purpose. Switching should be manual or motion sensitive, or ideally both.

Hospital beds are not the norm in a residential healthcare setting. There are many residential styles available from which to choose when specifying contract quality beds (see the example in Figure 16-10). Headboards, familiar items found in many homes, lend a homelike, residential quality; footboards are optional.

A word of caution when specifying single beds. There are twin beds and dormitory beds. They are both single beds, but they are not the same. Dormitory beds are not appropriate for the elderly. They are longer than a twin bed by 4 to 5 inches, and not as wide, rather about 3 inches narrower. This creates a dangerous situation for many elderly residents who are used to sleeping in a larger bed and are adjusting to sleeping in a smaller twin bed. A dormitory bed reduces the space that

Beds

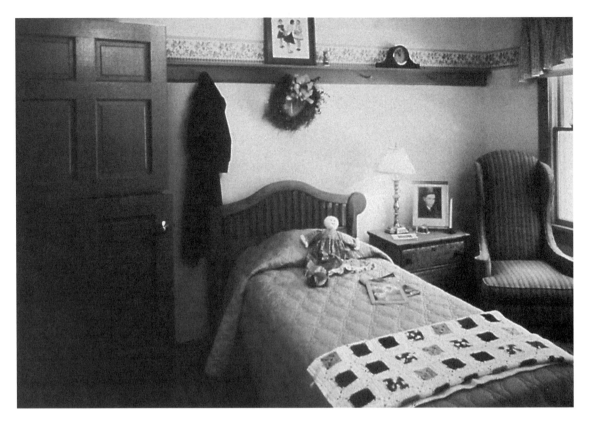

Figure 16-10 There are residential-style beds that give a more homelike feeling to residents' bedrooms. Woodside Place, Oakmont, PA. *Courtesy of Perkins Eastman Architects PC, Pittsburgh, PA. Photographer: Robert Ruschak.*

they are used to by several valuable inches. Since most residents are women, the extra length is usually unnecessary and takes valuable space away from the volume of the room. Residents with Alzheimer's disease are not able to make the normal adjustments that we take for granted, and for them the smaller bed size is a real danger. Unable to compensate for the smaller space, these individuals risk falling out of bed. Bed linens and mattress are also not standard sizes.

Products labeled for healthcare do not differentiate pediatrics from geriatrics, and healthcare labels do not mean products have been designed or adapted for the special needs of the elderly or the cognitively impaired. You must do your homework to be able to identify the selection criteria in order to measure whether a product meets the needs of your design. Manufacturers' sales representatives are not intentionally misleading, but usually don't know or understand the specific needs of geriatrics or of residents with Alzheimer's disease.

Residential care settings emphasize creating a homelike surrounding, but the materials used must still enhance function and have the "industrial strength" quality required to weather the use and abuse of assistive equipment and the routine application of strong cleaning agents. Products from manufacturers familiar with healthcare needs and use should be relied on to meet the important responsibility to good resident care.

Making appropriate fabric selections for healthcare settings requires information about the latest fabrics and finishes now available, maintenance and cleaning concerns, flammability requirements, infection control, and fabric enhancements. Upholstery fabrics specified for heavy-wear, high-stain areas must be increasingly stain-resistant to be cleaned effectively, preferably by in-house maintenance staff (see Figure 16-11).

In the last ten years the number of inherently flame-retardant fabrics available for healthcare use has increased immensely. Today there are numerous colors, patterns, and textures appropriate for draperies, bedspreads, shower curtains, cubicle curtains, and upholstery. Inherently flame-retardant polyester not only maintains its flame-retardant properties after continuous laundering, but it is dimensionally stable, so that drapery or bedspread measurements remain constant. Though flame-retardant fabrics are not required in many states for residential healthcare settings, they are very affordably priced and when they are used, resident safety is increased immeasurably.

Fabrics

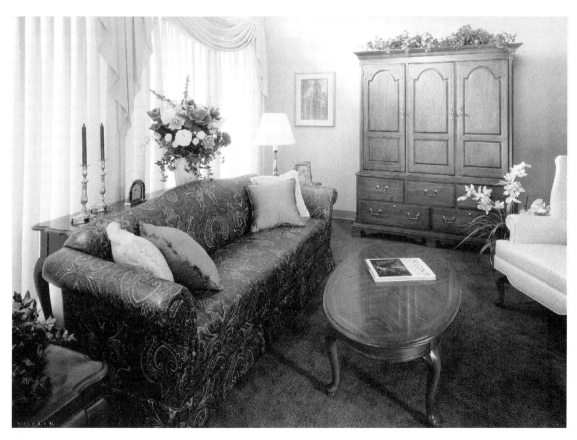

Figure 16-11 Making appropriate fabric selections for heavy-wear, high-stain areas in healthcare settings requires accurate information about fabrics and finishes. *Courtesy of Spruce Point Assisted Living Community, Florence, OR. Interior design: Cynthia Warner, Warner Design Associates. Photographer: Tom Rider.*

Fabrics may be inherently flame-retardant, as FR Trevira polyester and SEF modacrylic, or flame-retardant finishes may be topically applied.[7] It is important to be aware, however, that topical finishes must be applied and certified by professional finishers. Most designers are able to assist in this process.

One of the latest and most innovative introductions to the healthcare fabric market is Crypton, a totally new fabric that is water and stain resistant, antimicrobial, antifungal, antibacterial, extremely strong, and breathable. Crypton is not a coating or treatment sprayed on the fabric; instead each fiber is immersed so that Crypton becomes permanently encased in every fiber of the material.[8] The major advantages of this new fabric over vinyl is that the fabric breathes and fire blockers and moisture barriers are laminated to the back of the fabric, leaving the fabric face with the original texture. Fabrics retain the look and feel that is familiar and creating environments more like home is possible.

Crypton is ideal for use in healthcare settings and other high abuse areas. It is used for upholstery purposes. Many patterns are available and it passes TB 133. The fabric performs best when laminated to Intek Firegard or Kevlar.

Maintenance and Cleaning

How should healthcare textiles be cleaned? Fabrics should be sprayed with an upholstery prespray and allowed to sit for ten minutes. This step should be followed by wet extraction using a liquid rinsing and emulsifying agent. This approach represents a "steam cleaning" procedure, commonly the first step in upholstery stain removal. This method is effective in removing coffee, cola, urine, cough syrup, Maalox, mayonnaise, and blood. For oil-based and greasy stains, apply a solvent prior to steam cleaning. Always check for the manufacturer's recommended cleaning instructions.

Spills and cleaning solutions that bleed through fabric into cushions result in reoccurring spots and almost always mean reupholstering furniture. The largest fabric cleaning problems are blood, betadine, food grease, and dirt. Most healthcare settings want a vinylized fabric that is easy to clean, but has the look and texture of woven fabric, and textured fabric that has the stain-proof, leak-proof characteristics of vinyl.[9] With the new products coming on the market today, we are beginning to more effectively meet those needs.

Since today's upholstered fabrics must sometimes serve as fluid barriers, and still meet stringent new fire codes in complex assemblies, manufacturers are upgrading their healthcare textiles with high-tech finishes. The following is a list of some of the latest available enhancements.

- *Soil- and stain-resistant finishes and stain-repellent treatments*

  New types of machine-applied Scotchgard and Teflon treatments are environmentally compliant. Innovative, partial-clear face coatings can provide good, durable resistance to certain healthcare stains and easy cleaning of most stains.

- *Laminating*

  Teflon-coated fabrics, dark colors, chintzes, treviras can all be laminated with a matte vinyl finish. The process has now progressed to the point where even complex, textured weaves can be satisfactorily vinylized with durable vinyl films. These films are applied with high-bond strength that should not delaminate during normal wear.

- *Flammability*

  In addition to conventional topical flame-retardant treatments, inherently flame-retardant fibers, such as FR Trevira polyester and SEF modacrylic, and the wide use of fire barriers, potent new FR backcoatings have been developed. Fire barriers such as Firegard F187 and Kevlar Z-11 can be laminated to most upholstery fabrics to increase performance in meeting California TB 133. This option also eliminates the need for double upholstering.[10]

- *Fluid barriers*

  To preserve upholstery fabric, impermeable fluid barriers that prevent penetration of body fluids or spills into the upholstery are commonly applied to the fabric back. Established anti-microbial fluid barriers, such as Staph-Check, can also be laminated to virtually all upholstery fabrics. Trilaminates, involving fluid and fire barriers, can also be provided.

- *Anti-microbial finishes*

  Anti-microbial finishes inhibit the growth of microorganisms and, if not already standard, can be provided with most healthcare fabrics.

Creating settings that are familiar and bear a remarkable resemblance to home is complex, but becoming a less daunting challenge all the time. The enhanced range of options in fabric, furnishings, floorcovering, wallcovering, and finishes increases the possibility of providing aesthetically inviting environments while at the same time meeting the functional and healthcare needs of elderly residents.

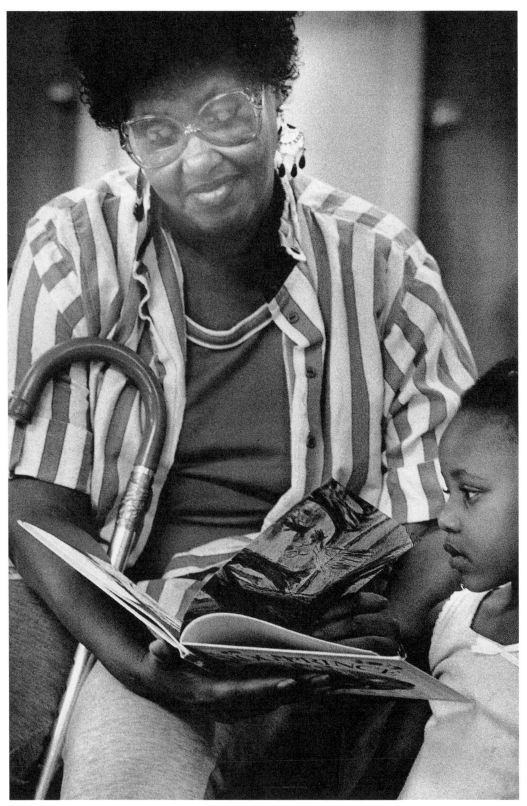

Courtesy of Nevins Family of Services, Methuen, MA.

CHAPTER 17

Floorcovering

Glare from overhead lighting and skylights, reflected on a highly polished floor surface, produces discomfort or disability glare, causing the elderly to squint, partially close their eyes when walking, or worse still, to become immobile. Good design can mitigate the risk of falls and disorientation with better lighting, reduction of glare, and the selection of nonslip and nonglare surfaces. This situation is easily rectified by using the appropriate carpet, which absorbs the light and eliminates the glare.

Flooring materials can be divided into three broad categories: resilient flooring, hard-surface flooring, and carpet. Resilient and hard surface flooring have been the traditional materials used in healthcare in the past. More recently, however, technical advances in the infection-control and stain-resistance properties of carpet have made it a viable alternative.

Carpet

Carpet adds visual warmth to a setting and improves the acoustical environment, making it seem more homelike (see Figure 17-1). Texture eliminates fatiguing glare produced by hard surfaces, provides better traction than hard flooring, and a softer surface in case of an unfortunate fall.

233

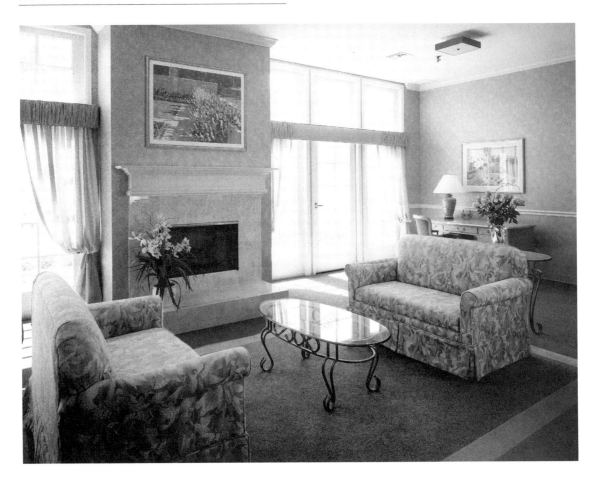

Figure 17-1 Carpet adds warmth and gives the setting a more residential look. It eliminates glare, improves the acoustical environment, and provides a safer walking surface. *Courtesy of Guardian of Rossmoor, Rossmoor, CA. Interior design: Cynthia Warner, Warner Design Associates. Photographer: Tom Rider.*

Thanks to advancements in technology and in fiber engineering, the long-term cost of maintaining high performance carpet is probably less than one-fifth the cost of caring for hard-surface floors. The initial installation costs can be higher, but with a sound maintenance program, savings can be significant.

Of all textile products used in healthcare settings, carpet is subjected to the most severe treatment in terms of foot traffic, soiling, and staining. Many factors have a strong influence on the performance, aesthetics, and value of carpet. In light of traffic, spills, and other severe environmental conditions to which carpet is subjected, it is not surprising that some carpets don't perform well. What is more surprising is how well some carpets do perform when they are: (1) well constructed of (2) fibers with superior engineering, (3) properly installed, and (4) properly maintained.[1]

Fiber/Yarn

A wide variety of polymers and natural fibers are used to produce carpet, but in healthcare the predominant fibers are nylon, olefin (polypropylene), and wool. Nylon is by far the most prevalent fiber in use and accounts for 70 percent of the market. The two types of nylon used as carpet fibers are Type 6.6 and Type 6. The main differences between the two are associated with the manufacturing and dyeing processes. Either is excellent for use in healthcare settings. All nylon fibers share certain characteristics that make nylon ideal for use in floorcovering:

- Exceptional strength and durability
- High abrasion resistance
- Excellent resilience
- Superior dyeing flexibility
- Smooth surface

Olefin, or polypropylene, does not have the high resilience of nylon or the flexibility in dyeing. While it does perform well in low traffic areas, it is primarily used when budget is more important than overall performance. Because wool is more expensive, it is used most often in board rooms or conference rooms.

The ultimate success of a carpet specification will depend on a proper balance of performance, aesthetics, and cost factors. Face construction, color, backing makeup, and proper cleaning are all important to long-term appearance retention or useful life. The factors of carpet construction that have the greatest impact on overall performance are yarn twist, pile height, and density, which is the amount of pile yarn in a given volume of carpet face. For a given carpet weight, lower pile height and higher pile yarn density will give the best performance for the money.

When color choice is important, better results can be achieved with yarn dyed nylon. When coupled with a nonflow–through vinyl backing, both yarn dyed and solution dyed floorcovering products can be cleaned equally well. Today's yarn dyed Type 6.6 nylon offers light fastness and performance equal to that of like-constructed products. Because the yarn is colored during the extrusion process, solution dyed nylon does offer some cost savings. Though yarn dyed nylon is less resistant to bleach, chlorinated cleaning products will cause severe fiber degradation with any nylon product.

Many carpets manufactured for specific use in healthcare settings now use antimicrobial carpet fibers, and other finishes that further reduce microbial buildup. The main advantage of these special finishes seems to be in preventing odors from bacterial decomposition caused by spills. Urine is the most serious problem if it penetrates the pile and soaks into the carpet backing.[2] Using an antimicrobial treatment does not eliminate maintenance. Cleaning can reduce microbial counts. Ideally, vacuum cleaning in healthcare settings should incorporate the use of a high-efficiency particulate air filter (HEPA) bag, so that bacteria which are picked up are not blown back into the air from machine exhaust.

All carpets sold in the United States must meet the federal flammability standards; local and regional standards also exist.

Floorcovering is one area where manufacturers have stepped up to the challenge of meeting special needs. There are excellent products now available for use in long-term care settings, which should inspire confidence. Nonflow–through moisture barriers keep moisture on the surface, where it can be readily cleaned.

Most of us have been victims of the unpleasant experience of NHO (nursing home odor). The greatest source of that odor is fluid that has penetrated the concrete slab or subflooring; in this case, surface cleaning is only wiping the surface and not removing the source of the problem. The subfloor must be sealed. If renovating, the floorcovering must be removed, and the underlayment must be first steam cleaned to remove the odor and bacteria and then sealed. A nonflow–through moisture barrier product and chemically welded seams provide additional protection. Every seam is another opportunity for seepage and when incontinence is an issue, minimizing the number of seams is essential. For this reason, carpet tiles are not a recommended solution in healthcare settings for the elderly.

Installation

Planning a quality new carpet installation is just as important as determining which carpet to purchase. For many years direct-glue has been the recommended method of installation, but again, technology has provided major improvement in installation methods. Products such as Collins and Aikman's Powerbond RS provide a clean, quick installation with no lingering odors. Powerbond incorporates its own unique tackifier and eliminates the need for wet adhesives. Installers just measure it, roll it up, peel the temporary protective plastic off, and roll it back out. A major source of offensive odor, carpet adhesive, is removed, and the carpet is traffic ready the moment it's rolled into place.

Resilient Flooring

Resilient flooring comprises sheet vinyl, vinyl tile, sheet rubber, and rubber tiles. Not only has resilient flooring made considerable advances in visual appeal, but the performance aspects in reducing sound transmission and improving slip resistance have improved. Resilient tile is one of today's most widely used resilient flooring materials.

Maintenance is perhaps the biggest drawback to the use of resilient flooring in residential settings for the elderly. As long as highly polished floors continue to be a standard, they continue to be a particular danger for older users. The glare generated from these highly buffed and polished surfaces could be classified as a form of passive restraint. The floor surface often appears wet or slick and is a source of anxiety, fear, and confusion for elderly residents. Their eyes can't adjust quickly enough when high levels of glare are present, and the resulting fear often keeps them immobile.

Toli Mature from Toli International combines the warm realistic look of wood in a heavy duty solid vinyl sheet flooring. This combination allows the look of hardwood floors in a low sheen, no-wax sheet vinyl, ideal for kitchens and small dining rooms. Another of their products, Spectraflors, introduces light texture in a sheet vinyl product that, when it remains unpolished as intended, helps to combat the problem of glare. A nice exapmle is shown in Figure 17-2.

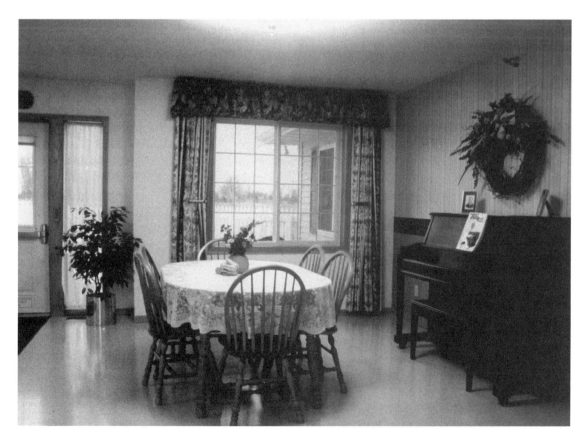

Figure 17-2 Resilient flooring with low sheen and improved slip resistance was used in this informal dining room. *Kensington Cottages at Mankato, Mankato, MN. Courtesy of Kensington Cottages Corporation, Golden Valley, MN.*

Rubber flooring is generally slip resistant, which helps to reduce falls in areas where water or other liquids may be present. The best rubber floors are soft and resilient, although raised patterns can present problems in walking for some residents, especially those who tend to shuffle.

Other Considerations in Floorcovering Selection

Strong contrast should be evident between the walls and the floor. Base trim molding should be matched to the wall color to give a clear, distinct contrast where the floor plane meets the vertical wall. When the flooring is coved or the base molding is matched to the floor, it can give a false sense of boundaries.

Often persons with Alzheimer's disease have impaired depth perception, which can cause a sharp contrast in color or pattern on the floor to be misunderstood as a change in depth. While pattern can be used in other areas, for the visually impaired and the mentally confused, pattern underfoot generates problems with perception and balance, which ultimately affects mobility.

Whatever the flooring selection, all floorcovering should be flush and even, with no frayed edges, loose strings, or loose tiles that might cause a resident to trip or fall. All floor surfaces should be wheelchair compatible, whether resilient flooring or carpet designed for healthcare.

Transitions from one type of flooring material to another must be as smooth and as level as possible. Because a transition may alter the color and texture of the floor, it can create the illusion, or the reality, of a difference in height, and can cause problems for older people with perceptual problems. To accommodate wheelchairs, shuffling feet, and walking aids, flooring transitions should be no greater than half an inch. Thresholds should be avoided whenever possible; they are a problem for older people who have difficulty adjusting their walking to the demands of different floor surfaces when they pass from one surface to another.[3] When they are unavoidable, their edges should be beveled, not abrupt or sharp. Area rugs are lovely but they are a trip hazard. For the visually impaired, the cognitively impaired, and the not so sure of foot, an uninterrupted walking surface is safer.

Carpet that has a nonflow–through moisture barrier, designed for use in healthcare settings, can be used in both hallways and resident bedrooms. Walking is easier for the resident when there is no transition from the hallway to the bedroom, and maintenance is easier when there is a single continuous surface to be cleaned. When surface transitions are made, for example between the bedroom and bathroom, if the same color intensity is maintained the visual perception is likely to be of a solid surface, even though the floorcovering is different.

It is important to have a consistent and thorough maintenance plan, plus a plan to address unusual spills. Proper and regular maintenance of any flooring material prolongs its life and maintains its appearance. The carpet maintenance plan should result from careful consideration of the carpet manufacturer's recommendations for cleaning methods.

Any floorcovering needs to be maintained and maintained properly, according to the manufacturers' recommended cleaning and maintenance methods. There are many new products on the market today that have been designed to meet specific needs. Floorcovering manufacturers have improved products immensely, but the improvements may be wasted if they are not maintained properly. No-wax resilient floors come with instructions on cleaning and specific instructions: Do Not Wax. It is up to consumers to read the instructions and make sure that the maintenance instructions are followed.

Reputable floorcovering manufacturer's representatives will provide on-site training sessions for maintenance teams on request. Particularly for new products, or for anyone using the products for the first time, this is a terrific advantage. Maintenance manuals or instructions for some products are available in Spanish, Chinese, and other languages as well as in English.

The only downside to using carpeting in any healthcare setting is the noisy extractor used for cleaning. Surely, in this day and age of technology revolution, someone can design a piece of equipment that minimizes the noise and the required drying time. Noise for the elderly, particularly those coping with Alzheimer's disease, is detrimental and dangerous. It is a major contributor to confusion, and causes agitation and sometimes catastrophic behavior. It seems so unnecessary. Solving this dilemma would not only win thanks from elderly residents, but kudos from others who have to deal with the noise and the results.

Maintenance

Checklist for Floorcovering Success

1. Correct Product Selection

☐ Select a product specifically designed to meet healthcare needs.

☐ Resilient floors:

    ☐ Look for nonslip surface.

    ☐ Choose a nonreflective finish.

☐ Carpet:

    ☐ Choose carpet with dense-face construction (level loop or dense cut pile twist construction).

    ☐ Choose carpet designed to withstand high traffic.

    ☐ Choose rolling-traffic friendly carpet.

    ☐ Specify nonflow–through vinyl moisture barrier back.

    ☐ Specify bound, nonleaching antimicrobial system.

    ☐ Choose Type 6.6 yarn dyed or solution dyed nylon.

    ☐ Make sure your choice is colorfast.

    ☐ Select a suitable color variety (clear, not grayed or muddy color).

    ☐ Minimize odor and fumes by minimizing use of wet adhesives.

2. Proper Preparation

    ☐ New construction: seal underlayment.

    ☐ Renovation: Remove floor covering and steam clean underlayment, more than once if necessary to remove odor, and seal.

3. Proper Installation

    ☐ Follow manufacturer's recommended directions.

    ☐ Minimize transitions and threshold heights.

4. Proper Maintenance

    ☐ Clean and maintain carpet on a regular basis.

    ☐ Use manufacturer's recommended cleaning methods.

NOTES

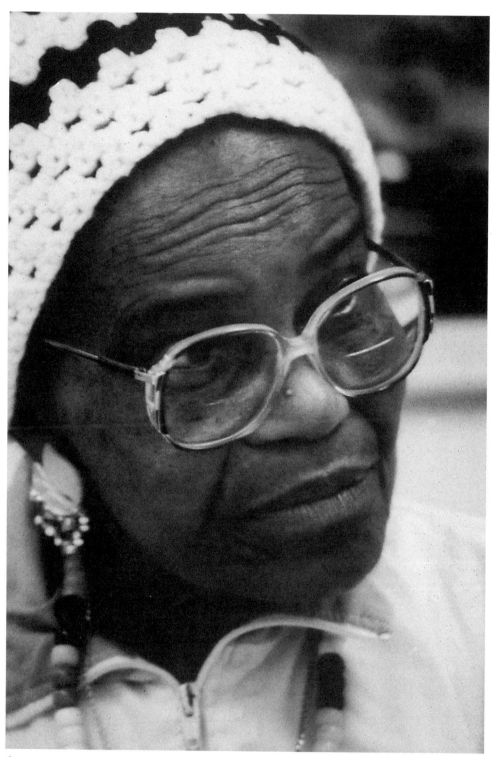

Courtesy of the Greater San Francisco Bay Area Alzheimer's Association. Photographer: Anna M. Rossi.

18

Wall Finishes and Ceiling Finishes

Paint colors, wallcoverings, floorcoverings, window treatments, and specialty decorative finishes are products carefully chosen to meet the unique requirements of healthcare settings. Designers have been instrumental in helping to change the role wallcoverings play in the design of today's healthcare environments. It wasn't so long ago that healthcare settings shied away from patterned wall coverings, fearing people would get tired of them; what they didn't consider was that people also tire of endless pale green painted walls or—even worse for sensory deprivation—pure white.

Wallcoverings

Wallcoverings have helped humanize healthcare environments, and are are one of the details that can make a setting more reminiscent of home, as shown in Figure 18-1. Pattern and color in both wallcovering and decorative border patterns have helped to enliven some otherwise unexciting settings. Living rooms, dining rooms, kitchens, and bathrooms are all familiar rooms where most people expect to find wallpaper used as a wall finish. Because of their durability and

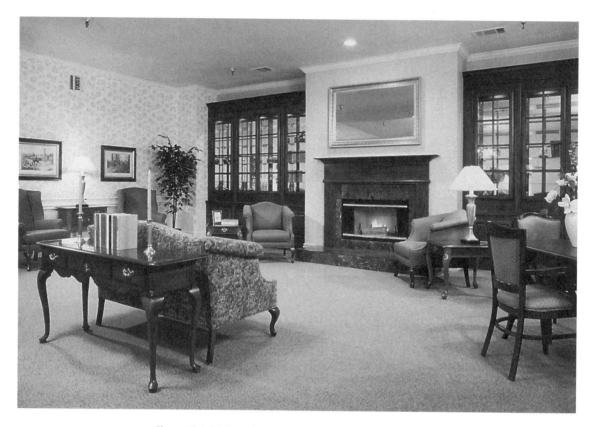

Figure 18-1 Wallcovering is one of the details that can make a setting more reminiscent of home. *Courtesy of Guardian of Concord, Concord, CA. Interior design: Cynthia Warner, Warner Design Associates.*

range of styles and colors, vinyl wallcoverings are used in residential healthcare environments to soften the setting.

In small areas, use wallpaper on all four walls to avoid visually breaking up the space and creating unintended confusion; using wallcovering on all walls provides consistency. In larger rooms, however, wallpapering only one wall can be successful. Kitchens, resident bathrooms, dining rooms, living rooms, alcoves, bathing rooms, and public bathrooms are all appropriate spaces where wallcovering adds to the residential quality and enhances the setting.

Vinyl wallcovering is fabric backed. The fabric backing provides stability and a bonding medium between the vinyl and the hanging surface so that it will retain adhesive. Vinyl wallcoverings should be specified by type and by weight:

- *Type I:* A light-duty wallcovering (7 to 13 ounces)
- *Type II:* A medium-duty wallcovering (13 to 22 ounces)
- *Type III:* A heavy-duty wallcovering (in excess of 22 ounces)

Protective coatings applied to vinyl wallcoverings help the product deliver maximum performance in terms of cleanability and long-lasting wear. Coated wallcoverings are especially good choices for installation in corridors where soiling is a serious problem.

Because so many of the greatest impact and soiling problems occur in corridors, this area demands high performance standards. Hallways and corridors are most often areas without windows or the ability to borrow illumination from another room, so an appropriate selection of light colors is essential. Corridors need 21- to 26-ounce vinyl with a protective coating.

Protective Finishes

One distinguishing breakthrough in vinyl wallcovering is the application of protective coatings, such as Tedlar film laminate, PreFixx protective finish, and Towercote and TEF acrylic coatings, to meet specific challenges that require extra protection. Each has distinct advantages, but common to all these protective coatings is their ability to retard staining. Their differences are the amount of time before staining occurs and the cleaning agents needed to remove the stains. Regular vinyl wallcoverings have a finishing coat with an added layer of acrylic that guards against routine soil.[1]

Most protective finishes can be cleaned with any nonabrasive household detergent without damage to the surface. If stains remain, solvents can be used on some finishes; it is important, however, to know the finish and the cleaning methods recommended. Not all protective finishes have the same recommended cleaning methods.

Regular unprotected vinyl offers limited protection against serious stains. Many of the patterns specified by designers are vinyl wallcoverings that would be found in the kitchens, bathrooms, and other areas where we use wallcovering in homes. The residential patterns we use in our own homes are still sadly lacking in the heavier wallcoverings normally specified for healthcare use. The result is that in many cases we specify Type I wallcovering to get the patterns and colors that remind us of home, instead of heavier Type II wallcovering designed for increased action and abuse. Protective finishes help to minimize the risk.

All of the protective finishes described contain an antimicrobial additive that's effective against the growth of many mold, mildew, fungal, and bacterial organisms. Some also have an antistaph protection. Mildew is a difficult problem in specific situations and in some areas of the country. Manufacturers can advise on preparations and protective measures for specific situations.

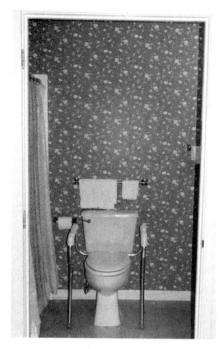

Figure 18-2 Wallpaper in the bathroom gives a more residential appearance and provides contrast between the toilet and the wall. *Courtesy of Tulip Garden, Decatur, GA.*

Many designers specify either Type I or Type II wallcoverings for residential healthcare, protected with a delustered acrylic protective finish. In many cases there is no added charge for the protective finish; it's simply a matter of knowing what to ask for or specify.

As healthcare moves toward more residential and homelike environments, wallcovering can be one of the most cost-effective ways to transform institutional settings to something more familiar, to breathe new life into the humdrum environments of residential and nursing care settings, to make them more like home. See, for example, the bathroom shown in Figure 18-2. It's one of the products we've traditionally used in our homes, and the visual appeal and the versatility of prints and textures, coupled with the benefits of protective finishes, can make it a preferable wall finish. With the trend of more residential looks in healthcare settings, particularly for the elderly, manufacturers of wallcovering could help by providing wallcovering patterns, currently produced for home use, in heavier weights suitable for use in residential healthcare settings.

Paint Selections for Healthcare

The selection of the right coating system or paint is an important element and an important step in updating residential healthcare settings. Today manufacturers offer a wide variety of architectural and industrial grade paints to meet almost every application need. Knowing how a paint will perform and matching those capabilities to the job requirements helps to narrow the choices. There are three basic paint ingredients—binder, pigment, and solvent—and the amount of these components in the paint has a direct impact on its performance.[2]

- *Binder:* This is the material that gives paint its ability to form a finishing film. The binder will affect durability, adhesion, and color retention.
- *Pigment:* Pigment is a powdery substance that gives paint its color and hiding capacities, along with thickness or "body."
- *Solvent:* This is the liquid component that gives paint its spreadability.

When selecting paint, it is important to consider performance characteristics. Top quality paint contains more solids (pigment and binder) than less expensive paints and offers superior durability and color retention. Less expensive paints often require multiple coats and generally do not perform as well.

Architectural paints are available in two types: latex (water based) and alkyd (oil based). Paint industry experts feel that vinyl acrylic binders in latex paint are superior in their ability to resist cracking, flaking, chipping, and fading. In addition, latex offers low odor, fast drying time, easy cleanup with soap and water, and smoother, easier application than alkyds.

The area where the paint is used will help determine the best choice for the job. The paint used in bathing rooms and showers must hold up to heat, humidity, and the expansion and contraction of surfaces, and that in hallways and corridors must endure constant cleaning with harsh, possibly abrasive agents. Semigloss and higher gloss finishes provide extra durability and stain resistance, but these benefits must be measured against the effects of glare in environments for the elderly. Even though high gloss paints are more durable, the benefits of an eggshell finish for elderly residents far exceed the durability of the paint, and consequently, it it a better selection. A nonglare eggshell finish used with a border print, possibly selected by the resident, individualizes a room and gives it a more personal look. Flat finishes should be used with a primer to maximize the performance of the top coat.

Surface Preparation

As with all finishes, preparation is key. Properly prepared surfaces ensure paint's ability to adhere and prolong the service life. Over 80 percent of all paint failures can be attributed to inadequate surface preparation. Surfaces must be clean and smooth and should be dry and free of mildew and other stains. For best results paint should be applied at temperatures between 50 and 85 degrees Fahrenheit.

Since paint is available in many grades and finishes, knowledge of the product and its capabilities and expectations based on the needs will help in making the most appropriate selection for the job.

Ceiling Finishes

One of the greatest differences between homes and institutional settings is the quality of the acoustic environment. Most healthcare settings have incorporated hard, smooth, nonporous surfaces that cause sound to bounce from one surface to another without being absorbed. Every design element contributes to a successful outcome, including the ceiling. An acoustical ceiling, in conjunction with other furnishing, will generally provide adequate sound absorption and noise reduction.

Design professionals recognize the importance of high performance products when designing for the healthcare environment. Acoustical ceilings and walls together absorbs sound reverberation and are the best way to control noise. Using carpet, in addition, will absorb footfall and some ambient noise.

A relatively new product in the American market, Eurostone Safety Ceiling, is an acoustical tile with no man-made mineral fibers to contribute to Sick Building Syndrome, and no organic binders to support growth of mold, mildew, fungus, or bacteria. It meets all fire safety codes, and best of all, Eurostone does not absorb moisture, which makes it ideal for use in bathing rooms and bathrooms, as well as the rest of the healthcare setting.

Another acoustical ceiling product is Armstrong's Cirrus ceiling, which offers a visual alternative with "Stars" and "Leaves." These patterns, designs carved into individual ceiling panels, can be interspersed with the selected acoustical ceiling. One star, for example, or many may be used and they can also be painted. This product demonstrates sensitivity and awareness of what a resident sees when lying in bed looking at the ceiling.

For painted ceilings, a color similar to the walls but lighter will make a small room seem larger. The ceiling should always be white, however, for higher reflectance qualities. Adding one-half gallon of the wall color to every five gallons of ceiling white gives the ceiling a soft tint, while still maintaining the reflectance quality, attaining both goals.[3]

Checklist for Wallcovering Success

1. Correct Product Selection
- ❏ Paint or wallcovering:
  - ❏ Choose a nonreflective finish.

- ❏ Wallcovering:
  - ❏ Use Type I or Type II (weight sufficient to withstand abuse).
  - ❏ Choose a wallcovering designed to withstand high traffic.
  - ❏ Specify protective finish if needed.
  - ❏ Specify antimicrobial backing.
  - ❏ Choose a pattern appropriate for elderly, low vision, and cognitive impairment.
  - ❏ Choose a clear, not grayed or muddy, color.
  - ❏ Make sure there will be no off-gassing odors.

2. Proper Preparation
- ❏ New construction: Seal underlayment and prime according to manufac-tur-er's instructions.
- ❏ Renovation: Remove old material, repair, seal, and prime.

3. Proper Installation
- ❏ Follow manufacturer's recommended directions.
- ❏ Use corner guards in high traffic areas; they are available in clear or color.
  - Match color as closely as possible to wall covering to avoid distraction.

4. Proper Maintenance
- ❏ Clean and maintain on a regular basis.
- ❏ Use manufacturer's recommended cleaning methods.

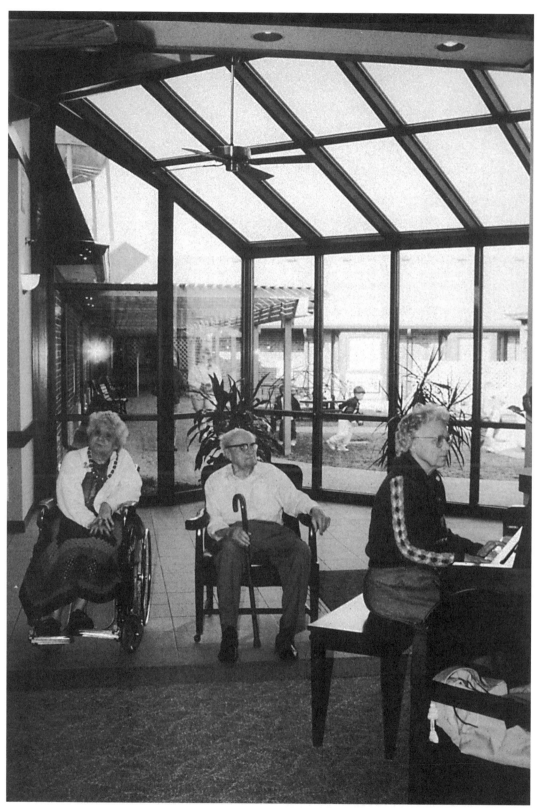

Courtesy of Foxwood Springs Living Centers, Raymore, MO.

19

Windows and Window Treatments

Many elderly people need a high level of illumination, without the hazard of painful, uncomfortable glare. Windows can be the source of natural light and pleasure if they are well placed and shielded to diffuse light and minimize daylight glare. By using light colors around windows, the reflective value can be increased by as much as 80 percent, and window treatments, such as translucent shades or sheer draperies, diffuse light and minimize daylight glare. Carpet dramatically reduces glare that can confuse an elderly person, and coupled with better lighting, minimizes the likelihood of falls and creates a safer environment.

Window Height

Lowering window sills to about 15 to 20 inches above the floor in the living room, dining room, or bedroom windows allows individuals who are seated to see outside (see Figure 19-1). Window seats can provide extra seating and keep individuals from walking into the window. In bedrooms for cognitively impaired residents, special precautions must be taken to use strong window frames and window stops. These

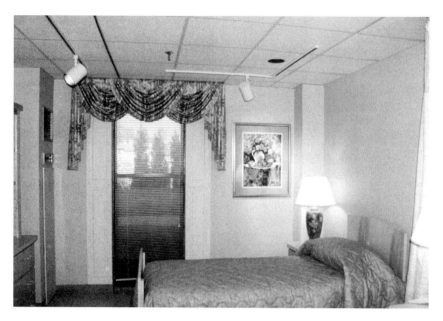

Figure 19-1 Lowering window sills will allow residents who are sitting or in bed to easily see outside. The attractive window treatment makes the window seem larger than it actually is. *Courtesy of Lenbrook Square, Atlanta, GA. Interior design: Linda Watson, ASID, Watson Limited Planning and Design.*

stops should allow a resident to open a window far enough for ventilation, but not enough to enable the resident to climb out.

The choices in window treatments are almost as broad and diverse as the varied number of sizes and shapes of windows themselves. Whether the windows are long or short, wide or narrow, flat or divided by mullions, most share one major requirement: the need for a window treatment that helps to regulate and control natural light. Adjustable window coverings help to control sunlight and glare.

Blinds

Horizontal blinds or mini blinds, with their tilting capability, will deflect the sun's light. With their ability to regulate the amount of natural light that permeates the room, horizontal blinds can greatly reduce energy requirements. Vertical blinds offer many of the same benefits for controlling natural light through their louver rotation operation. However, both the institutional appearance, and a more important drawback, the unprogrammed activity vertical louvers often provide for residents with cognitive impairment, cause vertical blinds not to be one of the better window covering solutions. In addition, horizontal and vertical blinds may create light patterns that can be quite disturbing visually. While it is not clear whether behavior problems are triggered by disturbing light patterns or lack of positive activity programming, there are still disturbed residents to be calmed.

For softer window treatments, light-filtering pleated shades feature a large selection of more translucent fabrics than either horizontal or vertical blinds, and offer some degree of light regulation. When combined with lambrequins or a variety of decorative valances, such as balloon or cloud shade valances, they also minimize hardness and the institutional look, as the attractive examples in Figures 19-2 and 19-3 demonstrate.

Pleated Shades

Pleated shades are available in fabrics that offer varying degrees of opacity and pleat width, as well as metalized backing that helps reflect the sun and provides the most energy-efficient window covering on the market. Room darkening or blackout linings can be added where necessary. Through the advancement of technology a wide range of flame resistant fabrics and finishes are available. Pleated shades can be custom sized to accommodate almost any window size and shape, and can even be manufactured to operate in reverse. Bottom-up shades allow windows to be exposed at the top and covered at the bottom for privacy.

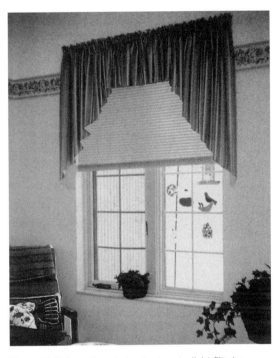

Figure 19-2 For softer window treatments, light-filtering pleated shades help to balance light and control glare. *Courtesy of Presbyterian Senior Care Green House, Oakmont, PA.*

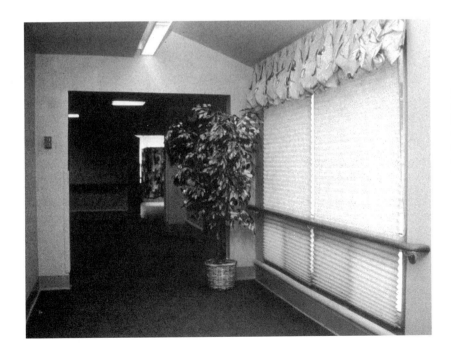

Figure 19-3 The soft valance minimizes the hard, institutional look. *Courtesy of On Lok Senior Health Services, San Francisco, CA. Interior design: Elizabeth Brawley, IIDA, Design Concepts Unlimited.*

Sunscreen Systems

Manual and motorized sunscreen systems are shades of woven FR vinyl sunscreens in a variety of densities that provide solar protection and control of glare and brightness, while maintaining a view to the outside. They look like roller shades and can be used with or without a valance for a decorative effect. These shades can be used to shade oversize windows, as well as custom sized for skylights and greenhouse windows. Even when open, draperies invariably cover part of the window. When attempting to expose the maximum window area to allow as much natural light as possible, these shades provide excellent light filtering qualities and glare control.

Draperies

Draperies are traditional window treatments that soften the window and the room. They can cover a window completely or be used as panels on either side, with or without a valance. They should be combined with either a pleated shade or sheer underdraperies to diffuse the natural light (see Figure 19-4). Fire-resistant (FR) lace is also available for old-fashioned lace curtains.

Traditional drapery hardware should be replaced with Break-A-Way wall-mounted or ceiling-mounted curtain hanging systems. This hardware has no metal pins and relies on Velcro to secure the drapery. This is a much safer system, particularly for confused residents. This same system is available for shower curtains with a selection of FR fabrics.

It is important to control heat and light, preserve privacy, and allow air to circulate. In addition to softening the aesthetics of a room, window treatments add a distinctively homelike quality, with the added advantage of durability, easy maintenance, and energy control.

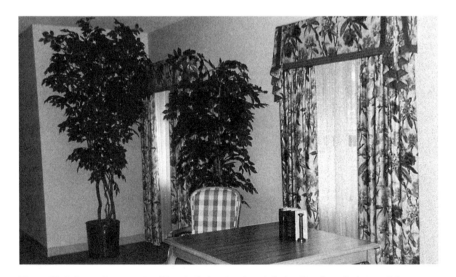

Figure 19-4 Draperies are a traditional window treatment that soften the window and the room.
Courtesy of The Hallmark at Palm Springs, Palm Springs, CA.

SECTION V

The Design Process

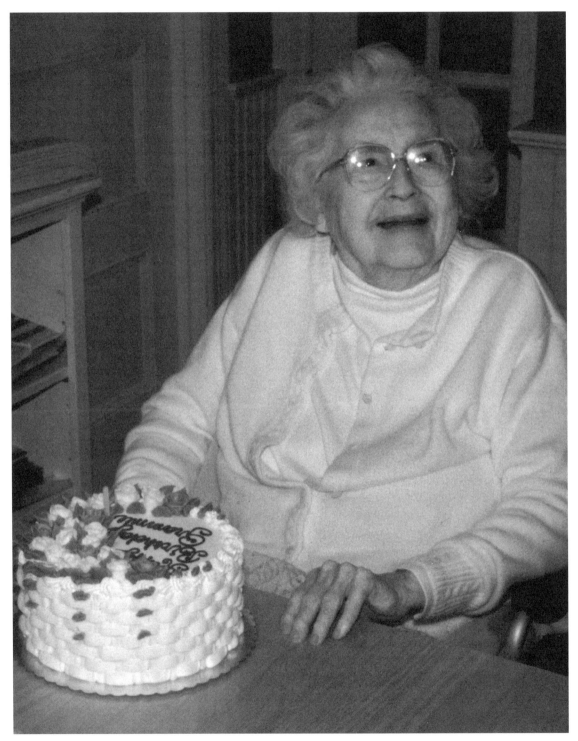

Courtesy of Paul Stevens.

CHAPTER 20

The Team Approach to the Design Process

Good design planning may take more time initially, involve more people, and require asking and debating some tough questions about how designs will function for users; however, if you design well in the first place, costly redesign can be avoided.

Responsible planning results in successful special care settings for individuals with Alzheimer's disease and for the elderly in general — settings that not only work for residents, but for staff, families, and visitors as well. Healthcare professionals who have worked with the frail elderly and with individuals with dementia will tell you that we are still learning, that we don't yet have all the answers. We need to continue to explore practical, innovative ideas based on the results of current research studies. Designing with flexibility and clear intention to accommodate change over time should be inherent in our process. By making an investment in sound planing, we create better environments and a more fulfilling experience for both aging residents and staff.[1]

257

How to Start the Design Process

Step One: Preparation—Creating the Program/Design Team (PDT)©

1. PDT© Selection

It's important to choose the team early to allow everyone to be part of the exploratory and planning process. For example, here's a list of possible team members you may want to consider:

- Architects
- Interior designers
- Administrators
- Nurses
- Maintenance and housekeeping staff
- Activities coordinators

A design project typically involves a team of professionals, and the players on the team might include the owner, the administrator, the architect, the interior designer, the director of nurses, a program or activity coordinator, and housekeeping and maintenance staff members. There may be others you wish to include, either on a permanent or consulting basis. Each person brings a particular expertise and perspective to the group, and it is important to acknowledge individual skills and the possibility that there may be some overlap in skill sets.

It is important that team members and consultants find a way to reach agreement about decision-making procedures and their various roles and responsibilities during the design and implementation process. Project goals and objectives, deciding whose needs should take precedence, are decisions that should be agreed upon early for the process to run smoothly. For the planning and design process to work, it should be shared by all involved.

This is a team process; don't design in a vacuum. The physical setting for this special population isn't just a building. The residents have special needs that, when planned and accommodated well, have a very positive effect on their ability to function and their quality of life. The residents and their activity programs should provide the foundation for the design and define how the building will look and function, not vice versa. The team will need to grapple with the problems presented by the existing building, the problems of the frail, aging residents, and the challenges presented by Alzheimer's disease; they will need to determine how best to support residents.

2. RESEARCH AND INFORMATION GATHERING

It is increasingly common for design professionals to work with behavioral scientists to explore special needs to design effective solutions. To discover solutions, it's essential to know and understand the problems at hand. Effective planning requires you to ask the following questions:

- Who are the residents?
- What are their needs?
- What are their abilities?
- What are their particular tastes and preferences?
- What activity programming will be needed?
- What are their families' expectations?

Today's communication and computer technologies make the process of gathering information much easier and faster than ever before. Literature searches and reviews are easily accessible. Literature reviews, interviews, and surveys, facility visits, renderings, drawings, simulation models, code reviews, and access to knowledgeable consultants are all tools available for your use.

Literature Reviews: Searches for relevant articles, books, reports, standards, and other materials will be valuable to your design process.

Interviews and Surveys: Providers and users can provide you with invaluable opinions and perspectives. Ask them about existing design features: what works, what doesn't? How might a design be improved, and what are good alternatives? Staff can be a bountiful resource of information—again, ask good questions and be willing to listen.

Facility Visits: Observing environments provides a wealth of information about how facilities work. Comparisons can be drawn about effective design features and behavior in similar settings. To prepare for a facility visit:

- Identify the specific environmental features and policies you want to investigate. Arrange for a knowledgeable facility guide.
- Be alert to "telling evidence" that environments may not be working as intended.
- Set realistic time estimates for the visit.[2]
- Document the visit with notes; don't rely on memory to remember what may be important details.
- Photographs and slides are useful to refresh your memory and share information with others. Be sure to secure permission

before taking any photographs. (Many settings are quite willing to allow photographs, but just as many, for a myriad of reasons, including residents' privacy, will not allow cameras.)

Renderings, Drawings, and Simulations: Proposed simulation drawings, renderings, computer-aided design (CAD), or models can be useful in examining design options — space layout, traffic patterns, walking areas, furniture layout, and outdoor spaces in relationship with the indoor setting.

Code Review: It is essential to review relevant codes and regulations. These include:

- Building codes
- Life safety (fire) codes
- Licensing
- Local codes and regulations

We must become familiar with and use the waiver process.

Building and life safety codes focus on safety and security issues only, to the exclusion of the social and psychological needs of residents. Since most codes are based on models for providing acute medical care, models that are not successful models for long-term care, if we are to implement innovative design, we must become familiar with and use the waiver process.

Our collaborative PDTeams© need to take an *active role* in educating regulatory agencies to better understand the relevant issues of design for long-term care facilities. Hiatt has suggested that rather than thrusting a project before them and putting them on the spot, we need to treat regulators as board members or as cautious, experienced colleagues in need of coaching.[3] Sit on the same side of the table — literally and figuratively. Develop ways of sharing what you have learned with these specialists as fellow professionals. Exploring new technologies and exchanging ideas is an opportunity to learn and provide a great service for all involved.

Step Two: Planning — Plan Before You Do!

1. ASSESSING THE SITUATION

In the assessment process it's important to define characteristics of the residents, programs, schedules, and the building design. To understand the residents it is important to understand normal age-related changes in vision, hearing, touch, smell, strength, and mobility, as well as those related more specifically to the stages of Alzheimer's disease.

For architecture and design to effectively respond to the comprehensive needs of older people, a clear understanding of the residents and the many ways they utilize environments is essential. Functional design must be understood by a decision-making group that includes board members, owners, designers (architects, engineers, interior designers), administrators, and representatives of each subspecialty that makes up a responsible caregiving team.[4] As a PDTeam© member, each of these participants should have a commitment to become more educated regarding the impact of environmental design and its potential for positive contribution to the quality of life. Utilize consultants, participate in workshops, read relevant materials, and tour facilities to broaden your experience.

You might also consider organizing a retreat or workshop, guided by an experienced facilitator, to grapple with issues that define the functional design characteristics of residents, programs, design implications, and design opportunities.[5] Retreats and professional workshops provide a forum for exploring and exchanging information, ideas, and techniques, and for developing tools to improve the design and overall understanding of what we're dealing with.

Be alert to the messages that the environmental design conveys and begin to plan changes that merge contemporary thinking with previous design. Make a fair and accurate appraisal of the current strengths and weaknesses of your program and your building. An assessment of the existing facility, its residents, and its current programs is useful planning information.

Create a vision statement. If you had the resources and opportunities, what would be your ideal setting? A clear vision drives good design and is immensely valuable in providing direction. Don't censor at this point; create the dream. It is amazing how often we ultimately create what we imagine. Don't get in your own way and limit what is possible. Even though you many not be able to do it all, you will, at the very least, be headed in the right direction with a map of how to get to your destination.

2. DEFINE PROBLEMS AND CHALLENGES

Good solutions require identifying the challenges and potential problems you'll encounter. Examples of these might include:

1. How can we optimize fitness at all levels of care and encourage exercise, motion, mobility? Examples of possible solutions might include access to outside areas, chairs that rock, and walking paths that go somewhere.

2. What features or props encourage people of varying capabilities to interact? As healthcare becomes more humanized, varying degrees of interaction are appealing and valuable to both the alert and the impaired, as well as the capable and the frail.[6]

3. What features obviously don't work well? Bathing and bathing rooms, for example, are particular problem areas. Might there be a connection between a cold, unfamiliar, frightening room and the resulting behavior? Does this remind you of home? I hope not! Did we ever refer to the bathroom as the "tub room"? I don't think so.

3. ESTABLISH A PRIORITY OF NEEDS; SET GOALS AND OBJECTIVES

Develop a philosophy statement, a written statement that recognizes the unique needs of elderly residents, or elderly residents with dementia. If this is an Alzheimer's special care setting, resident needs will likely be more complex. Guidelines for Dignity, available through the Alzheimer's Association, is an excellent guide.

Define the most critical goals that will direct the program. If the program is a therapeutic model care setting, then clearly define the therapeutic goals. Once the goals are identified, ask these questions:

- How will they be implemented?
- Where will the resources come from?
- Who will be responsible for implementation?

4. DEVELOP A PLAN

During this stage design an implementation plan. Be sure to incorporate the take-aways from each of the three previous steps: the assessment; the challenges; and a priority list of needs, the vision statement, and the goals and objectives.

Step Three: Functional Programming

Before preliminary design begins, programming is the critical phase when data about needs and preferences is obtained. An architect will typically use the data for analysis and then make recommendations for the preliminary design phase. Programming for elderly healthcare settings is more complicated because of the broad spectrum of needs. Architects and designers gain an understanding of these needs through programming and are then able to translate that information to designs that support abilities and help residents maintain their independence.[7]

For architecture to respond to the comprehensive needs of older people, a clear understanding of the people and the many ways they use an environment is needed. This phase of the design process identifies overall characteristics of the environment, for example, the residential quality, and the relationships between spaces (such as toilets adjacent to activity spaces and dining rooms). The process also addresses the sensory setting—lighting, acoustics and excessive noise—and the interior finishes and furnishings.

A balanced design addresses various impairments and varying levels of impairment, as well as the interaction of impairments. Individuals with cognitive impairment most likely also have vision and/or hearing impairments. Some may have mobility impairments. One of the most important challenges of environmental design is dealing with the interaction of multiple impairments. The solutions are typically complex.

> *One of the most important challenges of environmental design is dealing with the interaction of multiple impairments.*

Step Four: Facility Design

After the architectural programming that incorporates the activity program is completed, then specific design program features to support the activity program can be decided. When the team process functions well, the results are a building design that will have a complete behavioral and architectural program. This will include characteristics and details of each room by size, configuration, design features, adjacencies, use schedules, and furnishings. The designer's role is then to find creative design techniques to support this program

1. PARTICIPATORY DESIGN PROCESS

The participatory design process expands the decision-making responsibilities significantly, and although it is more complex, there are significant benefits. Rather than relying on just a few decision-makers, a participatory design process brings a team of people together to talk about common concerns and to clarify design objectives. With clear objectives designers are free to do what they do best— meet challenges with creative design approaches. Participation also helps to relieve anxieties about otherwise unknown changes ahead.[8]

There is no doubt that this process leads to better design decisions, for without the multidisciplinary participation, design decision-makers rely only on their own experience and intuition. The available written information on healthcare design for special needs and behavior is small, but growing. It is not, however, easily available to design professionals, and much of the information they do locate is based on opinion rather than objective data. Therefore, it is critical to collaborate to create the most effective designs.

The participatory process, for people who have been involved, tends to stimulate positive behavior and attitudes. There is more personal investment in the project, and staff tends to take better care of the resulting design.

2. DESIGN GUIDELINES

When all the information has been gathered, at this stage in the design process it is translated into design guidelines—also known as performance criteria. These guidelines clearly define how a particular design feature should function.

3. CONSULTANTS

Using credible consultants can be invaluable. They can contribute information from previous research on similar facilities. They often have skills in interpreting and reviewing design documents from a behavioral point of view, and can offer a clear perspective on the whole design process that "insiders" might not have. Consultation with experts can be costly; however, consultants may be able to quickly identify relevant design and behavior issues, resources, design guidelines, and other useful information, which will ultimately provide large cost savings.

4. WORKING GROUPS

The actual decision-making may often lie with a smaller group within the PDTeam$^©$. Working groups are one of the most common mechanism for design participation. They may meet only a few times to resolve specific problems, or they may meet more often to contribute ideas and track the design's progress. Working groups are an excellent way to respond to different design alternatives. They can review details of proposed designs and make design selections.

5. DESIGN REVIEW

Design review should not stop with the selection of a design, but instead should be an ongoing process. Systematic design review evaluates progress, provides ongoing opportunity to pick up missing details and improve on design solutions, and ultimately seeks to determine if the design will function the way it should. This process helps to avoid errors. It is much easier and far less expensive to make changes in the paper stage than during or after construction.

Computer-aided drawings show a design in three dimension; however, one of the biggest challenges in reviewing plans still remains. Reviewing floor plans in only one dimension and in a very small scale can be deceptive. Typically, there always appears to be more available space on a floor plan than in reality. Even seasoned professionals continually grapple with this. It is advisable to incorporate as many creative means of illustrating the design outcome as possible.

A design project for any healthcare special needs setting must be economically, physically, and politically feasible if it is to be implemented. What sets Alzheimer's special care settings apart is the emphasis placed on the social, psychological, and physical needs of residents, staff, families, and visitors. A resident's needs take priority. For example, the resident's need for mobility, to easily sit down and rise from a chair, carries more weight than the designer's need to select a particular chair that looks beautiful, but that may cause residents to need assistance in order to get up.

> *A resident's needs take priority.*

Step Five: Project Evaluation

Project or postoccupancy evaluation is a periodic, systematic evaluation of the completed project—a measurement and review process. The true test of the design of any healthcare setting is how well it performs over time. Flexible design periodically requires evaluating resident needs, and attending to any necessary changes in the environmental design to keep small problems from growing into larger ones. The data gathered in a postoccupancy evaluation is invaluable for improving residential settings.

Postoccupancy evaluations give a symbolic message to residents and their families that someone still cares about meeting their needs. Valuable information is available to the facility as a result of project evaluation; perhaps of even greater benefit is the information that can be used by other care providers to continue to improve residential healthcare settings.

Developing a reporting system and carefully documenting these evaluations not only allows those responsible for the special care setting to measure progress toward the goals, but also allows them to evaluate the reasons for success or failure in achieving the goals. We

Promote the drafting of building codes that put residents first.

are able to learn, move forward, and build on the strengths of what worked, while avoiding the weaknesses of what didn't, and learn why it didn't work. The information from evaluations must be shared with colleagues and with regulators to promote the drafting of building codes that put residents first. By making the evaluations more widely available, we can collectively improve the state-of-the-art of health-care design.

Woodside Place, an innovative and exceptionally well-designed Alzheimer's residential care setting, recently completed a three year study that included planning, program, and environmental design issues. The results of the study were recently published in the form of an evaluation. This is an extremely valuable contribution to all who learn from the information gathered and shared by Woodside Place.[9]

Postoccupancy evaluations provide an opportunity to answer questions about programming changes that may be of concern, and design issues that may appear to clash with programming objectives. For example, if a programming objective is to promote a residential, homelike ambiance, making a handicapped accessible bathroom look residential can be a challenge. Encouraging independence is crucial; using skill and creativity with interior finishes can meet the challenge. Design makes the impossible possible.

Design makes the impossible possible.

Special Care Settings Design Forms©

Currently, postoccupancy evaluation should be used to determine if design elements that are being incorporated into the facilities are truly enhancing the residents' quality of life.

The following forms are examples of ways to organize needed information. They can be changed or tailored to meet the specific needs of your project.

1. Design Guidelines: Figure 20-1

2. Predesign space programming: Figure 20-2 © Barker & Assoc.

3. Room finish/color schedule: Figure 20-3 © Barker & Assoc.

4. Interior product and color selections/approval: Figure 20-4 © Barker & Assoc.

5. Product information and specification: Figure 20-5 © Barker & Assoc.

Residential Living for Alzheimer Care
Pre-Design Space Programing

I. **Project Statement**
   A. *The Philosophy of Care is critical to define, as the environment needs to respond and support the approach to care.*
      1. *"Sense of ease"*
         Mastery of the surrounding environment while being comfortable in it.
         Encourage involvement with the surrounding environment.
         Provide flexibility within a completely safe environment.
      2. *"Let the individuals be themselves"*
         Maximize Resident independence by "guided choice and perceived freedom."
         Improve the quality of life for the Resident and Family by reducing frustration and stabilizing the mental and physical decline by providing the necessary support.
      3. *"Homelike environment"*
         Care Giver can participate with activities and care of Resident. Encourage and reinforce personal patterns of Daily Living.

II. **Alzheimer In-Patient Department**
   A. *General*
      1. *Function*
         a) Approximately 22 Alzheimer residents
            • Residents require only personal care, not medical care (not SNF model)
            • The program will run under the RCFE license, Title 22
            • The Residents can share daytime resources and programs with the Alzheimer Adult day care program
         b) A definition of the types of Residents that might be in the unit consists of:
            • Wandering, combative, disoriented, incontinent seniors over 65 years old.
            • Residents to be either - very physically active or quiet and depressed.
            • Only 25% maximum expected to be in wheelchair.
               • But make all space wheelchair accessible
               • Need to redefine wheelchair accessibility for this population
               • California code established based on Vietnam veteran physical capabilities, which are not applicable to these residents
      2. *Staffing*
         a) Program Assistants
            • 4 during day shift
         b) OTA or Recreation therapist
            • 1 person
            • OTR could be Director of Program also
         c) RN or LVN
            • 1 person
            • RN could be Director of Program
         d) Housekeeping
            • Part time (outside service presently)
               • Presently night shift only
               • Probably needs to be midmorning shift

Figure 20-1 Predesign space programming form example. *Courtesy of and copyright © by Barker Associates, Architects and Planners, Menlo Park, CA.*

3. Activities
  a) Services to be provided
  - Physical Diagnostic – Blood drawing for lab work and EKG.
  - Counseling – Care plans and conferences with relatives.
  - Therapy – including some physical therapy and speech (outside service), but mainly continuous Occupational therapy as part of Daily Living retraining.
  - Nutritional – Meals (constant food intake available), cooking groups (which is part of OT).
  - Daily Living – Dressing (over and under dressing issues), grooming.
  - Hygiene – Toileting (80% need assistance), every other day showering and bathing.
  - Activities – Conversation, eating, recreational therapy, art, music, housekeeping, walking, sitting and watching presentations or movies in groups (3 to 4 residents). Activities obviously overlap with Occupational therapy and Daily Living.

  b) Resident/Staff/Public Patterns
  - Daily patterns for residents
    - Wake up at near the same time
    - Toilet (with assistance if necessary)
    - Dress (with assistance if necessary)
    - Groom (with assistance if necessary)

    Breakfast in Family room
    - Respect person's original eating patterns
    - Allow flexibility

    Activities
    - Make beds and clean up room therapy (with assistance if necessary)
    - Make meals therapy with assistance
    - Do Laundry therapy
    - Current events
    - Activity program

    Lunch (repeat breakfast)
  - Daily Care providers (LVN) patterns and routines
  - Other daily activities and their patterns
    - Dietary
    - RN/Doctors

  c) Materials handling systems
  d) Internal communications
  e) Staff support systems
  f) Automation and technology

4. Interaction with Other Areas
  a) Adult Day Health will share the same floor
  - Adult Day Care for Alzheimer programs of 10 people will probably join the Residential Care program during the day
  - Residential Care Residents may use the specialized programs of Adult Day Health on occasion

  b) Some of the spaces can be shared between Programs
  - Library/Resources/Conference rooms
  - Bathing/Hygiene room
  - Gym/PT
  - Reception if Administration stays on floor

Figure 20-1 *Continued.*

268

- Physician exam rooms
- Quiet room/Den
- Staff lounge and restrooms

B. Specific Room Program

1. Resident rooms

- Type of space
  - Resident bedrooms
    - All Single rooms desirable but not practical
    - "L" shape is preferred to asymmetrical double
- Number and type of occupants
  - Single room – 1 Resident
  - "L" shaped or Double – 2 Residents
- Number of spaces
  - Mixed cluster of 5 residents with 4 cluster of rooms
  - Goal is 1 single to 1 "L" Shape to 1 double = 5 residents to a cluster
  - 20 to 22 beds goal
- Function/use of area
  - Sleeping
  - Privacy during daytime
  - Dressing
- Systems
  - Environmental needs
    - Outside window for light but without glare
    - Good ventilation (natural preferred) and heat
    - View outside preferred but need to reduce and limit outside noise
    - Residential finishes – Carpet on floors
  - Equipment/furnishing needs
    - Single bed for each resident
    - Personal possessions such as dressers and small chair
      - or supplied if resident doesn't have
    - Mirror over dresser
    - Built-in closet
      - 2 foot min., 4 foot more desirable
      - ½ locked or inaccessible
    - Wall space for personal pictures
    - Room for wheelchair accessibility
    - Space divider or separator if a shared room
  - Adjacencies required
    - Access to Family Room directly or just off corridor
    - Direct access to bathroom
      - Shared by no more than 2 people
      - Best to be visible from room

2. Resident "Bathroom"

- Type of space
  - Desired 1 for 2 residents
    - But building changes will have major cost for adding twice as many bathrooms

Figure 20-1 *Continued.*

269

- Number and type of occupants
  - 1 resident at a time with 1 assistant when required
- Number of spaces
  - 1 for each singles, "L" shape, or double = 3 per cluster
  - 1 for Respite room with roll-in shower?
- Function/use of area
  - Toilet and Lavatories only
    - Not a true bathroom
  - Supplies for Resident care
    - Supplies not to be in Resident's dresser drawers
- Systems
  - Environmental needs
    - Good air exchange
      - negative pressure
    - Good lighting levels
    - Cleanable walls and floors
      - Sheet vinyl flooring with cove base
      - Wainscot of plastic laminate or vinyl?
      - Smooth wall and ceiling finishes
    - Acoustics?
    - Floor drain?
    - GFI outlet?
  - Equipment/furnishing needs
    - Toilet (WC)
      - Adjustable height or Handicapped height (+18" high)
    - Lavatory
      - Counter with sink preferred for residential look over Handicapped wall hung sink
      - Contrast between sink and counter top
    - Grab bars as required by Title 24 Access
      - Best if both sides of the toilet could be part of toilet assembly
      - Can use towel racks if designed for weight
    - Supply cabinet for disposable gloves
    - Large door into bathroom for access
      - Might be accordion type or roll back
      - If swing type, swing out into bedroom (or hall)
    - Emergency Call
      - Wearable type preferred
  - Adjacencies required
    - In bedroom or directly off of bedroom
    - Also nice to be close to hall and family room to provide easy access to residents

3. Family room (lounges)
- Type of space
  - Family room like in a house
    - Room that people live in
    - Not a highly active space but a gathering area for 2 clusters of rooms
    - Tries to reflect "home" life

Figure 20-1 *Continued.*

270

- Number and type of occupants
    - 10 to 11 residents typical
        - May only have 5 to 6 at any one time
    - 2 Program Assistants
        - May not be in room but nearby, such as in Morning time
- Number of spaces
    - 2 similar but slightly different spaces
- Function/use of area
    - Social activity space for 2 clusters of residents
        - Informal
        - Modeled after a residential family room
    - Sitting areas
        - Small group of 2 to 4 residents
        - Single chair and lamp for single
    - "Breakfast bar" for early morning coffee and light snacks
    - Focus area such as fireplace or bay window area
    - Aquarium, stereo for listening or music chair
- Systems
    - Environmental needs
        - Good ventilation and heat
        - Good light (natural preferred) without glare
            - Indirect and lamps with shades
        - Good acoustics to reduce noise levels
    - Equipment/furnishing needs
        - Residential loveseats and comfortable chairs – seating for 10
            - Seating group with 2 loveseats and 2 side chairs or love seat
            - Wing chair with lamp for reading
            - Game table for 4
        - Fireplace or Bay window feature?
        - Carpet on floor
        - Acoustical ceiling and wall covering
        - Kitchenette to look like Home kitchen
            - Breakfast bar at 30 inches for 3 residents to sit at
            - Mini kitchen with refrigerator, microwave and sink
            - Should be able to be closed off when not supervised or being used
        - Desk for Program Assistance in lieu of a Nurses' station
        - Desk with lockable drawers for current paper work and personal items of PA's
    - Adjacencies required
        - Easy access and orientation from bedrooms and dining room/game room

4. Grooming area

- Type of space
    - Alcove space for personal grooming
- Number and type of occupants
    - 1 per each 5 Resident cluster
- Number of spaces
    - 1 per cluster = 4 total
- Function/use of area
    - Personal grooming in small group setting

Figure 20-1 *Continued.*

- Brushing and fixing hair
- Checking appearance
- Brushing teeth
- Washing face
- Systems
    - Environmental needs
        - Good indirect lighting
        - Ventilation and heating
            Exhaust for some odors?
        - Cleanable, washable walls and floors
            Sheet vinyl or lobo floor?
    - Equipment/furnishing needs
        - Vanity counter for 2 to 3 with
        - Mirror
            Full width of vanity
            Also need full length mirror
        - Lavatory for washing and teeth brushing – 2–3 sinks
            Separate from vanity to reduce mess
            Be able to close off when not supervised
    - Adjacencies required
        - Directly off bedroom on the way to the family room

5. Community activity spaces

- Dining room
    - Type of space
        - Dining room for 3 meals a day
        - Social day use room
    - Number and type of occupants
        - 10–15 residents typical
            5 people are from Day Care program for Lunch
        - 2 Program Assistants
        - OTA or Rec. therapist if Activity program
    - Number of spaces
        - 2 similar spaces
            Could be combined into larger room for group activities
    - Function/use of area
        - Dining room for formal meals 3 times a day
            3 small group seating areas
        - Social activity space for all residents
            Formal activities such as discussion, current events, cooking
            Activity that need use of tables
        - Party room for special occasions
    - Systems
        - Environmental needs
            - Good ventilation and heat
            - Good natural light without glare
                Indirect lighting
            - Good acoustical control on noise
            - Cleanable floors and walls surfaces

Figure 20-1 *Continued.*

- Equipment/furnishing needs
  - Chair and tables for dining groups of 4 with some groups of 2
  - Cleanable floors and walls
    Maybe a vinyl wood flooring, Lobo floor, or sheet vinyl
    Acoustical wallpaper with residential look
- Adjacencies required
  - Easy access and orientation from bedrooms and family room
  - Access to views and courtyard
  - Serving kitchen to be able to open up to space
  - Restroom for toileting after meals

- Energy or program room (game?)
  - Type of space
    - Activity room where everything is OK
      Maybe formal group activities or informal individual
  - Number and type of occupants
    - 1 room for 10–15 Residents
      If formal activity with 15 residents then will be staffed with
        2 Program Assistants
        1 Rec Therapist or OT
      If informal, may be only supervised by a night Program Assistant or RN
        while doing charting
  - Number of spaces
    1 room that can have many activities going on or different focuses
  - Function/use of area
    - Individual enrichment with touching, sounds, ADL such as folding clothes or
      trying on clothes
    - Group activities that require involvement and or movement
    - Music, physical activities, cooking if not done in dining
  - Systems
    - Environmental needs
      - Good ventilation and heat
      - Active exterior views
      - Good natural light without glare Indirect lighting
      - Good acoustical control on noise
      - Cleanable but soft floors and walls surfaces
    - Equipment/furnishing needs
      - Activity center for
        Music – Instruments and piano
        Color
        Touching
        Clothes
      - Chairs for group activities
  - Adjacencies required
    Easy access and orientation from family room
    Access to active views
    Serving kitchen to be able to open up to space if possible
    Restroom

Figure 20-1 *Continued.*

6. Corridors
- Type of space
    - Circulation space for
        - Residents to get to activity spaces
        - Staff to get between resident spaces and support spaces
    - Wandering path for residents
        - Must be secure, without dead ends
- Number and type of occupants
    - NA
- Number of spaces
    - Lengths to be as small as possible for access
    - Wandering path to go to different spaces rather than be a continuous loop
- Function/use of area
    - Access to spaces
    - Walking (wandering)[
- Systems
    - Environmental needs
        - Good indirect lighting
        - Low glare surfaces
        - Natural light wherever possible
        - Good ventilation, positive pressure
    - Equipment/furnishing needs
        - Should have benches for resting
            - Conflict with State Fire Marshall
        - Wander guard on corridor door
            - NO panic hardware if possible, use push plates on resident side
            - Paint to match walls where residents are restricted
        - Handrail at 41 inches height – oval design for resting elbows on
        - Wall surfaces that will not be damaged by wheelchairs
    - Adjacencies required
        - Connection to Resident bedrooms and dining room / family room
        - Connection for Staff service area to Resident areas

7. Restrooms
- Type of space
    - Toilet room
- Number and type of occupants
    - Single stall or multiple
- Number of spaces
    - 2–4 restrooms
- Function/use of area
    - To be used when Residents are in programs in lieu of going back to rooms
- Systems
    - Environmental needs
        - Good air exchange
            - negative pressure
        - Good lighting levels
        - Cleanable walls and floors
            - Sheet vinyl flooring with cove base

Figure 20-1 *Continued.*

274

Wainscot of plastic laminate or vinyl?

Smooth wall and ceiling finishes

- Acoustics?
- Floor drain?
- Equipment/furnishing needs
  - Toilet (WC)

    Adjustable height or Handicapped height (+18 inches high)
  - Lavatory

    Counter with sink preferred for residential look over Handicapped
    wall-hung sink

    Contrast between sink and counter top
  - Grab bars

    As required by Title 24 Access

    Best if both sides of the toilet

    Could be part of toilet assembly

    Can use towel racks if designed for weight
  - Large door into bathroom for access

    Might be accordion type or roll back

    If swing type, swing out into bedroom (or hall)
  - Emergency Call

    Wearable type preferred
- Adjacencies required

  In corridor or directly off of dining room / program room

  Also nice to be close to family room to provide easy access to residents

8. Bathing rooms

- Type of space

  Shower and bathing space
- Number and type of occupants

  1 resident

  1 Program Assistant and/or Beautician
- Number of spaces

  2 rooms
- Function/use of area

  Bathing twice a week

  Hair washing and fixing
- Systems
  - Environmental needs
    - Good air exchange

      negative pressure
    - Good lighting levels
    - Cleanable walls and floors

      Sheet vinyl flooring with 6 inches cove base or tile?

      Wainscot of plastic laminate or vinyl?

      Smooth wall wall and ceiling finishes
    - Acoustics
    - Floor drain
  - Equipment/furnishing needs
    - Roll-in shower

Figure 20-1 *Continued.*

275

- Bath tub
  Type and manufacturer?
- Toilet (WC)
- Lavatory
- Grab bars
- Emergency call
- Adjacencies required
  Off corridor and family room
  Accessible to Adult Day Health

9. Other related spaces
- Nurses lounge and restrooms
  - Type of space
  - Number and type of occupants
  - Number of spaces
  - Function/use of area
  - Systems
    - Environmental needs
    - Equipment/furnishing needs
    - Adjacencies required
- Outdoor spaces
- Quiet room/den
- Exam room
  Could be combined with the quiet room
  Shared with Adult Day Health
- Offices
- Conference room
- Entry lobby/reception
- Relatives living room
- Personal laundry room

Figure 20-1 *Continued.*

Examples of Design Principles

1. Single resident room with own toilet (shower, if feasible?)
2. Prefer cluster resident rooms around activity area
3. Multiple choices of activity areas (small to larger)
4. 2 units (neighborhoods) with intentional activity space and shared space between
5. Dining style: Dining space with kitchen
6. Entrance to unit and shared area ideally with visitors and separate entrance
      for service functions
7. Residential quality to environment
8. Separate exits to common outdoor space from neighborhood
9. Provide space for meds, ref, desk(s), but not a nurse's station
10. Create intimacy in space
11. Positive; secure, outdoor space with programmed activities
12. Need place for staff retreat
13. Visibility of outside from inside
14. Places for family visits that are intimate, not in room only
15. Lighting—Variable, properly designed, not obvious
16. Provide proper sound separation and audibility
17. Visual cueing:
      Patient room
      Unit (neighborhood)
      Entire suite'
18. Common bathing area—proper design for:
      Calm
      Privacy
      Comfort (humidity control)
19. Flexibility for change:
      Population changes
      Technology with care changes
      Interior design with FF&E changes
      Program changes
20. Acknowledge space for spiritual needs /mediation
21. Clear signage: unobtrusive, color, texture, coated

Figure 20-2 Design guidelines—example. Examples of design principles.

Room Finish Color Schedule

Room		Floor		Base		Wall		Wall/Upper Wall		Wainscot			Crown	Ceiling		Plas Lam	Paint	Countertop	Remarks
No.	Name	Material	Color	Material	Color	Material	Material	Color	Material	Color	Trim	Material	Material	Color	COLOR (2)	COLOR (3)	Material/Color	
101																		
102																		
103																		
104																		
105																		
106																		
107																		
108																		
109																		
110																		
111																		
112																		
113																		
114																		
115																		
116																		
117																		
118																		
119																		
120																		
121																		
122																		
123																		
124																		
125																		
126																		
127																		
128																		
129																		
130																		
131																		
132																		
133																		
134																		
135																		
136																		
137																		
138																		
139																		
140																		
141																		
142																		
143																		
144																		
145																		
146																		
147																		
148																		
149																		
150																		

Miscellaneous Item Finish Schedule

Item		Finish/Color	Remarks
1	Wood Light Valance Trim		
2	Wood Divider Strip		
3	Wood Chair Rail		
4	Wood Crown Molding		
5	Wood Base		
6	Wood Casework		
7	Wood Door trim		
8	Wood Stile & Rail Doors		
9	Wood Handrail		
10	Wood casing @ wdws		
11	Marble tile at gas burning appliance		

NOTES:
(1) See specifications for accent band tile colors.
(2) Includes Door and Cabinet plastic laminate colors.
    See Door Schedule to coordinate finish and finish color with appropriate door material.
    Plastic laminates are same color both sides of doors unless noted otherwise.
(3) Includes door frame and door paint color. See Door Schedule to coordinate finish and
    finish color with appropriate door material. Color indicated is on room side typical. Wood
    stile & rail doors are clear finish.
(4)
(5)
(6)

Figure 20-3 Room finish/color schedule form (two pages). *Courtesy of and copyright © by Barker Associates, Architects and Planners, Menlo Park, CA.*

Abbreviations

AC	Acoustical Ceiling	L	Plastic Laminate
BR	Bumper Rail Wall Guard	P	Paint
CP	Carpet	Plas Lam	Plastic Laminate
CR	Chair Rail	RB	Rubber Base
CT/Cer Tile	Ceramic Tile	SS	Synthetic Solid Surface Material
DS	Divider Strip	SV	Sheet vinyl
GB	Gypsum Board	WC	Wallcovering
		WD	Wood

Colors/Patterns

Code	Material	Manufacturer	Pattern	Color	Remarks
Floor Covering					
CP	Carpet				
SV1	Sheet vinyl				
SV2	Sheet vinyl				
SV3	Sheet vinyl				
CT1	Ceramic Tile / Grout				
CT2	Ceramic Tile / Grout				
Base					
Coved Base	Self-coved Vinyl Floor				
Cer Tile	Ceramic Tile Base				
R1	Rubber Base				
R2	Rubber Base				
R3	Rubber Base				
R4	Rubber Base				
Wall Finishes - Wallcovering/Wainscot/Ceramic Tile					
W3	Vinyl Wallcovering				
W6	Vinyl Wallcovering				
W7	Vinyl Wallcovering				
W8	Vinyl Wallcovering				
W9	Vinyl Wallcovering				
W10	Vinyl Wallcovering				
W11	Vinyl Wallcovering				
W12	Vinyl Wallcovering				
W13	Vinyl Wallcovering				
W14	Vinyl Wallcovering				
W15	Vinyl Wallcovering				
W17	Vinyl Wallcovering				
W18	Vinyl Wallcovering				
W19	Vinyl Wallcovering				
W20	Vinyl Wallcovering				
CT3	Ceramic Tile / Grout				
CT4	Ceramic Tile / Grout				
CT5	Ceramic Tile / Grout				
Paint					
P1	Paint				
P2	Paint				
P3	Paint				
P4	Paint				
P5	Paint				
P6	Paint				
P7	Paint				
Laminate					
L1	Plastic Laminate				
L2	Plastic Laminate				
L3	Plastic Laminate				
L4	Plastic Laminate				
L5	Plastic Laminate				
L6	Plastic Laminate				
Synthetic Solid Surface Material					
SS1	Syn. Solid Sur. Material				
SS2	Syn. Solid Sur. Material				
SS3	Syn. Solid Sur. Material				

Figure 20-3 *Continued.*

Interior Product and Color Selections / Approvals

Facility Name					Date	
Material	Location	Scheme	Manufacturer	Style/Pattern/Color	Approval	Remarks
Carpet						
Sheet Vinyl						
Floor Tile						
Wallcovering						
Paint						
Wainscot						
TSB						
Plastic Laminates				upper-		
				lower-		
				counter-		
				upper-		
				lower-		
				counter-		
Ceiling panels						
Door hardware						
Handrail brackets						

Figure 20-4 Interior product and color selection form. *Courtesy of and copyright © by Barker Associates, Architects and Planners, Menlo Park, CA.*

Product Information Memo

Project: _____   Date: _____

Job No.: _____   Research By.: _____

General Product Information

CSI No. _____

Product: _____

Spec. Section _____

General Description: _____

Where Used: _____

Review & Approved By *Other*	*In-House*	*Int Des/Arch*	*Client*	*User*
Preliminary Design	_____	_____	_____	_____
Construction Doc	_____	_____	_____	_____

Product Specification

Alternates or Options

Manufacturer: _____
_____

Model No.: _____

Size/Description: _____

Materials:
Sub-Component
/Model # _____
_____

Color/Finish: _____

Related Work/
Products: _____
_____

Rough-In / :
Fabrication
Requirements _____
_____
_____
_____

Installation/
Technical
Requirements: _____
_____
_____
_____

Reason for Choice:
Unit Cost: _____
_____
_____
_____

Rep.. or Dist. Name: _____   Referred by: _____
Phone _____   Past Project: _____
Fax

Figure 20-5 Product information and specification. *Courtesy of and copyright © by Barker Associates, Architects and Planners, Menlo Park, CA.*

*Architects,
Designers, and
Providers*

As the population ages, architects and designers will receive more requests to design residential healthcare settings. People are living longer and they want to live as independently and comfortably as possible. Design professionals are by definition problem-solvers, not just people who "make things pretty;" although that in itself would be a help. Aesthetics are vitally important, and if designers can create spaces that make someone feel good, then they are in fact improving that person's life. While improving aesthetics is an important contribution, imagine the satisfaction in knowing you have also enhanced the quality of someone's life, somone who up to now has been part of an almost invisible population.

The environment has a great impact on behavior. In designing for people with Alzheimer's disease or dementia, the designer's perspective and talent can be applied to one of the most challenging human conditions in the world. By focusing on the interior spaces and how residents experience them, by problem solving, and by analyzing every design decision, environments can be fashioned to provide support for residents' abilities and to enhance their quality of life. We either enable residents or disable them. We can empower residents through good design instead of limiting their choices.

Spend time in a long-term care setting—not merely as an observer. Try participating in actual hands-on caregiving experiences, such as feeding residents, helping them down the hall, or just take the time to talk with some residents. For designers and architects unfamiliar and inexperienced with long-term care, particularly the special needs of Alzheimer's disease and dementia, these can be both enlightening and moving experiences. They may also be among the most valuable career expanding experiences you will have. To the benefit of residents, staff, family, and providers, we can expect to see dramatically better design solutions in the hands of creative, experienced professionals with "real" firsthand understanding of the issues.

As unsettling as these experiences can be for those who have lived with a dementing illness, they can be emotionally overwhelming for someone unused to the mental, physical, and emotional challenges these illnesses caused. When arranging to spend time in a nursing home or on an Alzheimer's special care unit, arrange to have someone accompany you. The facility can provide an appropriate volunteer or staff escort. Your caregiver-companion can provide a wealth of information and support as you begin to experience what life with Alzheimer's is like. This person can be your "life preserver" as you learn, as a design professional, what a difference your talents can make when you truly understand the problems.

Many design professionals are unused to such an intimate experience of healthcare settings. It can be emotionally overwhelming and leave one feeling quite vulnerable. Healthcare professionals can express sensitivity to this situation by planning time to share experiences at the end of the day. This is time well spent, for it not only allows individuals to become more grounded, but through the experience and talking together, relationships of mutual respect and understanding are formed. It is a unique opportunity where everyone benefits. The project benefits, the team benefits, and most of all the residents benefit.

Listen and learn. Make the most of your own development by learning from the residents. What has worked in the past may or may not be working well today. It makes sense to reevaluate the extent to which residents needs are being served. Focus on resident's abilities, not on what they can't do.

> *Focus on resident's abilities, not on what they can't do.*

Design-enriched projects create a bridge. No matter whether the subject of design is interiors or products, graphics, or architecture, the basic processes and thinking are the same, as is the commitment to solve problems by blending function and form. Whether creating therapeutic environments for residents, or a satisfactory environment for the staff, healthcare designers have unique and demanding challenges. Most of these challenges concern space and budgetary constraints.

As I've mentioned throughout this book, design is a collaborative process. The design process is a strategy to try and insure everyone gets what he or she wants. It not only provides information, but helps to integrate that information, to meet challenges, and to enhance living environments.

> *Design is a collaborative process.*

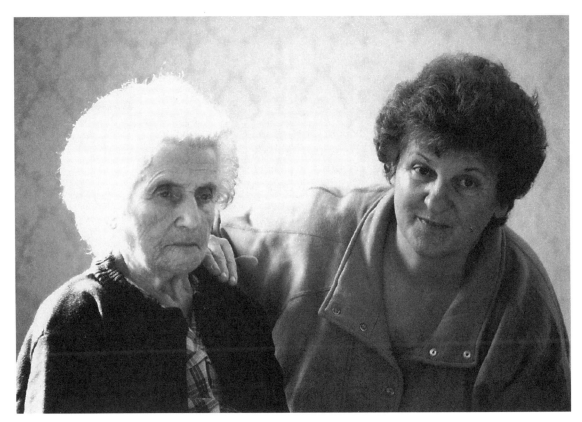

Courtesy of the Greater San Francisco Bay Area Alzheimer's Association. Photographer: Anna M. Rossi.

While improving aesthetics is an important contribution, imagine the satisfaction in knowing you have also enhanced the quality of someone's life, someone who up to now has been part of an almost invisible population.

Resource List

Alzheimer's Association
919 North Michigan Avenue, Suite 1000
Chicago, IL 60611-1676
(312) 335-8700
(800) 272-3900
FAX (312) 335-1110

Alzheimer's Association
Benjamin B. Green-Field National Alzheimer's
Library and Resource Center
919 North Michigan Avenue, Suite 1000
Chicago, IL 60611-1676
(312) 335-9602
FAX (312) 335-0214

Alzheimer's Association *Safe Return*
Program
Contact a local chapter or call
(800) 272-3900

Alzheimer's Association of Orange County
Memories in the Making
A Program of Creative Art Expression for Alzheimer
Patients
2540 North Santiago Boulevard
Orange, CA 92667
(714) 283-1111

Alzheimer's Disease Education and Referral
(ADEAR) Center
PO Box 8250
Silver Springs, MD 20907-8250
(301) 495-3311
(800) 438-4380
FAX (301) 495-3334

Alzheimer Society of Canada
1320 Yonge Street, Suite 201
Toronto, Ontario
M4T 1X2, Canada

American Association of Homes and Services
for the Aging (AAHSA)
901 E. Street NW, Suite 500
Washington, D.C. 20004-2037
(202) 783-2242

American Association of Retired Persons
(AARP)
601 E Street NW
Washington, DC 20049
(202) 434-2277

American Health Care Association
(AHCA)
1201 L Street NW
Washington, DC 20005
(202) 842-4444
FAX (202) 842-3860

American Institute of Architects (AIA)
Committees on Health Care,
Housing for Elderly, and Health Care Facilities
Research Program of the AIA Association of
Collegiate Schools of Architecture
1735 New York Avenue NW
Washington, DC 20006
(202) 785-5912
FAX (202) 628-0448

American Nurses Association (ANA)
600 Marylnad Avenue SW
Suite 100 W
Washington, DC 20024-2571
(202) 554-4444
(800) 274-4262
FAX (202) 651-7001

American Society on Aging (ASA)
833 Market Street, Suite 511
San Francisco, CA 94103
(415) 974-9600
FAX (415) 974-0300

American Society of Interior Designers (ASID)
608 Massachusetts Avenue, NE
Washington, DC 20002
(202) 546-3480

Arthritis Founation
1314 Spring Street NW
Atlanta, GA 30309
(404) 872-7100
(800) 283-7800

Assisted Living Facilities Association of America (ALFAA)
10300 Easton Place, Suite 400
Fairfax, VA 22031
(703) 691-8100
FAX (703) 691-8106

Canadian Association on Gerontology
1080 167 Lombard Avenue
Winnipeg, Manitoba
Canada R3B OT6

Canadian Long Term Care Association
204-124 Bloor Street East
Toronto, Ontario
Canada M4W 1B8

Center of Design for an Aging Society
6200 SW Virginia Avenue, Suite 210
Portland, OR 97201
(503) 246-8231

Center for Health Design, Inc.
4550 Alhambra Way
Martinez, CA 94553-4406
(510) 370-0345
FAX (510) 228-4018

Environmental Design Research Association
4977 Battery Lane #413
Bethesda, MD 20814
(301) 657-2657

Gerontological Society of America (GSA)
1275 K Street NW, Suite 350
Washington, DC 20005-4006
(202) 842-1275

Health Care Financing Administration (HCFA)
P.O. Box 340
Columbia, MD 21045
(410) 786-3000
Medicare Hotline (800) 638-6833

Help for Incontinent People
P.O Box 8310
Spartenburg, SC 29305-8310
(864) 579-7900
(800) 252-3337
FAX (864) 579-7902

Illuminating Engineering Society of North America (IESNA)
120 Wall Street, 17th Floor
New York, NY 10005-4001
(212) 248-5000
Recommended Practice for Lighting and the Visual Environment for Senior Living (IESNARP-28-96)

International Interior Design Association (IIDA)
Healthcare Forum
Chicago Merchandise Mart
Space 341
200 World Trade Center Chicago
Chicago, IL 60654
(312) 467-1950

ITT Hartford
The Hartford House — A Resource Guide
200 Executive Boulevard
Southington, CT 06489

The National Center for Access Unlimited (1992)
The Readily Achievable Checklist: A Survey for Accessibility
155 North Wacker Drive, #315
Chicago, IL 60606
(312) 368-0380

National Center for Vision and Aging
The Lighthouse, Inc.
Lighthouse National Information and Resource Service
111 East 59th Street
New York, NY 10022
(212) 821-9200
(800) 334-5497
FAX (212) 821-9705

The Lighthouse Inc. Educational Products Catalogue
The Lighthouse Inc. Consumer Products Catalogue
The Lighthouse Inc. Professional Products Catalogue

National Citizens' Coalition for Nursing Home Reform
1424 16th Street NW, Suite 202
Washington, DC 20036-2211
(202) 332-2275
FAX (202) 332-2949

National Council on the Aging (NCOA)
409 3rd Street SW, Suite 200
Washington, DC 20024
(202) 479-1200

National Fire Protection Association
470 Atlantic Avenue
Boston, MA 02210

National Geriatrics Society
212 West Wisconsin Avenue
Milwaukee, WI 53203

National Institute of Mental Health (NIMH)
Information Resources and Inquiries Branch
5600 Fishers Lane, Room 7C-02
Rockville, MD 20857
(301) 443-4513

National Institute on Aging (NIA)
Public Information Office
Building 31, Room 5C27
31 Center Drive MSC 2292
Bethesda, MD 20892-2292
(301) 496-1752
(800) 222-2225
FAX (301) 496-1072

Resource Directory for Older People
National Institute on Aging (see above)

Society for the Advancement of Gerontological Environments (SAGE)
13323 Borgman
Huntington Woods, MI 48070

Woodside Place
1215 Hulton Road
Oakmont, PA 15139
(412) 826-6500
Woodside Place Evaluation:
The First Three Years of a Residential Alzheimer's
Facility.

Product Manufacturers Resource List

Adden Furniture
26 Jackson Street
Lowell, MA 01852
(508) 454-7848

ADD Specialized Seating Technology
6500 South Avalon Boulevard
Los Angeles, CA 90003
(213) 752-0101
Long-term care seating

Akin Furniture
147 Commerce Street
Monticello, AK 71655
(501) 367-6263

Armstrong World Industries
PO Box 3001
Lancaster, PA 17604
(800) 448-1405
Ceiling systems

Art Research Institute, Ltd.
325 Kelson Drive
Atlanta, GA 30327
(770) 933-1733
Interior windows

Collins & Aikman Floorcoverings
311 Smith Industrial Boulevard
Dalton, GA 30720
(706) 259-2609
Floor covering systems

Essex Commercial Wallcoverings
3 University Plaza
Suite 200
Hackensack, NJ 07601
(201) 489-0100
Wallcovering

Fantagraph/Standard Textile Co., Inc.
One Knollcrest Drive
Cincinnati, OH 42537
(800) 888-5000
Crypton and FR fabrics

Formica Corporation
10155 Reading Road
Cincinnati, OH 45241
(513) 786-3039
Laminate surfacing material

General Electric
General Electric Customer Relations
Appliance Park
AP6-129
Louisville, KY 40225
(800) 626-2000

Hunter Douglas Window Fashions
1924 Chespark Drive
Gastonia, NC 28052
(800) 637-8610

Imperial Fastener Co., Inc.
1400 SW 8th Street
Pompano Beach, FL 33069
(954) 782-7130
Break-A-Way window drapery hardware

Intersign, Inc.
Box 710
Chattanooga, TN 37401
(800) 322-8426
FAX (423) 698-2864
Signage systems

Koroseal/Vicrtex Wallcoverings
3875 Embassy Parkway
Fairlawn, OH 44333
(800) 828-4556
Wallcovering

L&B Contract Industries West
PO Box 405
Perris, CA 92572
(800) 969-0777
Tables and seating

L&B Contract Industries
PO Box 303
Valley Cottage, NY 10989

The Lighthouse Inc.
111 East 59th Street
New York, NY 10022
(800) 334-5497
Products for low vision

MechoShade Systems, Inc.
42-03 35th Street
Long Island City, NY 11101
(718) 729-2020
Window shade systems

Philips Lighting
200 Franklin Square Drive
Somerset, NJ 08875
(908) 563-3000

Senior Style
4380 SW Macadam Avenue,
Suite 210
Portland, OR 97201
(503) 244-1719
Seating

Thomasville Furniture Industries
P.O. Box 339
Thomasville, NC 27360
(919) 472-4000
Furniture

Toli International
55 Mall Drive
Commack, NY 11725
(800) 446-5476
Solid vinyl sheet flooring

Wilsonart International
2400 Wilson Place
Temple, TX 76504
(817) 778-2711
Laminate surfacing material

Glossary

Abrasion Resistance—A measure of pile fiber's ability to withstand wear. Abrasion testing can be performed mechanically by a tetrapod or can be a visual rating or examination of actual floor test samples under regulated traffic conditions.

Aging in Place—A process whereby individuals remain in their living environment despite the physical and/or mental decline and growing needs for supportive services that may occur in the course of aging. For aging in place to occur, services are added, increased, or adjusted to compensate for the individual's physical and/or mental decline.

Ambient Light—The existing light found in a particular interior setting. The ambient light may be sunlight but, in a healthcare setting, is most likely to be fluorescent lighting.

American Society for Testing Materials—ASTM is an organization concerned with testing standards for a variety of materials. As the world's largest source of voluntary consensus standards for materials, products, systems, and services, ASTM is a resource for information on sampling and testing methods, health and safety of materials, safe performance guidelines, and effects of physical and biological agents and chemicals.

Antimicrobial—A chemical that prevents the growth of mold, bacteria, mildew, and so on, reducing their destructive action to carpet or wall-covering and eliminating accompanying odors.

Antistatic—Ability (natural or induced by chemical or conduction fiber) of a fiber to disperse electrical charge before buildup of static becomes noticeable to humans.

Assisted Living—"Assisted living" means a coordinated array of supportive personal and health services, available 24 hours per day, to residents who have been assessed to need those services, including residents who require formal long-term care.

Assisted living promotes resident self-direction and participation in decisions that emphasize independence, privacy, dignity, and homelike surroundings.

ASTM—See *American Society for Testing Materials.*

Blurred Vision—Can be caused by cataracts, corneal scars, and diabetes. Bright lights and glare make vision worse.

Board and Care Homes—Typically these are privately operated homes or facilities that provide living space, meals, and some personal care services. These may also be called assisted living or personal care homes, domiciliary homes, or homes for the aged. Medicare, Medicaid, and private insurance may not reimburse for these services. States may or may not license, inspect, or monitor these facilities.

Carpet—The general designation for fabric used as a floor covering.

Cataract—A clouding of the normally clear and transparent lens of the eye.

Central Vision Loss—People with macular degeneration have difficulty distinguishing facial features, reading, and eating (i.e., they have dificulty seeing food on a plate).

Chroma—The intensity or purity of a color is called its chroma. Adding a contrasting color (one opposite it on the color wheel) will decrease the chroma of a color.

Chronic Organic Brain Syndrome—A label sometimes applied to patients with a collection of symptoms such as memory loss, disorientation, confusion, personality changes, and inability to carry out normal daily activities. The preferred term for these symptoms is dementia or dementing illness.

Color Rendering Index—CRI is a scale used to measure the color rendering capabilities of lamplight: how much of the color spectrum is represented in the light and in what amounts. The color rendering index, which ranges from 1 to 100, measures the effect of light on colors and determines the suitability of light for any given purpose.

Color Temperature—Refers to the overall appearance of a light's color. It is usually measured directly from the source. Color temperature is measured in degrees Kelvin (K).

Contrast—The ability to discriminate light from dark.

Contrast Sensitivity—The ability of the eye to discern subtle degrees of contrast. The ability to discern an object against a background.

Cornea—The transparent part of the outer coat situated in the front of the eyeball, responsible for helping to focus light.

Coving—Used primarily with sheet goods and carpet, although tile can also be coved. The floor covering is installed up the wall to the desired height and finished at the top with capping.

CRI—See *Color Rendering Index.*

Cues—Verbal prompts or directions, signals, signs, or landmarks in the environment to help orient residents.

Delamination—The separation of layers in a laminate, through failure within the adhesive or the bond between the adhesive and laminate.

Dementia—The loss of intellectual function (such as thinking, remembering, and reasoning) of sufficient severity to interfere with a person's daily functioning. Dementia is not a disease in itself but a group of symptoms that characterize certain diseases and conditions. Symptoms may also include changes in personality, mood, and behavior. Dementia is irreversible when caused by disease or injury, but may be reversible when caused by drugs, alcohol, hormone or vitamin imbalances, or depression. Alzheimer's disease is the most common form of dementia.

Depression—The diagnostic criteria for major depression include symptoms such as depressed mood, marked diminished interest in everyday activities, change in appetite, insomnia or hypersommia, psychomotor agitation or retardation, fatigue or loss of energy, feelings of worthlessness or inappropriate guilt, diminished concentration or thinking abilities, and recurring thoughts of death and suicide. A diagnosis of major depression is made when at least five of these symptoms are present for at least two weeks.

Diabetic Retinopathy—A late complication of diabetes caused by a breakdown of the blood vessels of the retina. Damaged blood vessels may leak fluid or blood and develop scar tissue. Vision may fluctuate from nearly normal to blurred, distorted, or partially blocked.

Dimensional Stability—The ability to maintain the original intended dimensions when influenced by a foreign substance.

Direct-Glue Method—Installation technique in which carpet is glued directly to decking or subflooring.

Dry Foam Shampoo—Dry foam cleaning is a version of the shampoo method. The term "dry" is a relative term used to describe the low amount of liquid used (10% liquid, 90% air). Dry foam cleaning utilizes equipment with a foam generator that whips the shampoo liquid into a foam before it is applied to the carpet. It has a vacuum recovery system to extract the soiled foam solution.

Dry Powder Cleaning—A system in which an absorbent powder is worked into the carpet pile, then vacuumed out. The powder contains surfactants and solvents and is damp to the touch.

Environment—The whole of the external influences affecting the individual and determining his development.

Extractor—Wands used with steam cleaning equipment or any system that extracts moisture from the fabric or carpet.

Fabric Protector—Spray-on aftertreatment to protect treated fabric from rapid resoiling and staining.

fc—See *Foot Candle.*

Fifth Generation Stain-Resistant Fiber/Systems—After carpet is manufactured it is treated with a stain blocking process. A treatment is applied that fills the dye sites with a clear coating. This process blocks most fluids from actually reaching the dye surface, offering superior stain resistance, even after stains are allowed to dry.

Filament—A single strand of fiber. Natural filaments are grown as hair on animals or as part of a plant structure. Synthetic fibers are extruded with or without dye combined in the fiber.

Filament Yarn—A yarn made of two or more continuous monofilaments held together by twist or otherwise.

Fire Resistance—The ability of a material or assembly to withstand fire or to give protection from it.

Fire Retardant—A chemical or preparation of chemicals used to reduce flammability or to retard the spread of a fire over the surface.

Flame Resistance—The affinity of a carpet or fabric to factors involved in flame resistance, including the type and volume of pile fibers, the backing and adhesive systems, and any chemical additives that are topically applied.

Flame Retardant—A chemical compound that can be incorporated into a textile fiber during manufacture or applied to a fiber, fabric or other textile item during processing or use to reduce its flammability.

Flame Spread—The propagation of a flame away from the source of ignition across the surface of a liquid or solid, or through the volume of a gaseous mixture.

Flammability—A product's capacity for combustion with respect to flame spread, fuel contribution, smoke generation, and other factors.

Flanking Sound—Sound leakage. Some elements that can lead to flanking are improperly sealed floor and ceiling junctions, connecting ductwork, poor door seals, and electrical outlets.

Foot-candle—A measure of the light falling in an area and on a given object, abbreviated fc. Also known as illuminance. Different levels of illuminance are recommended for different tasks.

Formaldehyde—A chemical used in phenol-formaldehyde resin glue. Most furniture is held together by this glue, as is particleboard flooring. There is a good chance that small amounts of formaldehyde gas will collect on the carpet in dead air spaces, in corners, under furniture, and in closets. The presence of formaldehyde gas will manifest itself through a change in the carpet color, usually a loss of red dye. Therefore brown will turn to green and green to yellow. Formaldehyde is a deadly poison.

Glare—An intolerance to light.

Glaucoma—A buildup of fluid pressure (not tears) inside the eye resulting in damage to the optic nerve, which causes loss of peripheral vision and contrast.

Gluedown—A method of installation where the carpet is glued directly to the floor.

Hospice—A philosophy of care that focuses on relief of symptoms, pain control and providing personal, emotional, and spiritual support to patients and their families through the period of dying.

Hue—The name of a color. The primary colors are red, yellow, and blue. The secondary colors, made by mixing two primary colors, are orange, green, and violet.

Intraocular Pressure—The measurement of the pressure in the eyeball with a tonometer, done to rule out glaucoma.

Intervention and Care Strategies—Care methods and approaches that involve communication appropriate to the person with dementing illness, and plans that will meet that person's needs. Staff should be alert to the feelings expressed by the person with dementia, and should consider alternative actions, activities, or environmental stimuli that can serve to intervene, distract, or divert from potential problematic behavior.

Iris—The circular, colored portion of the eye that works as a shutter to control the size of the pupil in its center.

Jamb—The side of a door frame, doorway, or window; usually the side on which the opening for the lock is placed.

Lamp—a source of light; a bulb or capsule of any size or shape. Not to be confused with a lighting instrument.

Landmarks—Physical features of the environment that stand out and are memorable. Landmarks aid wayfinding by helping users to know where they are and to decide how to reach their destination.

Late Stage—Although determination of late, end, or terminal stage of Alzheimer's disease is highly individual, typically the dementia has progressed to the extent that the person has little capacity for self care, is usually incontinent, and may have difficulty with seizures, swallowing, infections, and communication.

Lens—The transparent structure in the eye behind the iris, which changes its shape to bring rays of light to focus on the retina.

Level Loop—A carpet style having all tufts in a loop form and of identical height. May be woven or tufted.

Licensure Certification—Each state licenses nursing homes on the basis of state standards. Six states currently have added requirements for special care units, and other states are developing such regulations. Federal regulations for Medicare and Medicaid certification are also done by the states and incorporate 1987 and 1990 OBRA nursing home reform requirements. The survey process determines which facilities meet standards to receive Medicaid or Medicare payments. State certificate of need regulations may also control the number of nursing home beds in a State. Local fire protection and life safety codes are also part of the regulatory structure.

Lightfastness—The ability of a material to resist color loss or fading due to exposure to light.

Low Vision—A significant reduction of visual function that cannot be corrected to the normal range by ordinary glasses, contact lenses, medical treatment, and/or surgery.

Lumen—The unit measuring the quantity of the actual light output of a lamp in all directions from the source.

Luminescence—Emission of light not caused by incandescence but rather caused by physiological processes, chemical action, friction, or electrical action.

Macula—An area in the center of the retina responsible for details, color, and daylight vision.

Macular Degeneration—The deterioration of the macula (center) of the retina, resulting in loss of the detail vision needed for reading small print and discerning facial features. This condition is generally considered to be age-related.

Masking Noise—Noise that covers up or masks other sounds. Masking noise may be naturally occurring background noise, such as that from HVAC systems, distant conversation, or outdoor sounds like traffic, or it may be produced intentionally. The most important consideration in electronic masking systems is to produce a sound spectrum that effectively masks intrusive noises without itself being intrusive.

Medicaid—A joint federal/state program intended to provide health-related services for low-income individuals. Eligibility requirements and services covered vary widely from state to state.

Medicare—Federal health insurance that pays for skilled care in a Medicare-certified skilled nursing facility for up to 100 days following hospitalization in a calendar year. Beneficiaries are required to make a coinsurance payment for the twenty-first through the hundredth day of care. There are no benefits provided for intermediate or custodial care.

Mildew—The growth of fungus, normally gray or black in color and having the appearance of small black specks of pepper. It is normally caused by exposure to excessive moisture.

Mission Statement—A written statement of the goals, intent, or purpose of the facility and/or care program, describing who the program serves, the location, characteristics of the environment, the staff, and their approach to care.

Mobility—The skill to travel safely, comfortably, and independently.

Moisture Barrier—Initial application of dry cleaning solvent to "waterproof" sensitive fabrics.

Noise Reduction Coefficient—The most popular laboratory rating for sound absorption. NRC makes it easier to compare different ceiling panels and other absorbent materials, and can range from 0.00 to 1.00—the higher the number, the more absorptive the material.

NRC—See *Noise Reduction Coefficient.*

Nursing Facility—A facility that provides skilled nursing care and related services for residents who require medical or nursing care; rehabilitation services for injured, disabled, or sick persons, and health-related care and services above the level of board and room and not primarily for the care and treatment of mental diseases. The distinction between intermediate care facilities (ICFs) and skilled nursing facilities (SNFs) has been eliminated for Medicaid payment differential.

Nylon—A thermoplastic polyamide resin derived from coal tar base, air, and water. Nylon was first discovered by DuPont chemists in 1938. Several years later it appeared in carpet and today is the most widely used carpet fiber. It is made either as staple or continuous filament. Characteristics: Rated as one of the longest wearing fibers, nylon is cleanable, dyeable, stain and soil resistant, abrasion resistant, able to recover resiliency, moth-proof, mildew-proof, nonallergenic, and fade resistant. It is usually acid dyed but may be solution dyed.

OBRA—See *Omnibus Budget Reconciliation Act of 1987.*

Occupational Safety and Health Administration OSHA—An agency of the U.S. Department of Labor. A federal regulatory agency with safety and health regulatory and enforcement authority for most U.S. industries.

Olefin—See *Polypropylene.*

Omnibus Budget Reconciliation Act of 1987—OBRA includes nursing home reform legislation focusing on residents' rights, assessment of a resident's cognitive status, identification of care needs, and other quality of care issues.

Optic Nerve—The nerve that carries impulses from the retina to the visual cortex of the brain.

Orientation—An awareness of self in relation to one's surroundings. This awareness is achieved through cognitive and sensory input.

OSHA—See *Occupation Safety and Health Administration.*

Peripheral Vision Loss—People with glaucoma or diabetes have loss of side vision. This affects the person's ability to move around safely in the environment.

Philosophy—The overall assumptions, values, attitudes, and ideas that influence the facility, staff, and program of a facility.

Pigment Dyeing—See *Solution Dyeing.*

Pile—The mass of raised tufts formed by the strands that have been cut at the carpet's surface; the pile provides the soft, compact, furry surface.

Polypropylene—A long-chain synthetic polymer that is composed of at least 85 percent by weight of propylene and that may be modified with several percents of another olefin, except amorphous (noncrystalline) polyolefins qualifying as rubber. The fiber is used for conventional carpet as well as indoor/outdoor carpets. Polypropylene is also being used in the manufacture of man-made backings. The fiber is produced in a continuous filament staple form, and solution dyed. Polypropylene is known for its outstanding stain resistance, easy cleanability, wearability, and low absorption factor. It is also abrasion resistant, mildew-proof, moth-proof, nonallergenic, resilient, and retains color.

Presbyopia—A significant loss of accommodation or focusing power.

Pupil—The round opening in the center of the iris that constricts and enlarges in response to light.

Resident Rights—In certified nursing facilities the rights of each resident are protected by law to safeguard and promote dignity, choice, and self-determination; the right to information; healthcare; transfer and discharge rights; handling of personal finances, and the right to be free from abuse and restraints. OBRA legislation requires each nursing facility "to care for its residents in such a manner and in such an environment as will promote maintenance or enhancement of the quality of life of each resident".

Restraints—Physical (attached or adjacent to the resident's body) and pharmacolgic (psychoactive drugs) methods that restrict a resident's movements and behavior. They have been most often used as a means to ensure an individual's safety as well as to minimize pacing, wandering, agitation, or combativeness.

Retina—The innermost layer of the eye containing nerve cells and fibers that extend from the eye to the visual cortex of the brain.

Seam Sealing—A procedure of applying a thin liquid adhesive to the two cut edges of a seam to lock in the tufts and prevent so-called edge ravel where the tufts are pulled out from the cut edge.

Seam Welding—Any stitchless procedure for joining fabrics based on the use of thermoplastic resins or the direct welding of thermoplastic materials. Seam welding is an alternative to conventional needle and thread seaming operations, and it is extremely popular in the nonwoven field.

Secondary Backing—Woven or nonwoven fabric reinforcement laminated to the back side of tufted carpet, usually with latex adhesive, to enhance dimensional stability, strength, strength resistance, lay-flat stiffness, and hand. Most secondary backings are woven jute, woven polypropylene, or nonwoven polypropylene.

Senility—This label often used to describe an individual 65 years of older with dementia. Senility used to be considered a normal part of aging. Today, physicians recognize that dementia is not a normal part of aging but the result of a disease such as Alzheimer's disease.

Solution Dyeing (or Pigment Dyeing)—Procedure producing one of the most steadfast and permanent colors in carpet. Solution dyeing is completely different and is only used with man-made fibers. The dye actually becomes part of the yarn fiber by adding the color to the fiber material when in a liquid state, prior to its being forced through the spinnerette.

Sound Movement—Direct sound is sound that reaches the listener in a straight path. Reflected sound is sound that reaches the listener after first being bounced off a hard surface, like a ball bouncing off a wall.

Sound Transmission Class—An STC rating tells you approximately how much sound will be reduced when traveling through the partition (wall or floor/ceiling). The rating range from 35 to over 60; the higher the rating, the less sound will be transmitted through the wall. The STC rating is designed to measure transmission of speech and some other sounds in a way that agrees with how the human ear perceives it.

Special Care Unit—Unit in a nursing home or residential facility that offers "special care" for people with dementia. These are also called dementia care units or Alzheimer's units.

Specialized Program for Alzheimer/Dementia Care—In this book, a special care unit, dedicated dementia care unit, or program for care for persons residing in a long-term care home or facility. An Alzheimer care program is provided by dementia-capable staff who structure the daily life of the care setting to meet the needs of their residents.

STC—See *Sound Transmission Class.*

Steam (Hot Water) Cleaning—The term steam cleaning is derived from the original concept of the equipment first utilized in the steam extraction process. Now manufacturers utilize high pressure pumps to deliver cleaning solutions to the cleaning tools and more efficient vacuum systems. The vacuum efficiency of steam extraction units is a combination of both airflow and lift. Most portable extractors utilize electric centrifugal vacuum systems. This system has superior cleaning results obtained by the flushing or rinsing ability.

Sundowning—Refers to an increase in confusion, restlessness, and/or agitation frequently experienced by the dementia patient in the late afternoon or early evening. Often sundowning occurs because the individual's internal clock is "out of sync" and he or she mixes up day and night. Sundowning may be precipitated by increased fatigue and decreasing ability to cope with a confusing environment.

Synthetic—Produced by chemical means.

Tackless Strip—Wood or metal strips fastened to the floor near the walls of a room, containing either two or three rows of pins angled toward the wall, on which the carpet backing is secured in a "stretch-in" installation.

Therapeutic Activities—Any activities that are found to be beneficial for the person with dementia.

Underlayment—Installed to cover subfloor irregularities and to absorb the movement of wood subfloors. A variety of underlayments are used to smooth and level irregularities: hardboard, particleboard, plywood, mastic with latex binders, mastic with asphalt binders, mastic with polyvinyl acetate, and so on.

Value—This describes the lightness or darkness of a color. Adding white to a color will lighten its value and give a tint of the color. Adding black to a color will darken it, producing a shade of the color.

Visual Acuity—The ability to see small details of objects, including print.

Visual Field—The total area seen by one or both eyes fixed in one position.

Watts—The power being consumed by a light source, not the light being emitted. Different from the quantity of light.

Wayfinding—Refers to what people see, what they think about, and what they do to find their way from one place to another. Wayfinding systems are the assistive mechanisms for persons to find their way from one place to another; these may be signs, arrows, or other environmental methods, including person-to-person assistance.

Yarn Dye—Topically applied color. Yarn dye is achieved most often through a vat dying process. Yarn dyed fibers offer the advantage of a wider range of available colors and design options.

References

Introduction

1 Census data, National Center for Health Statistics. Alzheimer's Association. Alzheimer's Disease Statistics (1991).

2 Alzheimer's Association. *The Alzheimer's Association National Public Policy Program to Conquer Alzheimer's Disease—1995.*

3 Fowles, D. G. Projections of Long-Term Care Needs. *Aging Magazine* (1992): 76.

4 Assisted Living Facilities Association of America (ALFAA), Senior Statistics.

5 National Center for Health Statistics.

6 Alzheimer's Association. Alzheimer's Disease Statistics (1991).

7 Alzheimer's Association. State Policy Clearinghouse. Washington, DC (1994).

8 Alzheimer's Association. *The Alzheimer's Association National Public Policy Program to Conquer Alzheimer's Disease—1995.*

Chapter 1

1 Kaufman, M. Universal Design in Focus. *Metropolis: The Urban Magazine of Architecture and Design* (November 1992).

2 Schneider, E. The Scientific Director of the Buck Center for Research in Aging to Marin County Board of Supervisors. *HealthSpan.* Vol. 6, No. 1 (Summer 1995): 3–6.

3 Schneider, E. The Scientific Director of the Buck Center for Research in Aging to Marin County Board of Supervisors. *HealthSpan.* Vol. 6, No. 1 (Summer 1995): 3–6.

4 Liberman, J. Take Off Your Glasses and See. *Universal Light Technology News* (Winter/Spring 1995).

5 The Lighthouse Headquarters in New York: A National Model of Accessibility for People with Impaired Vision. Presented at NEOCON, Chicago (1994).

6 Bedell, T. The Scent of a Memory. *Age Wave: More Life.* Vol. 1, No. 3 (1994): 4–5.

7 Bedell, T. The Scent of a Memory. *Age Wave: More Life.* Vol. 1, No. 3 (1994): 4–5.

8 AIA Foundation. *Design for Aging: An Architects Guide.* Washington, DC: The AIA Press (1985): 1–9.

9 Forer, A. Heading Off Osteoporosis. *AgeWave: Get Up and Go* (September 1994): 5.

10 Healing Motions. *AgeWave: More Life.* Vol. 1, No. 3 (September 1994).

11 Injection Spells Relief for Arthritic Joints. *HealthSpan, Buck Center for Research in Aging.* Vol. 6, No. 1 (Summer 1995).

12 American Academy of Orthopedic Surgeons.

13 Streim, J. and I. Katz. Treating Depression. *Provider* (May 1994).

14 Differential Diagnosis of Dementing Diseases. National Institutes of Health Consensus Development Conference Statement. Vol. 6, No. 11 (July 6–8, 1987): 17–24.

15 A Special Report: Alzheimer's Disease. *Harvard Health Letter.* Boston: Harvard Medical School Health Publication Group (1994): 1–5.

16 A Special Report: Alzheimer's Disease. *Harvard Health Letter.* Boston: Harvard Medical School Health Publication Group (1994): 1–5.

17 U.S. Congress, Office of Technology Assessment. *Losing a Million Minds: Confronting the Tragedy of Alzheimer's Disease and Other Dementias.* Washington, DC: U.S. Government Printing Office. OTA-BA-323 (1987): 9.

18 A Special Report: Alzheimer's Disease. *Harvard Health Letter.* Boston: Harvard Medical School Health Publication Group (1994): 1–5.

19 Differential Diagnosis of Dementing Diseases. National Institutes of Health Consensus Development Conference Statement. Vol. 6, No. 11 (July 6–8, 1987): 17-24.

20 Bachman, D. L., P. A. Wolf, R. Linn, J. E. Knoefel, J. Cobb, A. Belanger, R. B. D'Agostino, and R. White. Prevalence of Dementia and Probable Dementia: Senile Dementia of the Alzheimer's Type in the Framingham Study. *Neurology.* Vol. 42 (1992): 115–119.

21 Differential Diagnosis of Dementing Diseases. National Institutes of Health Consensus Development Conference Statement. Vol. 6, No. 11 (July 6–8, 1987): 17–24.

Chapter 2

1 Alzheimer's Association. *The Alzheimer's Association National Public Policy Program to Conquer Alzheimer's Disease — 1995.*

2 Alzheimer's Association. Memory and Aging (1991).

3 Discoveries in Health for Aging Americans: Progress Report on Alzheimer's Disease 1994. National Institutes of Health, National Institute on Aging (1994).

4 Alzheimer's Association. Memory and Aging (1991).

5 Discoveries in Health for Aging Americans: Progress Report on Alzheimer's Disease 1994, National Institutes of Health, National Institute on Aging (1994).

6 Discoveries in Health for Aging Americans: Progress Report on Alzheimer's Disease 1994. National Institutes of Health, National Institute on Aging (1994).

7 The Alzheimer's Association. *The Alzheimer's Association National Public Policy Program to Conquer Alzheimer's Disease — 1995.*

8 Alzheimer's Association. Is It Alzheimer's? Ten Warning Signs (1994).

9 A Special Report: Alzheimer's Disease. *Harvard Health Letter.* Boston: Harvard Medical School Health Publication Group (1994): 1–5.

10 Discoveries in Health for Aging Americans: Progress Report on Alzheimer's Disease 1994. National Institutes of Health, National Institute on Aging (1994).

11 Alzheimer's Association. Is It Alzheimer's? Ten Warning Signs (1994).

Chapter 3

1 Lindheim, R. and S. L. Syme. Environments, People, and Health. *Annual Reviews Public Health.* Vol. 4 (1983): 335–359.

2 Lindheim, R. and S. L. Syme. Environments, People, and Health. *Annual Reviews Public Health.* Vol. 4 (1983): 335–359.

3 Lindheim, R. and S. L. Syme. Environments, People, and Health. *Annual Reviews Public Health.* Vol. 4 (1983): 335–359.

4 Hiatt, L. *Nursing Home Renovation Designed for Reform.* Boston: Butterworth Architecture (1991): 2.

5 U.S. Public Health Service. Vital and Health Statistics. *Characteristics of Nursing Home Residents Health Status and Care Received.* National Nursing Home Survey United States. May–December 1977. Pub. No. (PHS) 81-1712, Washington, DC: The Services (1981).

6 Hiatt, L. *Nursing Home Renovation Designed for Reform.* Boston: Butterworth Architecture (1991): 7.

7 Brawley, E. Form Versus Function. Presented at the Alzheimer's Association National Education Conference, Chicago (1994).

8 Hiatt, L. *Nursing Home Renovation Designed for Reform.* Boston: Butterworth Architecture (1991): 2, 4.

9 Liebrock, C. *Beautiful Barrier-Free.* New York: Van Nostrand Reinhold (1993).

10 Syme, S. Leonard, Professor Emeritus of Epidemiology, School of Public Health, University of California, Berkeley. The Contribution of Roslyn Lindheim. Presented at the Conference on Blueprint for Aging, University of California, Berkeley, Oakland (June 1995).

11 Hiatt, L. *Nursing Home Renovation Designed for Reform.* Boston: Butterworth Architecture (1991): 7.

12 Hiatt, L. *Nursing Home Renovation Designed for Reform.* Boston: Butterworth Architecture (1991): 4.

13 Brawley, E. Alzheimer's Disease: Designing the Physical Environment. *The American Journal of Alzheimer's Care and Related Disorders & Research* (January/February 1992): 3–8.

14 Fowles, D. G. Projections of Long-Term Care Needs. *Aging Magazine* (1992): 76.

15 Kleeman, W. *The Challenge of Interior Design.* Boston: CBI Publishing (1981): 149.

16 Rickman, L. and C. Soble. *Home for a Lifetime: A New Market Niche for NAHB Builders/Remodelers.* Washington, DC: National Association of Home Builders National Research Center (1988): 11.

Chapter 4

1 Kirk, T., Vice-President, Patient & Family Services, Alzheimer's Association. *Assisted Living Today.* Vol. 1, No. 3 (Spring 1994): 32–36.

2 Young, Diane, Chairperson, Patient & Family Services Committee, Alzheimer's Association. *Assisted Living Today.* Vol. 1, No. 3 (Spring 1994): 32–36.

Chapter 5

1 U.S. Congress, Office of Technology Assessment. *Losing a Million Minds: Confronting the Tragedy of Alzheimer's Disease and Other Dementias.* Washington, DC: U.S. Government Printing Office. OTA-BA-323 (1987): 9.

2 U.S. Department of Health and Human Services, Centers for Disease Control, National Center for Health Statistics. The National Nursing Home Survey, 1985: Summary for the United States. DHHS Pub. No. (PHS) 89-1758, Hyattsville, MD (January 1989).

U.S. Congress, Office of Technology Assessment. *Special Care Units for People with Alzheimer's and Other Dementias*. Washington, DC: U.S. Government Printing Office. OTA-H-543 (1992): 10.

3 U.S. Congress, Office of Technology Assessment. *Special Care Units for People with Alzheimer's and Other Dementias*. Washington, DC: U.S. Government Printing Office. OTA-H-543 (1992): 58.

4 U.S. Congress, Office of Technology Assessment. *Special Care Units for People with Alzheimer's and Other Dementias*. Washington, DC: U.S. Government Printing Office. OTA-H-543 (1992): 16.

5 Discoveries in Health for Aging Americans: Progress Report on Alzheimer's Disease 1994. National Institutes of Health, National Institute on Aging (1994).

6 Rockey, A. The Exceptional Environment: Preparing for Dementia Care. *Provider* (July 1993): 25–36.

7 Berg, L., K. C. Buckwalter, P. K. Chafetz, L. P. Gwyther, D. Holmes, K. Koepke, M. P. Lawton, D. A. Lindeman, J. Magaziner, K. Maslow, J. Morley, M. Ory, P. Rabins, P. D. Sloane, and J. Theresi. Special Care Units for Persons with Dementia. *Journal of American Geriatrics Society.* Vol. 39, No. 12 (December 1991): 1229–1236.

8 Gold, D. T., P. D. Sloane, L. Matthew, M. Bledsoe, and D. Konanc. Special Care Units: A Typology of Care Settings for Memory-Impaired Older Adults. *Gerontologist.* Vol. 31, No. 4 (August 1991): 467–475.

9 Ohta, R. J.and B. M. Ohta. Special Units for Alzheimer's Disease Patients: A Critical Look. *Gerontologist.* Vol. 28, No. 6 (December 1988): 803–808.

10 Weisman, G., M. Calkins, and P. Sloane. The Environmental Context of Special Care. *Alzheimer's Disease and Associated Disorders,* Vol. 8, Supplement 1. New York: Raven Press (1994): S308–320.

11 Ohta, R. J. and B. M. Ohta. Special Units for Alzheimer's Disease Patients: A Critical Look. *Gerontologist.* Vol. 28, No. 6 (December 1988): 803–808.

Gold, D. T., P. D. Sloane, L. Matthew, M. Bledsoe, and D. Konanc. Special Care Units: A Typology of Care Settings for Memory Impaired Older Adults. *Gerontologist.* Vol. 31, No. 4 (August 1991): 467–475.

12 Ohta, R. J. and B. M. Ohta. Special Units for Alzheimer's Disease Patients: A Critical Look. *Gerontologist.* Vol. 28, No. 6 (December 1988): 803–808.

Berg, L., K. C. Buckwalter, P. K. Chafetz, L. P. Gwyther, D. Holmes, K. Koepke, M. P. Lawton, D. A. Lindeman, J. Magaziner, K. Maslow, J. Morley, M. Ory, P. Rabins, P. D. Sloane, and J. Theresi. Special Care Units for Persons with Dementia. *Journal of American Geriatrics Society.* Vol. 39, No. 12 (December 1991): 1229–1236.

Gold, D. T., P. D. Sloane, L. Matthew, M. Bledsoe, and D. Konanc. Special Care Units: A Typology of Care Settings for Memory-Impaired Older Adults. *Gerontologist.* Vol. 31, No. 4 (August 1991): 467–475.

13 Weisman, G., Calkins, M., & Sloane, P. The Environmental Context of Special Care. *Alzheimer's Disease and Associated Disorders, Supplement 1.* New York: Raven Press, Ltd. (1994): S308-320.

14 Ohta, R. J. and B. M. Ohta. Special Units for Alzheimer's Disease Patients: A Critical Look. *Gerontologist.* Vol. 28, No. 6 (December 1988): 803–808.

15 Ohta, R. J. and B. M. Ohta. Special Units for Alzheimer's Disease Patients: A Critical Look. *Gerontologist.* Vol. 28, No. 6 (December 1988): 803–808.

Berg, L., K. C. Buckwalter, P. K. Chafetz, L. P. Gwyther, D. Holmes, K. Koepke, M. P. Lawton, D. A. Lindeman, J. Magaziner, K. Maslow, J. Morley, M. Ory, P. Rabins, P. D. Sloane, and J. Theresi. Special Care Units for Persons with Dementia. *Journal of American Geriatrics Society.* Vol. 39, No. 12 (December 1991): 1229–1236.

16 Boling, K. and L. Gwyther. Defining Quality for Nursing Home Residents with Dementia. *Dementia Units in Long Term Care,* ed(s). Sloane, P. and L. Matthew. Baltimore: Johns Hopkins Press (1991): 3–22.

17 Sloane, P. and Matthew, L. The Therapeutic Environment Screening Scale. *The American Journal of Alzheimer's Care and Related Disorders & Research.* (November/December 1990): 22.

18 Rockey, A. The Exceptional Environment: Preparing for Dementia Care. *Provider* (July 1993): 25–36.

19 Alzheimer's Association Patient and Family Services. *Guidelines for Dignity: Goals of Specialized Alzheimer/Dementia Care in Residential Settings* (1992): 7.

20 Alzheimer's Association Patient and Family Services. *Guidelines for Dignity: Goals of Specialized Alzheimer/Dementia Care in Residential Settings* (1992): 7.

21 U.S. Congress, Office of Technology Assessment. *Special Care Units for People with Alzheimer's and Other Dementias*. Washington, DC: U.S. Government Printing Office OTA-H-543 (1992): 10–11.

22 U.S. Congress, Office of Technology Assessment.

Special Care Units for People with Alzheimer's and Other Dementias. Washington, DC: U.S. Government Printing Office OTA-H-543 (1992): 18.

23 Lawton, M. P. Environmental Approaches to Research and Treatment of Alzheimer's Disease. *Alzheimer's Disease Treatment and Family Stress: Directions for Research.* E. Light and B. D. Lebowitz (Eds.). Rockville, MD: National Institute of Mental Health, U.S. Department of Health and Human Services (1989).

24 U.S. Congress, Office of Technology Assessment. *Special Care Units for People with Alzheimer's and Other Dementias.* Washington, DC: U.S. Government Printing Office OTA-H-543 (1992): 19.

25 Robinson, A., B. Spencer, and L. White. *Understanding Difficult Behaviors.* Ypsilanti, MI: Eastern Michigan University (1992).

26 Rabins, P., E. Morril, L. Johnson, S. Smith, and R. Low. Perspectives on a Special Care Unit. *The American Journal of Alzheimer's Care and Related Disorders & Research* (September/October 1990): 13–21.

27 Robinson, A., B. Spencer, and L. White. *Understanding Difficult Behaviors.* Ypsilanti, MI: Eastern Michigan University (1992).

28 Namazi, K., P. J. Whitehouse, L. Rechlin, M. Calkins, B. Johnson, B. Brabender, and S. Hevener. Environmental Modifications in a Specially Designed Unit for the Care of Patients with Alzheimer's Disease: An Overview and Introduction. Article 1. *The American Journal of Alzheimer's Care and Related Disorders & Research* (November/December 1991): 3–9.

29 Hiatt, L. *Nursing Home Renovation Designed for Reform.* Boston: Butterworth Architecture (1991): 4.

30 Hiatt, L., J. P. Rupprecht, S. Brekhus, and T. Moss. Wandering. *The Gerontologist.* Vol. 18, No. 3 (1978).

31 Mace, N. and P. Rabins. *The 36 Hour Day.* Baltimore: The Johns Hopkins University Press (1991).

32 Rabins, P., E. Morril, L. Johnson, S. Smith, and R. Low. Perspectives on a Special Care Unit. *The American Journal of Alzheimer's Care and Related Disorders & Research* (September/October 1990): 13–21.

33 Rabins, P., E. Morril, L. Johnson, S. Smith, and R. Low. Perspectives on a Special Care Unit. *The American Journal of Alzheimer's Care and Related Disorders & Research* (September/October 1990): 13–21.

34 Coons, D. Wandering. *The American Journal of Alzheimer's Care and Related Disorders and Research.* Vol. 3, No. 1 (1988).

35 Namazi, K., T. Rosner, and M. Calkins. Visual Barriers to Prevent Ambulatory Alzheimer's Patients from Exiting Through an Emergency Door. *Gerontologist.*

Vol. 29 (1989): 699–702.

36 Williams, M., G. Doyle, E. Feeney, P. Lenihan, and S. Salisbury. Alzheimer's Unit by Design. *Geriatric Nursing* (January/February 1991).

37 Namazi, K., T. Rosner, and M. Calkins. Visual Barriers to Prevent Ambulatory Alzheimer's Patients from Exiting Through an Emergency Door. *Gerontologist.* Vol. 29 (1989): 699–702.

38 Sanford, J. Design Research for Older Adults: Implications for the Design of Long Term Care Facilities for People with Dementia. *The Journal of Healthcare Design* (1995): 79-84.

39 Dickinson, J., J. McLain-Kark, and A. Marshall-Baker. The Effects of Visual Barriers on Exiting Behavior in a Dementia Care Unit. *The Gerontologist.* Vol. 35, No. 1 (1995): 127–130.

40 Namazi, K., P. J. Whitehouse, L. Rechlin, M. Calkins, B. Johnson, B. Brabender, and S. Hevener. Environmental Modifications in a Specially Designed Unit for the Care of Patients with Alzheimer's Disease: An Overview and Introduction. *The American Journal of Alzheimer's Care and Related Disorders & Research* (November/December 1991): 3–9.

41 Brawley, E. The Impact of the Environment on People with Alzheimer's Disease. Presented at the Alzheimer's Association Education Conference, Kansas City (1994).

42 Rabins, P., E. Morril, L. Johnson, S. Smith, and R. Low. Perspectives on a Special Care Unit. *The American Journal of Alzheimer's Care and Related Disorders & Research* (September/October 1990): 13–21.

Chapter 6

1 Hiatt, L. G. Designing for Mentally Impaired Persons: Integrating Knowledge of People with Programs, Architecture and Interior Design. Presented at the Annual Meeting of the American Association of Homes for the Aging, Los Angeles (1985).

2 Calkins, M. Proper Environment May Be Therapeutic to Influence Dementia Patients' Behavior. *Group Practice Journal* (July/August 1991): 58–66.

3 Cohen, U. and G. Weisman. *Holding on to Home:* Baltimore, MD: The Johns Hopkins University Press (1991): 28–35.

4 Calkins, M. P. *Design for Dementia.* Owings Mill, MD: National Health Publishing (1988).

5 Weisman, G., M. Calkins, and P. Sloane. The Environmental Context of Special Care. *Alzheimer's Disease and Associated Disorders,* Vol. 8, Supplement 1. New York: Raven Press (1994): S308–320.

6 Wimberly, E. and N. Kutner. Atlanta Case Study: Determining What Is "Special" in an Alzheimer

Disease Special Care Unit. *Alzheimer's Disease and Associated Disorders,* Vol. 8, Supplement 1. New York: Raven Press (1994): S115–125.

7 Mace, N. and P. Rabins. *The 36 Hour Day.* Baltimore: The Johns Hopkins University Press (1991).

Chapter 7

1 Clark, L. *The Ancient Art of Color Therapy.* New York: Pocket Books (1975): 21.

2 Clark, L. *The Ancient Art of Color Therapy.* New York: Pocket Books (1975): 26.

3 Edmunds, L. N., *Cell Cycle Clocks.* New York: Marcel Dekker (1984): 121–122.

4 Clark, L. *The Ancient Art of Color Therapy.* New York: Pocket Books (1975): 27.

5 Weininger, J. Sun: Nutrition Tips for Summer. *The San Francisco Chronicle* (June 15, 1994).

6 Tinetti, M. and M. Speechley. Prevention of Falls Among the Elderly. *The New England Journal of Medicine.* Vol. 320, No. 16 (April 1989): 1055.

7 Wurtman, R. J. The Effects of Light on the Human Body. *Scientific American.* Vol. 233 (July 1975): 3.

8 Singer, C. and R. Hughes. Clinical Use of Bright Light in Geriatric Neuropsychiatry. *Lighting for Aging Vision and Health* (1995): 143–146.

9 Lewy, A., T. Wehr, F. Goodwin, D. Newsome, and S. Markey. Light Suppresses Melatonin Secretions in Humans. *Science.* Vol. 210 (1980): 1267–1269.

10 Lewy, A. and D. Newsome. Different Types of Melatonin Circadian Secretory Rhythm in Some Blind Subjects. *Journal of Clinical Endocrinology and Metabolism.* Vol. 56, No. 6 (1983): 1103–1107.

Singer, C. and R. Hughes. Clinical Use of Bright Light in Geriatric Neuropsychiatry. *Lighting for Aging Vision and Health.* (1995): 143–146.

11 Ubell, E. Lighten Up Winter Sadness. *Parade Magazine* (November 3, 1991): 12–14.

12 Singer, C. and R. Hughes. Clinical Use of Bright Light in Geriatric Neuropsychiatry. *Lighting for Aging Vision and Health* (1995): 143–146.

13 Rae, S. Bright Light, Big Therapy. *Modern Maturity* (February/March 1994).

14 Gallagher, W. Solar Power. *American Health* (January/February 1991).

15 Hollowich, F. *The Influence of Ocular Light Perception on Metabolism in Man and in Animal.* New York: Springer-Verlag. Vol. 2 (1979): 13–14.

16 Wurtman, R. J. The Effects of Light on the Human Body. *Scientific American.* Vol. 233 (July 1975): 3.

17 Black, D. Does Sunlight Heal or Harm? *The Health Consumer's Health & Wellness Report.* Springville, UT: Tapestry Communications. Vol. 3, No. 6 (1993).

18 Campbell, S., D. Kripke, J. Gillin, and J. Hrubovcak. Exposure to Light in Healthy Elderly Subjects and Alzheimer's Patients. *Physiological Behavior.* Vol. 42 (1988): 141–144.

19 Singer, C. and R. Hughes, Clinical Use of Bright Light in Geriatric Neuropsychiatry. *Lighting for Aging Vision and Health* (1995): 143–146.

20 Singer, C. and R. Hughes, Clinical Use of Bright Light in Geriatric Neuropsychiatry. *Lighting for Aging Vision and Health* (1995): 143–146.

21 Campbell, S., D. Dawson, and M. Anderson. Alleviation of Sleep Maintenance Insomnia with Timed Exposure to Bright Light. *Journal of American Geriatric Society.* Vol. 41 (1993): 829–836.

22 Rae, S. Bright Light, Big Therapy. *Modern Maturity* (February/March 1994).

23 Rae, S. Bright Light, Big Therapy. *Modern Maturity* (February/March 1994).

24 Rae, S. Bright Light, Big Therapy. *Modern Maturity* (February/March 1994).

25 Satlin, A., L. Volicer, V. Ross, L. Herz, and S. Campbell. Bright Light Treatment of Behavioral and Sleep Disturbances in Patients with Alzheimer's Disease. *American Journal of Psychiatry.* Vol. 149, No. 8 (1992): 1028–1032.

26 Singer, C. and R. Hughes. Clinical Use of Bright Light in Geriatric Neuropsychiatry. *Lighting for Aging Vision and Health* (1995): 143–146.

27 Marberry, S. and L. Zagon. *Color as Light and Energy.* New York: Wiley (1995).

28 *The Lighthouse National Survey on Vision Loss: The Experience, Attitudes and Knowledge of Middle-Aged and Older Americans.* New York: The Lighthouse (1995).

29 Boling, R. Eye on the Aging Eye. *Modern Maturity* (January/February 1996).

30 Crews, J. E. and R. G. Long. Critical Concerns and Effective Practices Among Programs for Older People Who Are Visually Impaired, Part II: A Preliminary Report of the Findings of Three Focus Groups. *Aging & Vision News.* Lighthouse National Center for Vision and Aging. Vol. 7, No. 1 (Spring 1995).

31 National Center for Health Statistics (1986), R. J. Havlik. Aging in the Eighties: Impaired Senses for Sound and Light in Persons 65 Years and Over. Preliminary data from the Supplement on Aging to the National Health Interview Survey, United States, January–June 1984. *Advance Data from Vital and Health Statistics.* No. 125. DHHS Pub. N. (PHS) 86–1250, Public Health Services. Hyattsville, MD (September 19, 1986).

Stuen, C., *Aging & Vision News.* Lighthouse National Center for Vision and Aging. Vol. 7, No. 1 (Spring 1995).

32 U.S. Senate Special Committee on Aging, the American Association of Retired Persons, the Federal Council on Aging, and the U.S. Administration on Aging. Aging America—Trends and Projections. Washington, DC: U.S. Department of Health and Human Services (1991): 252.

33 National Center for Health Statistics (1986), R. J. Havlik. Aging in the Eighties: Impaired Senses for Sound and Light in Persons 65 Years and Over. Preliminary data from the Supplement on Aging to the National Health Interview Survey, United States, January–June 1984. *Advance Data from Vital and Health Statistics*. No. 125. DHHS Pub. N. (PHS) 86–1250, Public Health Services. Hyattsville, MD (September 19, 1986).

34 Fangmeier, R. *The World Through Their Eyes: Understanding Vision Loss*. New York: The Lighthouse (1994): 8.

35 Fangmeier, R. *The World Through Their Eyes: Understanding Vision Loss*. New York: The Lighthouse (1994): 9.

36 American Optometric Association.

37 Fangmeier, R. *The World Through Their Eyes: Understanding Vision Loss*. New York: The Lighthouse (1994): 19.

38 Fangmeier, R. *The World Through Their Eyes: Understanding Vision Loss*. New York: The Lighthouse (1994): 26.

39 Fangmeier, R. *The World Through Their Eyes: Understanding Vision Loss*. New York: The Lighthouse (1994).

40 Cronin-Golomb, A. Vision in Alzheimer's Disease. *The Gerontologist*. Vol. 35, No. 3 (1995): 370–376.

41 Cronin-Golomb, A., R. Sugiura, S. Corking, and J. H. Growdon. Incomplete Achromatopsia in Alzheimer's disease. *Neurobiology of Aging*. Vol. 14 (1993): 471–477.

Kurylo, D., et al. Broad-Band Visual Capacities Are Not Selectively Impaired in Alzheimer's Disease. *Neurobiology of Aging*. Vol. 15 (1994): 305–311.

42 Cronin-Golomb, A., S. Corkin, and J. H. Growdon. Visual Dysfunction in Alzheimer's disease: Relation to Normal Aging. *Annals of Neurology*. Vol. 29 (1991): 41–52.

43 Cronin-Golomb, A., S. Corkin, and J.H. Grodon. Visual Dysfunction Predicts Cognitive Deficits in Alzheimer's Disease. *Optometry and Vision Science*. Vol. 72 (1995): 168–176.

44 Horowitz, A. Vision Impairment and Functional Disability Among Nursing Home Residents. *The Gerontologist*. Vol. 34 (1994): 316–323.

Cronin-Golomb, A. Vision in Alzheimer's Disease. *The Gerontologist*. Vol. 35, No. 3 (1995): 370–376.

45 Fangmeier, R. *The World Through Their Eyes: Understanding Vision Loss*. New York: The Lighthouse (1994).

46 Cronin-Golomb, A. Vision in Alzheimer's Disease. *The Gerontologist*. Vol. 35, No. 3 (1995): 370–376.

Chapter 8

1 Guth, S. K. Effects of Age on Visibility. *American Journal of Optometry*. Vol. 34 (1957): 463–477.

2 McFarland, R. A. and M. B. Fisher. Alteration of Dark Adaptation as a Function of Age. *Journal of Gerontology*. Vol. 10 (1955): 424–428.

3 Noell, E. Long Term Care Design: Lighting. *Journal of Healthcare Design*. Vol. IV (1991): 65–69.

4 Dana, A. Glare. *Interiors* (March 1992): 81.

5 Noell, E. Long Term Care Design: Lighting. *Journal of Healthcare Design*. Vol IV (1991): 65–69.

6 Noell, E. Long Term Care Design: Lighting. *Journal of Healthcare Design*. Vol. IV (1991): 65–69.

7 Birren, F. *Color and Human Response*. New York: Van Nostrand Reinhold (1978): 35–41.

8 Dana, A. *Interiors* (March 1992): 81.

9 Wurtman, R. J. The Effects of Light on the Human Body. *Scientific American*. Vol. 223 (July 1975): 3.

10 Colby, B. *Color and Light: Influences and Impact*. Glendale, CA: Chroma Productions (1990).

11 Brainard, G. The Future Is Now: Implications of the Effect of Light on Hormones. Brain & Behavior. *Journal of Healthcare Design*. Vol. VII(1994): 49–56.

12 Childs, K. The Daylighting Option. *Perspective* (Summer 1995): 20–21.

13 Noell, E. Issues, Problems and Opportunities. *Lighting for Aging Vision and Health* (1995): 149–157.

14 Noell, E. Issues, Problems and Opportunities. *Lighting for Aging Vision and Health* (1995): 149–157.

15 Childs, K. The Daylighting Option. *Perspective* (Summer 1995): 20–21.

16 Seliger, S. The Right Light. *Home Office* (Fall 1986): 84–86.

17 Colby, B. *Color and Light: Influences and Impact*. Glendale, CA: Chroma Productions (1990): 51.

18 Blecker, N. The Benefits of Energy Efficient Lighting. *Interiors & Sources* (January/February 1992).

19 Benya, J. R. Advanced Health Care Facility Lighting Design. *Journal of HealthcareDesign*. Vol. VI (1993): 185–191.

20 Schwartz, B. Watching Your Back. *Interiors* (September 1992): 65.

21 Schwartz, B. Off-Site System Maintenance. *Interiors* (February 1994): 20.

22 *Shades of Light*. Richmond (1995).

23 *Shades of Light.* Richmond (1995).

24 Benya, J. R. Advanced Health Care Facility Lighting Design. *Journal of Healthcare Design.* Vol. VI (1993): 185–191.

25 Noell, E. Issues, Problems and Opportunities: Appropriate Lighting for Aging Vision and Health. *Lighting for Aging Vision and Health* (1995): 149–156.

Chapter 9

1 Colby, B. *Color and Light: Influences and Impact.* Glendale, CA: Chroma Productions (1990).

2 Birren, F. *Color & Human Response.* New York: Van Nostrand Reinhold (1978): 91.

3 Birren, F. Color and Psychotherapy. *Interior Design* (December 1983): 166–169.

4 Colby, B. *Color and Light: Influences and Impact.* Glendale, CA: Chroma Productions (1990).

5 Birren, F. *Color & Human Response.* New York: Van Nostrand Reinhold (1978).

6 Colby, B. *Color and Light: Influences and Impact.* Glendale, CA: Chroma Productions (1990).

7 Calkins, M. *Design for Dementia.* Owings Mills, MD: National Health Publishing (1991).

8 Cooper, B. A. Long-Term Care Design: Current Research on the Use of Color. *The Journal of Healthcare Design.* Vol. VI (1993): 61–67.

9 Hughes, P. and R. Neer. Lighting for the Elderly: A Psychobiological Approach to Lighting. *Human Factors.* Vol. 23, No. 1 (1981): 65–85.

10 Cristarella, M. Visual Functions of the Elderly. *American Journal of Occupational Therapy.* Vol. 31, No. 7 (1977): 432–440.

11 Cooper, B. A. Long-Term Care Design: Current Research on the Use of Color. *The Journal of Healthcare Design.* Vol. VI (1993): 61–67.

12 Cristarella, M. Visual Functions of the Elderly. *American Journal of Occupational Therapy.* Vol. 31, No. 7 (1977): 432–440.

13 Nebes, R. D. and S. Corkin. *Handbook of Neuropsychology.* Vol. 4 (1991).

14 Cooper, B., M. Ward, C. Gowland, and J. McIntosh. The Use of the Lanthony New Color Test in Determining the Effects of Aging on Color Vision. *Jourrnal of Gerontology.* Vol. 46, No. 6 (1991): 320–324.

15 Cooper, B. Long-Term Care Design: Current Research on the Use of Color. *The Journal of Healthcare Design.* Vol. VI (1993): 61–67.

16 Cooper, B. Long-Term Care Design: Current Research on the Use of Color. *The Journal of Healthcare Design.* Vol. VI (1993): 61–67.

17 Cristarella, M. Visual Functions of the Elderly. *American Journal of Occupational Therapy.* Vol. 31, No. 7 (1977): 432–440.

Boynton, R. *Human Color Vision.* New York: Holt, Rinehart and Winston (1979).

Tetlow, K. Contrasting Colors. *Interiors* (September 1993): 42.

18 Fozzard, J., E. Wolf, B. Bell, R. McFarland, and Podolsky. *Behavioral Processes.* L. Poon (Ed.) (1980): 497–534.

19 Cooper, B., M. Ward, C. Gowland, and J. McIntosh. The Use of the Lanthony New Color Test in Determining the Effects of Aging on Color Vision. *Jourrnal of Gerontology.* Vol. 46, No. 6 (1991): 320–324.

20 Arditi, A. *Color Contrast and Partial Sight: How to Design with Colors that Contrast Effectively for People with Low Vision and Color Deficiencies.* New York: The Lighthouse (1995).

21 Pastalan, L. The Empathic Model: A Methodological Bridge Between Research and Design. *Journal of Architecture Education.* Vol. 31 (1977): 14–15.

Cooper, B. Long-Term Care Design: Current Research on the Use of Color. *The Journal of Healthcare Design.* Vol. VI (1993): 61–67.

22 Brawley, E. Alzheimer's Disease: Designing the Physical Environment. *The American Journal of Alzheimer's Care and Related Disorders & Research* (January/February 1992): 3–8.

23 Knoblauch, K. and A. Arditi. Choosing Color Contrasts in Low Vision: Practical Recommendations. Sighted, Vision Research. *The Lighthouse Research Institute.* New York: The Lighthouse (1993): 1.

24 Arditi, A. *Color Contrast and Partial Sight: How to Design with Colors that Contrast Effectively for People with Low Vision and Color Deficiencies.* New York: The Lighthouse (1995).

25 Knoblauch, K. and A. Arditi. Designing Effective Color Contrasts for the Partially-Sighted. Technical Report VR02. *The Lighthouse Research Institute.* New York: The Lighthouse (1993): 4.

26 Arditi, A. *Color Contrast and Partial Sight: How to Design with Colors that Contrast Effectively for People with Low Vision and Color Deficiencies.* New York: The Lighthouse (1995).

27 Knoblauch, K. and A. Arditi. Designing Effective Color Contrasts for the Partially-Sighted. Technical Report VR02. *The Lighthouse Research Institute.* New York: The Lighthouse (1993): 5.

28 Colby, B. *Color and Light: Influences and Impact.* Glendale, CA: Chroma Productions (1990).

29 Trent, L. Putting Color to Work. *Interiors & Sources.* (May/June 1992) 100–103.

30 Trent, L. Putting Color to Work. *Interiors & Sources.* (May/June 1992) 100–103.

31 Brawley, E. Alzheimer's Disease: Designing the Physical Environment. *The American Journal of Alzheimer's Care and Related Disorders & Research* (January/February 1992): 3–8.

32 Brawley, E. Alzheimer's Disease: Designing the Physical Environment. *The American Journal of Alzheimer's Care and Related Disorders & Research* (January/February 1992): 3–8.

33 Birren, F. *Color & Human Response*. New York: Van Nostrand Reinhold (1978).

34 Hiatt, L. Breakthroughs in Long Term Care Design. *Journal of Healthcare Design*. Vol III (1991): 205–215.

35 Schultz, D. J. Special Design Considerations for Alzheimer's Facilities. *Contemporary Long Term Care*. (November 1987): 48–56.

36 Calkins, M. Designing Special Care Units: A Systematic Approach. *The American Journal of Alzheimer's Care and Research* (March/April 1987): 16–22.

37 Cooper, B., A. Mohide, and S. Gilbert. Testing the Use of Color in Long-Term Care Settings. *Dimensions in Health Service*. Vol. 66, No. 6 (1989): 22–26.

38 Cooper, B. A Model for Implementing Color Contrast in the Environment of the Elderly. *American Journal of Occupational Therapy*. Vol. 39, No. 4 (1985): 253–258.

39 Cooper, B. Long-Term Care Design: Current Research on the Use of Color. *The Journal of Healthcare Design*. Vol. VI (1993): 61–67.

40 Hiatt, L. G. Architecure for the Aged: Design for Living. *Inland Architect*. Vol. 23 (1978): 6–17.

41 Birren, F. Color and Psychotherapy. *Interior Design* (December 1983): 166–169.

Chapter 10

1 Trent, L. On the Importance of Color. *Interiors & Sources* (September 1994): 48–49.

2 Hiatt, L. The Color and Use of Color in Environments for Older People. *Nursing Homes*. Vol. 30, No. 3 (1981): 18–22.

3 Schultz, D. J. Special Design Considerations for Alzheimer's Facilities. *Contemporary Long Term Care* (November 1987).

4 Dobbs, M. and C. Nagy. Alzheimer's Disease: The Relationship Between Selected Wallcoverings Patterns and Resident Behaviors in a Special Care Unit (1990).

5 Brawley, E. Alzheimer's Disease: Designing the Physical Environment. *The American Journal of Alzheimer's Care and Related Disorders & Research* (January/February 1992): 3–8.

6 Hiatt, L. G. Touchy About Touching? *Nursing Homes*. Vol. 29, No. 6 (1980): 42–46.

7 Brawley, E. Alzheimer's Disease: Designing the Physical Environment, *The American Journal of Alzheimer's Care and Related Disorders & Research* (January/February 1992): 3–8.

8 Ulrich, R. S. Effects of Interior Design on Wellness: Theory & Recent Scientific Research. *Journal of Healthcare Design*. Vol. III (1990): 97–109.

9 The Pet Connection. *Alzheimer's Association National Newsletter*. Vol. 15, No. 4 (Winter 1995).

10 Bedell, T. The Scent of a Memeory. *Age Wave: More Life*. Vol. 1, No. 3 (1994): 4–5.

11 Bedell, T. The Scent of a Memory. *Age Wave: More Life*. Vol. 1, No. 3 (1994): 4–5.

12 Gappell, M. *Interiors & Sources* (January/February 1995): 67.

13 Birren, F. *Color and Human Response*. New York: Van Nostrand Reinhold (1978): 97.

14 Birren, F. Color and Psychotherapy. *Interior Design* (December 1983): 166–169.

15 Birren, F. *Color & Human Response*. New York: Van Nostrand Reinhold (1978): 99–100.

16 Birren, F. *Color & Human Response*. New York: Van Nostrand Reinhold (1978).

17 Birren, F. *Color & Human Response*. New York: Van Nostrand Reinhold (1978): 99.

18 Birren, F. Color and Psychotherapy. *Interior Design* (December 1983): 166–169.

Chapter 11

1 Glass, L., Professor Emeritus of Anatomy and Psychiatry, University of California at San Francisco. Maybe the Walls Have Ears: I'm Not Sure I Do. Presented at the Blueprint for Aging Conference, Berkeley, CA (June 1995).

2 Payne, S. The Problem with Privacy. *Interiors & Sources* (September 1994): 74–77.

3 Glass, L., Professor Emeritus of Anatomy and Psychiatry, University of California at San Francisco. Maybe the Walls Have Ears: I'm Not Sure I Do. Presented at the Blueprint for Aging Conference, Berkeley, CA (June 1995).

4 Payne, S. The Problem with Privacy. *Interiors & Sources* (September 1994): 74–77.

5 Payne, S. The Problem with Privacy. *Interiors & Sources* (September 1994): 74–77.

6 Payne, S. Home Is Where the Sound Is. *Interiors & Sources* (October 1994): 79–81.

7 Payne, S. Sound Plans for Open-Plan Offices. *Interiors & Sources* (July/August 1994): 70–73.

8 Payne, S. The Problem with Privacy. *Interiors & Sources* (September 1994): 74–77.

9 Payne, S. Home Is Where the Sound Is. *Interiors & Sources* (October 1994): 79–81.

10 Goodfriend, L. Acoustics. In A. Bush-Brown and D. Davis (Eds.). *Hospitable Design for Healthcare and Senior Communities*. New York: Van Nostrand Reinhold (1992): 181–182.

11 Payne, S. The Problem with Privacy. *Interiors & Sources* (September 1994): 74–77.

12 Payne, S. The Problem With Privacy. *Interiors & Sources* (September 1994): 74–77.

13 Grumet, S. Sounding Board: Pandemonium in the Modern Hospital. *The New England Journal of Medicine.* Vol. 328 (February 11, 1993): 433–437.

14 Noell, E. Design in Nursing Homes: Environment as a Silent Partner in Caregiving. *Generations* (Winter 1995–1996): 14–17.

14 Payne, S. and D. Stover. Sound 2000. *Interiors & Sources* (January/February 1995): 68–69.

Chapter 12

1 AIA Foundation. *Design for Aging: An Architect's Guide.* Washington, DC: The AIA Press (1987): 145.

2 Carpman, J. Wayfinding: The Sign of the Times. *Group Practice Journal* (July/August 1991): 42–44.

3 Calkins, M. *Design for Dementia.* Owings Mills, MD: National Health Publishing (1988).

4 Weisman, G. D. Wayfinding and Architectural Legibility: Design Considerations in Housing Environments for the Elderly. In V. Regnier and J. Pynoos (Eds.). *Housing for the Elderly: Satisfaction and Preferences.* New York: Garland Publishing (1982).

5 Carpman, J. Wayfinding: The Sign of the Times. *Group Practice Journal* (July/August 1991): 42–44.

6 Weisman, G., M. Calkins, and P. Sloane. The Environmental Context of Special Care. *Alzheimer's Disease and Associated Disorders,* Vol. 8, Supplement 1. New York: Raven Press (1994): S308–320.

7 Calkins, M. Designing Special Care Units: A Systematic Approach. *The American Journal of Alzheimer's Care and Research* (March/April 1987): 16–22.

8 AIA Foundation. *Design for Aging: An Architect's Guide.* Washington, DC: The AIA Press (1987): 145.

9 Marberry, S. and L. Zagon. Color as Light and Energy. *The Power of Color: Creating Healthy Interior Spaces.* New York: Wiley (1995).

10 Weisman, G., M. Calkins, and P. Sloane. The Environmental Context of Special Care. *Alzheimer's Disease and Associated Disorders,* Vol. 8, Supplement 1. New York: Raven Press (1994): S308–320.

11 Namazi, K., T. T. Rosner, and L. Rechlin. Long-Term Memory Cueing to Reduce Visuo-Spatial Dis-orientation in Alzheimer's Disease Patients in a Special Care Unit. *American Journal of Alzheimer's Care and Related Disorders & Research.* Vol. 6 (1991): 16–21.

12 Namazi, K. and B. Johnson. Physical Environmental Cues to Reduce the Problems of Incontinence in Alzheimer's Disease Units. *The American Journal of Alzheimer's Care and Related Disorders & Research.* Vol. 6 (1991): 22–28.

13 Namazi, K. and B. Johnson. Physical Environmental Cues to Reduce the Problems of Incontinence in Alzheimer's Disease Units. *The American Journal of Alzheimer's Care and Related Disorders & Research.* Vol. 6 (1991): 22–28.

14 Fangmeier, R. *The World Through Their Eyes: Understanding Vision Loss.* New York: The Lighthouse (1994): 19.

Chapter 13

1 Mace, N. and P. Rabins. *The 36 Hour Day.* Baltimore: The Johns Hopkins University Press (1991).

2 Calkins, M. P. *Design for Dementia.* Owings Mills, MD: National Health Publishing (1988): 32.

3 Klages, K. Tailor-Made for Alzheimer Patients. *The Chicago Tribune* (October 2, 1994).

4 Cohen, U., G. Weisman, K. Day, W. Robinson, J. Dicker, and G. Meyer. *Illustrative Designs: Environments for People with Dementia.* Milwaukee: The School of Architecture and Urban Planning at The University of Wisconsin (1990): 35–36.

5 Noell, E. Issues, Problems, and Opportunities. *Lighting for Aging Vision and Health* (1995): 149–157.

6 AIA Foundation. *Design for Aging: An Architect's Guide.* Washington, DC: The AIA Press (1987): 145–146.

7 Colby, B. *Color & Light: Influences and Impact.* Glendale, CA: Chroma Productions (1990): 15–16.

8 Hunt, R. Complete Color Prescription. *The Ancient Art of Color.* Los Angeles: Devorss and Co. (1962): 55.

9 Bailey, I., H. Dornbusch, P. Harvey, and G. Nash-Kirton. Modifications of the Visual Environment for the Elderly. Presented at the Blueprint on Aging Conference, University of California at Berkeley (1995).

10 Cohen, U. and G. Weisman. *Holding on to Home: Designing Environments for People with Dementia.* Baltimore: The Johns Hopkins University Press (1991).

11 Cohen, U., G. Weisman, K. Day, W. Robinson, J. Dicker, and G. Meyer. *Illustrative Designs: Environments for People with Dementia.* Milwaukee: The School of Architecture and Urban Planning at The University of Wisconsin (1990): 37.

12 Cohen, U. and G. Weisman. *Holding on to Home: Designing Environments for People with Dementia.* Baltimore: The Johns Hopkins University Press (1991).

13 Kershner, C. and A. A. MacKay. "Town Meeting" on Environmental Needs in a Long Term Care Facility. A report prepared for the Maryland Association of Nonprofit Homes for the Aging (1992).

14 Ohta, R. and B. Ohta. Special Units for Alzheimer's Disease Patients: A Critical Look. *Gerontologist*. Vol 28, No. 6 (December 1988): 803–808.

15 Alverman, M. Towards Improving Geriatric Care with Environmental Interventions Emphasizing a Homelike Atmosphere: An Environmental Experience. *Journal of Gerontological Nursing*. Vol. 5, No. 3 (1979): 13–17.

16 Roach, M. Reflections in a Fake Mirror. *Discover* (1985): 76–85.

17 Namazi, K. and B. Johnson. Designing Independently: A Closet Modification Model for Alzheimer's Disease Patients. *The American Journal of Alzheimer's Care and Related Disorders & Research*. Vol. 7 (1992): 22–29.

18 AIA Foundation. *Design for Aging: An Architect's Guide*. Washington, DC: The AIA Press (1987): 72–74.

19 Liebrock, C. *Beautiful Barrier-Free*. New York: Van Nostrand Reinhold (1993): 161.

Chapter 14

1 Hellen, C. *Alzheimer's Disease Activity-Focused Care*. Stoneham, MA: Butterworth-Heinemann (1992).

2 Cohen, U. and K. Day. Emerging Trends in Environments for People with Dementia. *The American Journal of Alzheimer's Care and Related Disorders & Research* (January/February 1994): 3–11.

3 Cohen, U. and K. Day. Emerging Trends in Environments for People with Dementia. *The American Journal of Alzheimer's Care and Related Disorders & Research* (January/February 1994): 3–11.

4 Mace, N. and L. Gwyther. Selecting a Nursing Home with a Dedicated Dementia Care Unit. *Alzheimer's Association* (1988).

5 Calkins, M. Proper Environment May Be Therapeutic to Influence Dementia Patients' Behavior. *Group Practice Journal* (July/August 1991): 58–66.

6 Rovner, B. What Is Therapeutic About Special Care Units?: The Role of Psychosocial Rehabilitation. *Alzheimer's Disease and Associated Disorders, Journal*. Vol. 8, Supplement 1. New York: Raven Press (1994): S355–359.

7 Mayers, K. and C. Block. Specialized Services for Demented Residents in Washington State Nursing Homes: Report of a Survey. *The American Journal of Alzheimer's Care and Related Disorders & Research* (July/August 1990): 17–21.

8 Gold, M. Bringing Focus to the Mind of Dementia. *Provider* (May 1994).

9 Semans, D. Individual Perspectives: Personal Experiences of Alzheimer's Disease. Presented at the Alzheimer's Association National Education Conference, Chicago (July 1995).

10 Alzheimer's Association of Orange County. "Memories in the Making." Orange, CA (1995).

11 Gold, M. Bringing Focus to the Mind of Dementia. *Provider* (May 1994).

12 Mayers, K. and C. Block. Specialized Services for Demented Residents in Washington State Nursing Homes: Report of a Survey. *The American Journal of Alzheimer's Care and Related Disorders & Research* (July/August 1990): 17–21.

13 Boling, R. Health Extra. *Modern Maturity* (September/October 1995): 22.

14 Bush-Brown, A. Activity and Membership vs. Confinement and Isolation. In Bush-Brown, A. and D. Davis, (Eds.) *Hospitable Design for Healthcare and Senior Communities*. New York: Van Nostrand and Reinhold. (1992): 22.

15 Halloin, J. Application of Current Knowledge in Lighting. *Lighting for Aging Vision and Health* (1995): 159–166.

16 Noell, E. Long Term Care Design: Lighting. *Journal of Healthcare Design*. Vol. IV (1991): 65–69.

17 AIA Foundation. *Design for Aging: An Architect's Guide*. Washington, DC: The AIA Press (1987): 84.

18 Peppard, N. Effective Design of Special Care Units. *Provider* (May 1986).

19 Beck, C., B. Baldwin, T. Modlin, and S. Lewis. Caregivers' Perception of Aggressive Behavior in Cognitively Impaired Nursing Home Residents. *Journal of Neuroscience Nursing*. Vol. 22 (1990): 169–172.

Cohen-Mansfield, J. Agitated Behavior. *Journal of the American Geriatric Society*. Vol 34 (1986): 722–727.

20 Sloane, P. D., V. Honn, S. Dwyer, J. Wieselquist, C. Cain, and S. Meyers. Bathing the Alzheimer's Patient in Long Term Care: Results and Recommendations from Three Studies. *The American Journal of Alzheimer's Disease* (July/August 1995).

21 Sloane, P. D., V. Honn, S. Dwyer, J. Wieselquist, C. Cain, and S. Meyers. Bathing the Alzheimer's Patient in Long Term Care: Results and Recommendations from Three Studies. *The American Journal of Alzheimer's Disease* (July/August 1995).

22 Foltz-Gray, D. Rough Waters. *Contemporary Long Term Care* (September 1995): 66–70.

23 Sloane, P. D., V. Honn, S. Dwyer, J. Wieselquist, C. Cain, and S. Meyers. Bathing the Alzheimer's Patient in Long Term Care: Results and Recommendations from Three Studies. *The American Journal of Alzheimer's Disease* (July/August 1995).

24 Sloane, P. D., V. Honn, S. Dwyer, J. Wieselquist, C. Cain, and S. Meyers. Bathing the Alzheimer's Patient in Long Term Care: Results and Recommendations from Three Studies. *The American Journal of Alzheimer's Disease* (July/August 1995).

25 Sloane, P. D., V. Honn, S. Dwyer, J. Wieselquist, C. Cain, and S. Meyers. Bathing the Alzheimer's Patient in Long Term Care: Results and Recommendations from Three Studies. *The American Journal of Alzheimer's Disease* (July/August 1995).

26 Cohen, U., G. Weisman, K. Day, W. Robinson, J. Dicker, and G. Meyer. *Illustrative Designs: Environments for People with Dementia.* Milwaukee: The School of Architecture and Urban Planning at The University of Wisconsin (1990):

Chapter 15

1 Gilleard, C. J. *Living with Dementia: Community Care of the Elderly Mentally Infirm.* Philadelphia, PA: The Charles Press (1984).

2 Weisman, G. Improving Way-Finding and Architectural Legibility in Housing for the Elderly. *Housing the Aged: Design Directives and Policy Considerations.* New York: Elsevier. V. Regnier and J. Pynoos, Eds. (1987): 441–464.

3 Randall, P., S. Burkhardt, and J. Kutcher. Exterior Space for Patients with Alzheimer's Disease and Related Disorders. *American Journal of Alzheimer's Care and Related Disorders & Research* (July/August 1990): 31–37.

4 Stephens, P. Outdoor Environments for People with Dementia. Presented at the National Alzheimer's Design Assistance Project, San Diego (January 1996): 1–13.

5 Lovering, M. J. Alzheimer's Disease and Outdoor Space: Issues in Environmental Design. *American Journal of Alzheimer's Care and Related Disorders & Research* (May/June 1990): 33–40.

6 Randall, P., S. Burkhardt, and J. Kutcher. Exterior Space for Patients with Alzheimer's Disease and Related Disorders. *American Journal of Alzheimer's Care and Related Disorders & Research* (July/August 1990): 31–37.

7 Hall, G., M. V. Kirschling, and S. Todd. Sheltered Freedom—An Alzheimer's Special Care Unit in an ICF. *Geriatric Nursing* (May/June 1986): 132.

8 Namazi, K. H. and B. D. Johnson. Pertinent Autonomy for Residents with Dementias: Modification of the Physical Environment to Enhance Independence. *The American Journal of Alzheimer's Care and Related Disorders & Research* (January/February 1992): 16–21.

9 Stephens, P. Outdoor Environments for People with Dementia. Presented at the National Alzheimer's Design Assistance Project, San Diego (January 1996): 1–13.

10 Lovering, M. J. Alzheimer's Disease and Outdoor Space: Issues in Environmental Design. *American Journal of Alzheimer's Care and Related Disorders & Research* (May/June 1990): 3–40.

11 Stephens, P. Outdoor Environments for People with Dementia. Presented at the National Alzheimer's Design Assistance Project, San Diego (January 1996): 1–13.

12 Hoover, R. Healing Gardens and Alzheimer's Disease. *American Journal of Alzheimer's Disease* (March/April 1995): 1–9.

13 Calkins, M. *Design for Dementia.* Owings Mills, MD: National Health Publishing (1988): xi.

14 Randall, P., S. Burkhardt, and J. Kutcher. Exterior Space for Patients with Alzheimer's Disease and Related Disorders. *American Journal of Alzheimer's Care and Related Disorders & Research* (July/August 1990): 31–37.

15 Hoover, R. Healing Gardens and Alzheimer's Disease. *American Journal of Alzheimer's Disease* (March/April 1995).

16 Skolaski-Pelliteri, T. Environmental Adaptations Which Compensate for Dementia. *Physical and Occupational Therapy in Geriatrics.* Vol. 3 (1983): 31–44.

17 Lovering, M. J. Alzheimer's Disease and Outdoor Space: Issues in Environmental Design. *American Journal of Alzheimer's Care and Related Disorders & Research* (May/June 1990): 3–40.

18 Lovering, M. J. Alzheimer's Disease and Outdoor Space: Issues in Environmental Design. *American Journal of Alzheimer's Care and Related Disorders & Research* (May/June 1990): 33–40.

19 Hoover, R. Residential Care: Design Enhancements Including Therapeutic Gardens. Presented at the Alzheimer's Association National Education Conference, Chicago (July 1995).

20 Marcus, C. C. and M. Barnes. *Gardens in Healthcare Facilities: Use, Therapeutic Benefits, and Design Recommendations.* Martinez, CA: The Center for Health Design (1995): 61–63.

Chapter 16

1 Leib, R. and K. Abelbeck. Promoting Patient Mobility in Long-Term Care Settings. ADD Specialized Seating Technology (1992).

2 Leib, R. and K. Abelbeck. Promoting Patient Mobility in Long-Term Care Settings. ADD Specialized Seating Technology (1992).

3 Leib, R. The Changing Face of Health Care. *Interiors & Sources* (July/August 1993).

4 Claman, E. Personality of the Chair in A. Bush-Brown and D. Davis (Eds.). *Hospitable Design for Healthcare and Senior Communities.* New York: Van Nostrand Reinhold (1992): 186–187.

5 Noell, E. The Environment: Silent Partner in Caregiving. *Generations.* (Winter 1995–1996): 14–19.

6 California Technical Bulletin 133: Questions and Answers. A Fire Test for Seating Furniture in Public Buildings. State Department of Consumer Affairs Bureau of Home Furnishings and Thermal Insulation (January 1992).

7 Gurian, M. and B. Little. Textiles at the Limits. *Contract Design* (October 1993): 90–94.

8 Crypton: Specifier. End User Information Packet. Fantagraph (1996).

9 Gurian, M. and B. Little. Textiles at the Limits. *Contract Design* (October 1993): 90–94.

10 Gurian, M. and B. Little. Textiles at the Limits. *Contract Design* (October 1993): 90–94.

Chapter 17

1 Armstrong, J. E., D. J. Jose, and V. Ramachandran. Specifying Carpet for Health Care Environments. *Interiors & Sources.* (Nov/Dec 1991): 74–77.

2 Armstrong, J. E., D. J. Jose, and V. Ramachandran. Specifying Carpet for Health Care Environments. *Interiors & Sources.* (Nov/Dec 1991): 74–77.

3 Weinhold, V. Flooring Options: Carpet Now a Major Contender. *Health Facilities Management* (May 1992): 96–100.

Chapter 18

1 Protective Finishes: A Look at Some Clear Choices. *Technical Quarterly* (Spring 1992).

2 Wilson, A. J. Paint Selections for Health Care Environments. *Interiors & Sources* (March 1994): 70–73.

3 Colby, B. *Color and Light: Influence and Impact.* Glendale, CA: Chroma Productions (1990).

Chapter 20

1 Carpman, J. R. Socially Responsible Health Facility Design: The Direction for the New Millennium. *Group Practice Journal* (July/August 1991): 32–39.

2 Carpman, J. R. Socially Responsible Health Facility Design: The Direction for the New Millennium. *Group Practice Journal* (July/August 1991): 32–39.

3 Hiatt, L. G. The Environment's Role in the Total Well-Being of the Older Person. In G. G. Magam and E. L. Haught (Eds.) *Well-Being and the Elderly: An Holistic View.* Washington, DC: American Association of Homes for the Aging (1986): 23–38.

4 Hiatt, L. G. The Environment's Role in the Total Well-Being of the Older Person. In G. G. Magam and E. L. Haught (Eds.) *Well-Being and the Elderly: An Holistic View.* Washington, DC: American Association of Homes for the Aging (1986): 23–38.

5 Hiatt, L. G. The Environment's Role in the Total Well-Being of the Older Person. In G.G. Magam and E. L. Haught (Eds.) *Well-Being and the Elderly: An Holistic View.* Washington, DC: American Association of Homes for the Aging (1986): 23–38.

6 Hiatt, L. G. The Environment's Role in the Total Well-Being of the Older Person. In G.G. Magam and E. L. Haught (Eds.) *Well-Being and the Elderly: An Holistic View.* Washington, DC: American Association of Homes for the Aging (1986): 23–38.

7 Eggert, R. Programming Your Way to Successful Design. *Spectrum* (September/October 1994).

8 Carpman, J. R. Socially Responsible Health Facility Design: The Direction for the New Millennium. *Group Practice Journal* (July/August 1991): 32–39.

9 Woodside Place Evaluation: The First Three Years of a Residential Alzheimer's Facility. Prepared by Silverman, M., E. Ricci, C. McAllister, and C. Keane, Department of Health & Human Services, University of Pittsburgh; Saxon, J., Alzheimer's Disease Research Center University of Pittsburgh Medical Center; Ledewitz, S., Carnegie Mellon University. Prepared for the Presbyterian Association on Aging (January 1995).

Index